Frontiers in Bioactive Compounds

(Volume 3)

(Therapeutic Implications of Natural Bioactive Compounds)

Edited by

Dr. Mukesh Kumar Sharma
Department of Zoology,
SPC Government College,
Ajmer -305001, Rajasthan,
India

&

Dr. Pallavi Kaushik
Department of Zoology,
University of Rajasthan,
Jaipur-302004, Rajasthan,
India

Frontiers in Bioactive Compounds

Volume # 3

Therapeutic Implications of Natural Bioactive Compounds

Editors: Mukesh Kumar Sharma & Pallavi Kaushik

ISSN (Online): 2468-6409

ISSN (Print): 2468-6395

ISBN (Online): 978-981-5080-02-5

ISBN (Print): 978-981-5080-03-2

ISBN (Paperback): 978-981-5080-04-9

©2022, Bentham Books imprint.

Published by Bentham Science Publishers Pte. Ltd. Singapore. All Rights Reserved.

First published in2022.

need for a court order if at any point you breach any terms of this License Agreement. In no event will any delay or failure by Bentham Science Publishers in enforcing your compliance with this License Agreement constitute a waiver of any of its rights.

3. You acknowledge that you have read this License Agreement, and agree to be bound by its terms and conditions. To the extent that any other terms and conditions presented on any website of Bentham Science Publishers conflict with, or are inconsistent with, the terms and conditions set out in this License Agreement, you acknowledge that the terms and conditions set out in this License Agreement shall prevail.

Bentham Science Publishers Pte. Ltd.
80 Robinson Road #02-00
Singapore 068898
Singapore
Email: subscriptions@benthamscience.net

**BENTHAM
SCIENCE**

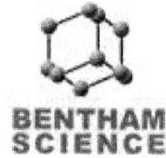

CONTENTS

FOREWORD

We take the opportunity to communicate with you, through this foreword message of the book series with thematic focus on **'Frontiers in Bioactive Compounds (Volume 3) Title: Therapeutic implications of Natural Bioactive Compounds'**.

The nature has provided us enormous genetic potential which has evolved through ages and appears not only in form of biological diversity but also in form of biologically active molecules called bio-active compounds. Many bioactive compounds obtained from natural sources include, phenolics, alkaloids, tannins, saponins, lignin, glycosides, terpenes etc. have been studied thoroughly for therapeutic applications with potential use in pharmaceutical industry.

The assessment of wide-ranging therapeutic potentials of these bioactive compounds has led to the discovery of many modern drugs in recent times. In the present era, it is believed that the natural product-based medicine is considered as the most suitable and safe to be used as an alternative medicine due to their low or no side effects at the effective doses. Moreover, World Health Organization aims to increase the integration of traditional medicine in order to improve health care system. Therefore, natural products research has become a thrust area among scientific community aimed toward understanding the chemistry, analytical methodologies, biosynthetic mechanisms, and pharmacological activities of several natural bioactive compounds. Thus, it is prime interest of researchers to develop understanding about various natural bio-active compounds in order to promote the drug discovery research and to complement the medical world by developing novel drug molecules with superior bioactivities.

The present book series entitled **'Frontiers in Bioactive Compounds (Volume Title: Therapeutic implications of Natural Bioactive Compounds)'** includes 13 chapters contributed by many academicians, scientists, and researchers from various leading institutes from India and abroad. The editors have made enormous and successful effort to assemble a huge variety of knowledge on structures and therapeutic potential of various natural bioactive compounds present in plants, fungi, algae, marine organisms etc. Chapter contributors have extensively reviewed the therapeutic role of various bioactive compounds against many health disorders in human such as COVID-19, cancer, diabetes, immuno-modulators, neurodegenerative changes and many diseases of farm animals.

We believe this book surely provides updated information on the structure, properties and much therapeutic application of various natural bioactive compounds to graduate, undergraduate students, teachers, food scientists, nutritionists, pharmaceuticals, physicians, food industrials, as well as for health-conscious consumers. We congratulate the editors **Dr. Mukesh Kumar Sharma** and **Dr. (Mrs.) Pallavi Kaushik**, and all contributing authors for bringing the collection of their noble piece of work and also for the grand success of this book.

Prof. Ashok Kumar
President
Nirwan University, Jaipur
Former Vice Chancellor
CSJM University, Kanpur and
DDU University, Gorakhpur (UP), India

&

Dr. Yoshihisa Matsumoto
Professor (PI)
Tokyo Institute of Technology,
Institute of Innovative Research
Laboratory for Zero-Carbon Energy, Tokyo, Japan

PREFACE

Bioactive compounds have been used as traditional medicines since ancient times. Therefore, the study of therapeutic potential of various bioactive compounds against many diseases and health disorders has been an important area for scholars, academicians, doctors and pharmaceutical industry people.

There are very few books available currently to cover such a wide spectrum of topics. Therefore, this book is a definitive compilation of chapters which are mainly focused on the therapeutic implications of bioactive compounds derived from natural sources like bacteria, algae, fungi, plants and animals. Various chapters in the book incorporate the knowledge based on traditional medicine with recent advances in bioactive molecular research and their pharmaceutical and industrial importance.

A brief note on the 13 chapters of this book is given as follows:

Chapter 1 highlights the recent development strategies of flavonoids prevailing in the field of neurodegenerative diseases like Alzheimer's, Parkinson's, and multiple sclerosis, along with their limitations and strategies to encounter the challenges.

Chapter 2 deals with recently discovered plant and marine originated natural compounds for cancer therapeutics. This is an attempt to consolidate data on various bioactive compounds concerning with more targeted and innoxious approach along future outlook.

Chapter 3 gives a comprehensive idea about natural bioactives from plants and other sources with antibiofilm activity. Clinical validation of these bioactives will aid the medical field with alternate preventive and treatment methods against pathogenic biofilms.

Chapter 4 is a compilation of research on SARS CoV-2 with its life cycle, pathogenesis, and currently used drugs for treatment, including the synthetic ones, medicinal herbs and the specific bioactive compounds found efficacious against COVID- 19.

Chapter 5 discusses the common groups of plant derived bioactive compounds with anti-diabetic potential by virtue of their potential to modulate various pathways involved in the regulation of blood glucose levels.

Chapter 6 focuses on therapeutics and industrial application of the algae derivatives' primary and secondary metabolites.

Chapter 7 presents an overview of the traditional uses, phytochemical constituents and various pharmacological properties of F.vulgare and T.ammi seeds.

Chapter 8 is an attempt to consolidate information on recently observed bioactive compounds which have aided in unrelenting research to explore their potential use for the treatment of various livestock diseases.

Chapter 9 provides an overview on the isolation and characterization of the bioactive compounds derived from Indian medicinal plant H. indicus, their biological properties with particular emphasis on anti-diabetic potential.

Chapter 10 deals with different works and approaches employed for utilizing tea polyphenols against pesticide induced toxicity carried out internationally and nationally, along with their future prospects.

Chapter 11 emphasizes upon the role of various bioactive compounds derived from fungal sources with their pharmacological importance.

Chapter 12 focuses on a few extensively scrutinized immunomodulatory phytocompounds from medicinal plants such as Tinospora cordifolia, Andrographis paniculata, Curcuma longa, Zingiber officinale, Allium sativum, Terminalia chebula and Piper longum which have been studied in experimental (in vitro and in vivo) models and few compounds have exhibited good therapeutic potential in clinical trials also.

Chapter 13 describes the bacteria-derived bioactive compounds like antibiotics, enzymes and other secondary metabolites like Gallic acid, Amicoumacin, Prodigiosin, Nystatin, Spinosad, Milbemycin, Lipstatin, Subtilin, Albaflavenone, Mollemycin A which have been studied for their inhibitory action against bacteria, fungi, insects, pests, *etc.*

We appreciate the tremendous efforts of the authors from renowned institutions of India, Japan and China for sharing their pieces of expertise in the contributed chapters. We shall also extend a hearty thanks to Bentham Science Publishers for providing the opportunity to contribute as editors of this book.

Dr. Mukesh Kumar Sharma
JSPS (Japan) Fellow
Associate Professor
Department of Zoology
SPC Government College
AJMER-305001
(Raj.) India

&

Dr. Pallavi Kaushik
Assistant Professor
Department of Zoology
University of Rajasthan
Jaipur-302004
Rajasthan, India

List of Contributors

Amit Kumar Dixit	Central Ayurveda Research Institute-CCRAS, Kolkata, India
Amrita C. Bhagwat	Symbiosis School of Biological Sciences, Lavale, Pune, Maharashtra, India
Amrita M. Patil	Symbiosis School of Biological Sciences, Lavale, Pune, Maharashtra, India
Avijit Banerji	Central AyurvedaResearch Institute-CCRAS, Ministry of Ayush, Kolkata, India Formerly of Chemistry Department, Kolkata, India
Damodar Gupta	Institute for Nuclear Medicine and Allied Sciences, DRDO, New Delhi, India
Deepti Dixit	School of Biochemistry, Madhya Pradesh, India
Devojit K. Sarma	ICMR-National Institute for Research in Environmental Health, Bhopal, India
Julie Banerji	Formerly of Chemistry Department, Kolkata, India
Manoj Kumar	ICMR-National Institute for Research in Environmental Health, Bhopal, India
Mayank Handa	National Institute of Pharmaceutical Education and Research-Raebareli, Lucknow, U.P., 226002, India
Meenakshi Samartha	Department of Zoology, Bhopal, India
Mukesh Kumar Sharma	SPC Government College, Department of Zoology, Ajmer-305001, India
Nandini Goswami	IIS (deemed to be University) Jaipur, Rajasthan, 302020, India
Neetu Kachhwaha	Department of Zoology, University of Rajasthan, Jaipur-302004, India
Neha Jain	University of Rajasthan, Department of Zoology, Jaipur-302004, India
Pallavi Kaushik	University of Rajasthan, Department of Zoology, Jaipur, Rajasthan, India
Parvathy G. Nair	National Ayurveda Research Institute for Panchakarma, Thrisuur, Kerala, India
Prachi Jain	University of Rajasthan, Department of Zoology, Jaipur, Rajasthan, India
Pritom Chowdhury	Department of Biotechnology, Tea Research Association, Jorhat, Assam, India
P.V.V. Prasad	Central Ayurveda Research Institute-CCRAS, Kolkata, India
Qadir Alam	Central Ayurveda Research Institute-CCRAS, Kolkata, India
Rahul Shukla	National Institute of Pharmaceutical Education and Research-Raebareli, Lucknow, U.P., 226002, India
Rajani Sharma	SMS Medical College, Department of Microbiology, Jaipur, India
Ravindra M. Samarth	ICMR-National Institute for Research in Environmental Health, Bhopal, India ICMR-Bhopal Memorial Hospital & Research Centre, Bhopal, India
Renu Khandelwal	Department of Zoology, University of Rajasthan, Jaipur-302004, India
S.J.S. Flora	National Institute of Pharmaceutical Education and Research-Raebareli, Lucknow, U.P., 226002, India
Shalini Jain	IIS (deemed to be University) Jaipur, Rajasthan, 302020, India
Sicheng Liu	Department of General Surgery, Innovation Center for Minimally Invasive Techniques and Devices, Zhejiang, 310019, Hangzhou, China

Sneha Keelka University of Rajasthan, Department of Zoology, Jaipur-302004, Rajasthan, India

Sreemoyee Chatterjee IIS (deemed to be University) Jaipur, Rajasthan, 302020, India

Sunil D. Saroj Symbiosis School of Biological Sciences, Lavale, Pune, Maharashtra, India

Swasti Shubham ICMR-National Institute for Research in Environmental Health, Bhopal, India

Yoshihisa Matsumoto Tokyo Institute of Technology, Institute of Innovative Research, Tokyo, Japan

CHAPTER 1

Flavonoid Based Bioactive for Therapeutic Application in Neurological Disorders

S.J.S. Flora[1,*], Rahul Shukla[1] and **Mayank Handa[1]**

[1] *National Institute of Pharmaceutical Education and Research-Raebareli, Lucknow, U.P., 226002, India*

Abstract: Flavonoids belong to a class of natural, polyphenolic dietary compounds which modify the neuropathological state of the brain. Some flavonoids like quercetin and other, reduce the inflammation, carcinogenicity, and oxidation promotes neuroprotection and comprises the major component of cosmetics, medicinal and dietary supplements. Daily intake of flavonoids helps to mitigate the risk of several neurological disorders like Alzheimer's disease, Parkinson's disease, multiple sclerosis, *etc*. Flavonoids exhibit their pharmacological effect through various mechanisms like cholinesterase inhibition, scavenging free radicals, memory enhancement *via* attenuation of amyloid plaques, tau targeting detoxification and neural antiinflammation. Administration of flavonoids to biological system has to pass through several biological checkpoints like first pass metabolism, intestinal absorption, and entry into blood brain barrier. Flavonoids exhibit difference in pharmacokinetic and pharmacodyanmic profile due to difference in their structures. Recent literature reports have proved promising therapeutic potential in neurological disorders. This chapter highlights the recent development of flavonoids prevailing in the field of neurodegenerative, its limitations and drug delivery approaches to encounter the challenges.

Keywords: Flavonoids, Alzheimer's, Parkinson's, Natural Biological, Neurodegenerative disorder.

INTRODUCTION

Flavonoids are plant derived secondary metabolites [1]. Flavonoids are long-serving in treatment of diseases [2]. Flavonoids have been considered as good therapeutic agents due to their easy extraction, diversification, and abundance. To date, around 7,000 or more different types of flavonoids have been discovered from plants (vegetables and fruits). These naturally occurring metabolites possess numerous beneficial effects and mitigate plenty of health problems thus plays a

---

[*] **Corresponding author S.J.S Flora:** National Institute of Pharmaceutical Education and Research-Raebareli, Lucknow, U.P., 226002, India; Tel: +91-94254 82305; E-mail: sjsflora@hotmail.com

Mukesh Kumar Sharma and Pallavi Kaushik (Eds.)

significant role in drug designing and discovery [3, 4]. Flavonoids own good affinity for several body proteins, excellent antioxidant activity, metal chelation ability, and additionally can alter enzymes, receptors, and transporters [3, 5, 6]. There are ample amount of research studies advocating its anti-cancer, anti-inflammatory, anti-diabetic, neuroprotective, antimicrobial activities, and as cardiovascular drugs [6 - 10]. Some studies reported it as a cognitive enhancer, while others claim flavonoids as therapeutic against Alzheimer's disease (AD). These results were observed in preclinical evaluation [11 - 13]. It was also reported that flavonoids and its derivative metabolites can interact with several subcellular targets [14] for example, interaction of flavonoids with PI3-kinase/Akt and ERK signalling pathways receptors can accelerate the neuroprotective proteins expression and increase neuronal count [15 - 18]. Flavonoids enhance cerebrovascular functionality thus improving blood flow the brain and triggers the generation of neurons that ultimately results in better cognition. There are numerous other mechanisms that reported the beneficial effects of flavonoids.

Flavonoids have ability to suppress the inflammation mediated neuronal apoptosis, inhibition of abnormal β and γ secretase and curb the oxidative stress, thus can debilitate the progression and onset of AD [19, 20]. Thus, flavonoids can act as neuroprotectants by improving the quality and quantity of neurons.

Flavonoids Chemistry and its Classification

Flavonoids are polyphenols with chemical structure involving two benzene rings interconnected with a pyran ring, one is amalgamated with pyran ring while the other is attached as a substitute in pyran ring. On the basis of benzene ring substitution, saturation of pyran ring, derivatization can be possible that owned physicochemical properties suitable for neuroprotectant.

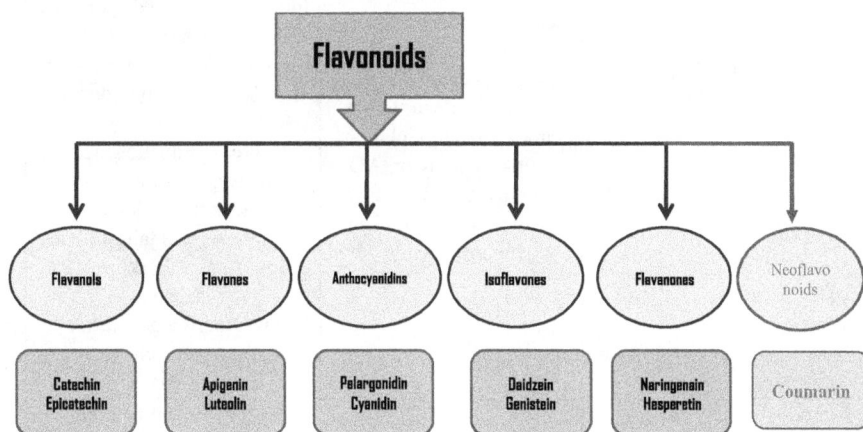

Fig. (1). (a) Flow chart presentation of flavonoids.

Flavonoids Classification

Depending on the benzene ring position and pyran attachment along with extent of oxidation and unsaturation of pyran ring, flavonoids are chemically classified into different groups having different pharmacological properties discussed below (Fig. **1** and Table **1**).

Table 1. Summary of flavonoids obtained from medicinal plants' with potential neuropharmacological properties.

Flavonoids	Source	Study Design	Results	References
Anthocyanin flavonoids	Blackberry extract Grape juice	Male wistar rats/APP/PS1 model of AD Male Wistar rats/ Lipopolysaccharide/ interferon-γ-induced glial cells activation	Behavioral and motor improvements, Decrease (TNF-α and IL-1β), nitric oxide production, Down-regulation of CNTF, CINC-3, IL-10. Antioxidants, scavengers of reactive oxygen species (ROS) and reactive nitrogen species (RNS).	[70-73]
Epigalocatechin Galate (EGCG) Genistein	Green tea	Anti-amyloid study Secretases inhibition assays EGCG mediated estrogen receptors (Estrogen receptor-α Phosphoinositide 3-kinase, Ak) modulation. Anti-tau study on AD Transgenic animals Antioxidant studies in neuronal cells	Suppress the expression of oxidative stress factors, and reduce neuronal apoptosis and later protein expression in PI3K, p-AKT and eNOS signaling pathway. Reduced ERK and NF-kB pathways Suppressed Ab induced lipid peroxidation Inhibit Ab-induced apoptosis, Caspase activity Improve Neuronal survival Increase Non-amyloidogenic APP Decrease Fibrillogenesis decrease Formation of sarkosyl-soluble phosphorylated tau isoforms low Risk of Parkinson's disease low Neurodegeneration decrease ischemic hippocampal injury high PI3-kinase activity Increase Nigral damage *via* scavenging of free radicals	[74-77] [78-80] [81-83]

(Table 1) cont.....

Quercetin Curcumin Cyanidin-3-O-glucoside (Cy3G)	Citrus Flavonoid Edible Plants Curcuma longa Hibiscus sabdariffa	APP Tg neuronal cells AD animal model Tg2576 model	Decrease the formation of Ab peptides Decrease BACE1 activity Increase Soluble Ab Decrease GSK-3 activity Lower Association of PS1-APP Modulation of GSK-3b/tau Decrease Cognitive dysfunctions	[84, 85] [86, 87]
Myricetin Indirubins Morin	Vegetables Fruits, Berries Nuts, Tea Edible Plants	AChE inhibition assay Protein kinases study Ab induced Cytotoxicity in neuroblastoma cells 3xTg-AD mice	Decrease BACE1 activity, Interrupt fibrillization reduced Heparin-induced tau formation decrease CDK5/p25, GSK-3b activity reduced Tau hyperphosphorylation decrease Ab-induced cytotoxicity	[61, 88]
Blueberry Flavonoids	Blueberry	Chronic animals study Activated microglia cells Anti-inflammatory action	Increase HC Akt phosphorylation increase Downstream mTOR activation increase Arc/Arg3.1 decrease TNF-a decrease NO Production, IL-1b Decrease Cox-2, iNOS, and IL-1β	[89, 90]
Isoflavones Flavanols, Anthocyanins rich food/ Compounds/ Extracts	Soy foods Grapes juice, Cocoa Blueberry, Pomegranate	AD animal models Brain estrogen study Behavioral Tasks Memory tasks Locomotor tasks	Increase BDNF Increase NGF Increase CREB Increase AChE Increase Cognition Decrease Working memory deficits Mimic Brain estrogens activity	[91-93] [94, 95]
128 Flavonoids including, Silibinin Genistein, Apigenin, kaempferol, Naringin, Quercetin, Diosmin, Silymarin	Foods Citrus Fruits Natural Products	Cholinesterase inhibition assays	Decrease AChE activity Decrease BChE activity	[96] [97]

BACE1, Beta amyloid cleaving enzyme-1; BDNF, Brain derived neurotrophic factor; NGF, Nerve growth factor; NO, Nitrous Oxide; AD, Alzheimer's disease; ACh, Acetylcholine.

Isoflavones

Flavonoids benzene ring attachment to pyran ring at 3rd position is called isoflavones. Soybean is a major natural source of isoflavones [23]. Isoflavones are biodegradable and possess good antioxidant activity. A research study claimed to synthesize its derivative by Suzuki coupling reaction [24] while others used triazin for derivatization of isoflavone. It was reported that application of enzymes or heterogonous catalyst are promising methods for isoflavone synthesis [25, 26]. Structures of few isoflavones are:

Neoflavonoids

When benzene ring is attached to 4th position of pyran ring then the compound is called neoflavonoids. Neoflavonoids exhibit potential antidiabetic pharmacological activity [27]. Neoflavonoids are comprised of neoflavenes and neoflavones. Neoflavonoids can be obtained from both natural as well as synthetic source. Natural sources of this heterocyclic compound are *Dalbergia odorifera* [28], *Echinops niveus* [29], *Polygonum perfoliatum* [30], and *Nepalese propolis* [31].

Flavones

Chemical structure of flavones contains carbonyl group attached to pyran ring at position 4 and double bond between positions 2 and 3. Flavones have two hydroxyl groups at each aromatic ring. This compound can obtain by both natural and synthetic source although natural is more common source [32].

Flavonols

Flavonols, also known as 3-hydroxyflavones, contain hydroxyl group on pyran ring at 3rd position. Flavonols are synthesized chemically by derivatizing flavones using oxidation, followed by cyclization by chalcones. Further, replacing hydrogen associated with hydroxyl group of glucose that yields flavonol glycoside.

Pachypodol is a unique example of flavonol as it does not actually belong to this group but considering its chemical structure, pachypodol comes under flavonols.

Flavanones and Flavanonols

Flavanones are 2,3-dihydroflavones and flavanonols are 3-hydroxy flavanones. Chemically flavanonols have saturated pyran ring with hydroxyl group at 3rd position and 4th position for carbonyl.

Flavanols

Flavonoids that do not contain carbonyl group at position 4 are called flavanols. Chemically, flavanols have saturated pyran ring and di-substitution at positions 2 and 3 allowing 4 possible diastereomers. Position 2 of pyran ring is substituted by the benzene ring while 3 is attached with hydroxyl group. The prominent difference between flavonoids and flavanol is the absence of hydroxyl group at position 3. For this reason, flavonoids classified under this group without being fit in definition of flavanols.

Anthocyanidins

These are the pigmented flavonoids widely available in cationic form (as chloride salt). Anthocynadins are salt forms of 2-phenylchromenylium (flavylium) cation. Anthocyanidins group contains petunidin, capensinidin, hirsutidin, aurantinidin, delphinidin, cyaniding, pelargonidin, malvidin, europinidin, pulchellidin, peonidin, and rosinidin. All are different due to their substitution.

Chalcones

Chalcones do not contain pyran ring but due to the same synthetic approach, these are classified under flavonoids. Chalcones have pyran moiety present as an open structure. The carbonyl group of this open structure conjugated with double bond yields α,β- unsaturated ring. This can act as Michael acceptor for several organic reactions.

Flavonoids and its Abundancy in Nature

Flavonoids are secondary products widely distributed in plant kingdom. Most of the flavonoids contain colour and promote some essential pharmacological functions such as pollination. Flavonoids are classified based on aglycone ring and state of oxidation and reduction (see Fig. **2**). Some other criteria for differentiation of flavonoids are hydroxylation degree of aglycon, saturation of pyran ring, hydroxyl group position, derivatization of hydroxyl group. Generally, fruits, vegetables, juices, cereals are major sources of flavonoids [21].

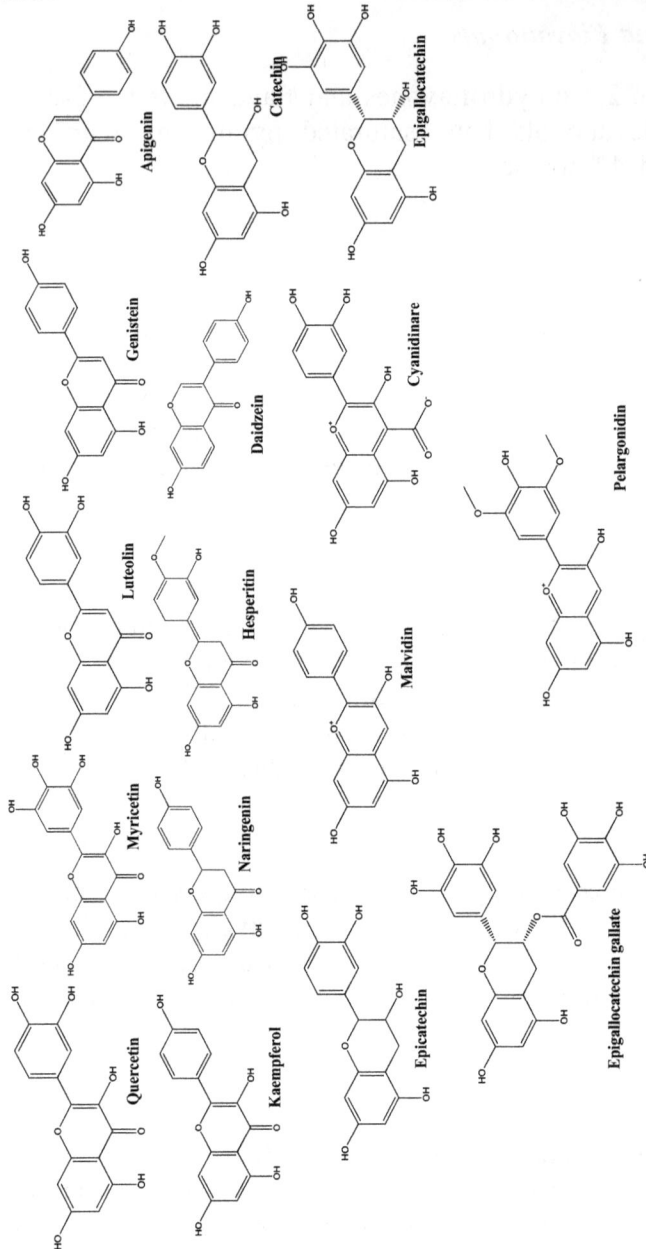

Fig. (2). Chemical structure of some common flavonoids.

Quercetin, myricetin, and kaempferol (flavonols) are few examples of flavonoids obtained from vegetables whereas luteolin and apigenin are found in celery, chamomile, and green peppers. Genistein and daidzein are isoflavones naturally present in soy and its products; flavanones such as, naringenin and hesperidin are found in tomatoes and citrus fruits. Some other flavans like epicatechin, epigallocatechin gallate (EGCG), epigallocatechin and catechin are present in green tea, chocolate and red wine. Berry fruits and red wine are enriched with anthocyanidins like malvidin, cyanidinare, and pelargonidin [22].

Flavonoids and its Pathological Targets in Neurological Disorders

Cholinesterase Inhibitors

Enzymes cholinesterases like AChE (acetylcholinesterase) and BChE (butylcholinestrase) cause the hydrolysis of acetylcholine (ACh) neurotransmitter, which regulates the impulse neurotransmission between different neuron synapses. As the AD pathogenesis includes scarceness of ACh, the cholinesterase inhibitors are being one of the essential therapeutics for maintaining the neurotransmitter levels at the synapse for longer durations [33]. The clinical data available currently shows that using this method is the most effective treatment for AD symptoms, thus reducing clinical approval at the end of the four drugs [34]. It was effectively applied in the treatment of ataxia and dementia, Parkinson's disease (PD). Due to adverse effects and inadequate effectiveness of available marketed drugs, more effective and safer drugs are to be developed in urge.

Various flavonoid compounds like naringin, apigenin, quercetin, kaempferol, diosmin, genistein, silibinin, and silymarin have shown anti-cholinesterase effects. Quercetin, was being most effective with 76.2% anti-cholinesterase activity against AChE while, other flavonoids have shown genistein -65.7%, luteolin - 54.9% and silibinin - 51.4% inhibitory activity against enzyme BChE [35].

As per the published reports of 2011 by Uriarte-Pueyo and Calvo co-workers report 128 flavonoids in relation to their ability to inhibit AChE. Depending on their potential as ChE inhibitors, they are considered therapeutic potential for AD [97].

Scavengers of Free Radical

Aerobic respiration causes the formation of free radicals, which get countered by the various antioxidants present in the body. If free radicals are formed in excess amounts, oxidative stress occurs leading to the disturbances in physiological functions of essential body elements like proteins and lipids [36]. Together with the part of free radicals in diseases, they are well prone to inflammation of neurons leading to AD development. Oxidative stress markers with their increased levels confirmed that oxidative stress is the main feature of AD [36]. The lower antioxidant levels and activity was observed in plasma of AD diagnosed patients

[37]. It was also detected that there was increased levels of various protein and lipid oxidation byproducts in the preclinical AD based transgenic animal models [38]. The higher amounts of pathogenic markers for AD like neurofibrillary tangles (NFTs) and Aβ in animals containing oxidative stress indication of free radicals as the initiating agents of AD [39]. Almost all reactive oxygen species (ROS) are formed in mitochondria [40]. The lack of cytochrome c oxidase in AD patients causes mitochondrial dysfunction and leads to the formation of excess ROS [41]. In the metal ions Aβ presence leads to an overrun of the free radicals and is known as mitochondrial poison [42]. In response to this, the usage of ions such as clioquinol in AD mimicked transgenic animal models is known to provide beneficial effects. Neurodegenerative disorders and AD have other characteristics like glial cells activation [43, 44]. By using NADPH oxidase (NOX), there is generation of pro-inflammatory cytokines and enhanced production of superoxide anions by the microglia activation. The occurrence of increased amounts of NOX subunits and removal of NOX gene in transgenic animals lead to improved cognitive and cerebrovascular functions indicating its role in the pathophysiology of AD [45]. In addition, glial cells activation releases NO from inducible nitric oxide synthase (iNOS) and reacts with superoxide along with the production of peroxinitrite thereby causing nitrosative stress. Their involvement was based on the genetic removal of iNOS leading to improved gliosis, reduced Aβ load and the reduced phosphorylation of tau protein in mutant animals. Components of green tea like catechins and polyphenols are stronger antioxidative agents that scavenge free radicals by chelating metal ions [46]. EGCG prevention from DNA induced stress damage by transference of electron to active ROS-induced areas [46]. Green tea components suppress the lipid peroxidation in chain reaction and origination by iron ascorbate in brain components of mitochondria. Amongst catechins, EGCG is considered to be the most effective compound [47]. EGCG suppresses fibrils production during Aβ synthesis and reduces lipid peroxidation which was formed by Aβ [48, 49]. It also inhibits apoptosis induced by Aβ, caspase activity, thereby increasing the surviving capacity of hippocampal neurons [49].

Memory Enhancers

Certain literature reports that the flavonoids are effective in preventing AD and impairment of cognition in animal models, which makes them potential therapeutics for treatment of neurological diseases. Anti-amyloidogenic effect of flavonoids was intermediated by targeting the key enzymes, which caused the pathogenesis and accumulation of amyloid plaques (Aβ). It was currently stated that anthocyanin-rich flavonoid compounds available in bilberry and black currant have the ability of preventing behavioural changes and altering APP dispensation in APP/PS1 AD induced mouse model [50]. Similarly, chronic treatment with tannic acid by means of the AD transgenic induced animal model of PS/APP for cerebral amyloidosis with improvements in transgene between animal behaviour and memory. Nobiletin, a citrus flavonoid was reported that it has the ability to reduce Aβ load and suppress Aβ induced memory deficits in the hippocampus of mutated animals [51]. In addition, chronic delivery of grape polyphenols leads to increased memory as well as decreases solubilised oligomer levels in Tg2576 animal's brain tissue [52]. Luteolin, a flavonoid based citrus, is shown to reduce the Aβ peptides formation in transgenic APP neuronal cells and reduce BACE1 activity (see Figs. **3** and **4**) [53].

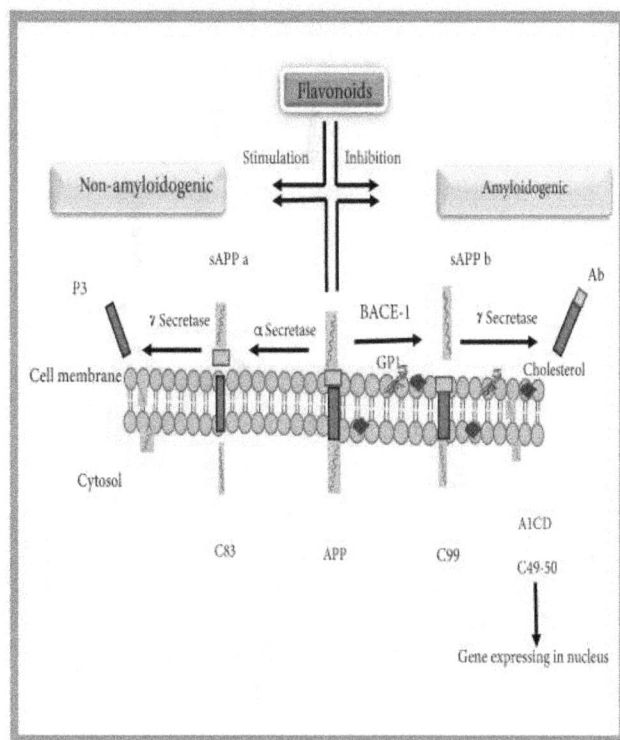

Fig. (3). Schematic presentation of molecular ways of Flavonoid action.

In addition, continuous polyphenol administration containing curcumin and grape seed extract for 9 months inhibits Aβ placement in the brains of AD induced animals [53]. Numerous studies report various beneficial properties of green tea due to the presence of EGCG. EGCG, a green tea-based polyphenol reduces the Aβ load by inhibiting the APP-converting enzyme [54, 55]. Naturally available flavonoids like EGCG and curcumin are reported to inhibit the modification of BACE1-mediated Aβ neuronal cultures [56]. Isorhamnetin reports neuroprotective activity against memory impairment induced by Aβ [57]. It improves comprehension and memory by building defence system of cholinergic signalling, antioxidant, and synaptic plasticity [58]. Kaempferol reduces cognitive deficits by monitoring neuro-inflammation and antioxidants [59], and increases retaining of memory and proliferation of CA1 neurons in hippocampus [60]. Quercetin, another flavonoid, has proficient therapeutic applications in AD. It produces a decrease in plaque load and mitochondrial impairment through AMPK activation and it improves brain function [61].

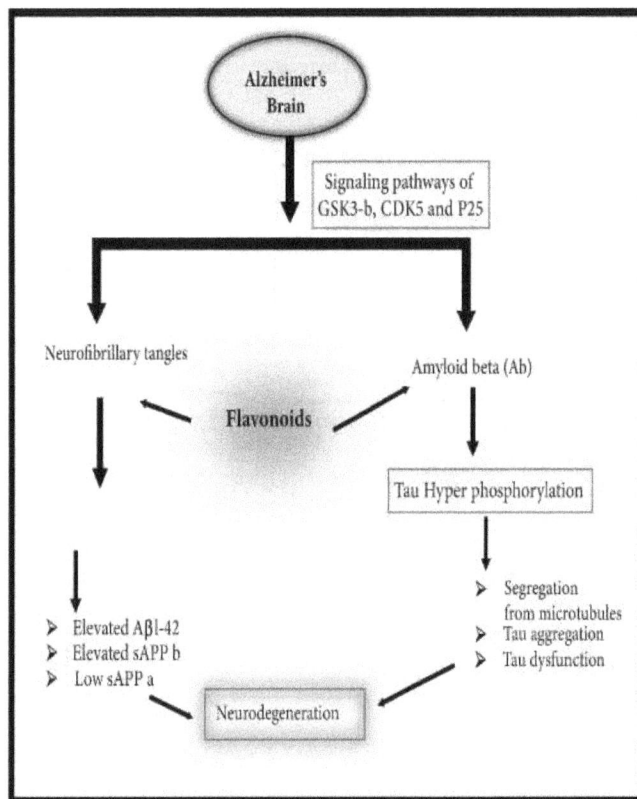

Fig. (4). Signaling pathway for Flavonoids mechanism in Alzheimer's brain.

The increase in EGCG production of APP processing non-amyloidogenic shows that phosphoinositide 3-kinase/ estrogen receptor-a/ Ak-transforming based processes. Depletion of post-menopausal estrogen is interlinked with the enhanced risk of AD in the patients, where selective receptor modulates AD therapeutic approach. EGCG regulated estrogen receptor modulation may be a substitute for estrogen-based treatment in managing AD [62]. It also provides beneficial effects of neuroprotection by inhibiting amyloid fibrils sheets rich in Aβ and inhibits fibrillogenesis. This fibrillogenesis reticence is regulated through binding with unopened polypeptides and suppressing their conversion into intermediate neurotoxic compounds [63]. In addition, EGCG is able to differentiate large amounts of Aβ fibrils into smaller proteins and as a result, they are unable to synthesize and thus have no toxic effects [64]. Myricetin has prominent potency as an *In-vitro* anti-amyloid and therefore has a potential therapeutic effect on neurodegeneration-related psychiatric disorders [65, 66]. In general, literature suggests flavonoids have the potential to disrupt the Aβ fibrillization formation process, inhibiting the important enzyme BACE1 involved in the Aβ formation, leading to Aβ product inhibition. However, more research is needed to determine neuromodulatory potency and lower processes of flavonoids in use of clinics.

Tau Targeting

Several studies indicate the effects of flavonoids on the production of highly phosphorylated tau protein, an important characteristic of AD [67, 68]. For example, epicatechin-5-gallate (EG) and myricetin have been stated to hinder the formation of heparin-mediated tau [69]. EG treatment in AD-induced transgenic animal models predicted modified tau profiles by inhibiting the generation of tau isoforms of sarkosyl-soluble phosphorylated [70]. In some projects working with grape seed proanthocyanidin extract (GSPE) and tau based neuropathology was considerably decreased in AD animal models by inhibiting tau peptide synthesis, its termination and its final clearance [71]). NFTs and accumulation of hyperphosphorylated tau proteins are chief majorly contributes the impairment of brain. The phosphorylation of tau proteins is mainly catalysed by various kinases such as GSK-3b, thus involved in the pathophysiology of AD. Flavonoids suppress the activity of different enzymes like kinases and hence help prevent AD. For example, indirubins inhibit the activity of protein kinases along with GSK-3b as well as CDK5 / p25, which are involved in the hyperphosphorylation of tau proteins seen in AD patients.

Morin, a flavonoid, is stated with the activity of constraining GSK-3b activity and tau protein phosphorylation. It also reduces Aβ-induced phosphorylation based on tau protein and prevents cytotoxicity induced by Aβ in human neuroblastoma cells. Additionally, morin treatment has decreased tau protein hyperphosphorylation in hippocampal neurons AD mice mutant animals of 3xTg [72]. Cyanidin 3-O-glucoside (Cy3G) protects significantly against abnormalities caused by Aβ administration in GSK-3b / tau mutations mediated animal models [73].

Neuro Anti-inflammation and Detoxifier

Neurodegenerative outcomes, which are observed in several neurological disorders appear to be provoked by numerous events neuro-inflammation, glutamatergic excitotoxicity, endogenous antioxidants depletion as well as neurotoxicity, which are mediated by different metabolic products [74]. There are various scientific pieces of evidences suggest flavonoids might also respond to internalise neuronal injuries mechanism and could basket the development of neurodegenerative disorders [17, 75]. Green tea consumption was reported to reduce PD threat, and deteriorate ischemic hippocampal injury and neurodegeneration that could be attributed to EGCG presence [76]. It was found that EGCG is known for modulating numerous signalling pathways basically PI3-kinase and protein kinase C role in neuroprotection and minimizes nigral damage by chelation of free radicals [76, 77]. Some of the *in vitro* studies also substantiated that flavonoid prevents the Parkinson's disease pathological aspects by obstructing the endogenous neurotoxin formation thus inhibits the nitric oxide production in activated microglia cells. It was found that blueberry flavonoids also exhibit TNF-α, nitric oxide, IL-1b production in microglia cells [78]. Some other flavonoids like wogonin, quercetin, EGCG, baicalein modulates neuro-inflammation and production of astrocyte/ microglial-mediated nitric oxide [79, 80]. The above actions are arbitrated by lipid kinase based signalling pathways, transformation of protein, pro-inflammatory based transcription factors, nitric oxide production, cyclooxygenase (COX-2) expression and iNOS downstream regulation, scavenging of free radicals, liberation of cytokine and NOX activation [81]. It was also reported that genistein and EGCG enhances the glutathione production by PI3-kinase-reliant based nuclear factor erythroid 2–related factor 2 (Nrf2)-induced antioxidant pathway regulation [82].

Targeting Other Pathways

It was found that flavonoids bind preferentially with neuronal receptors which include tyrosine receptor kinase B (TrkB), GABA-A, d-opioid, nicotinic, testosterone, estrogen, adenosine receptors and mediate numerous neuropharmacological actions [55, 83]. There were many reports related to good flavonoids neuroprotective effects and their metabolites by interacting with neuronal signalling pathways [84]. All the above interact with several lipid kinase, protein kinase signalling pathways like mitogen-activated kinase (MAPK), tyrosine kinase, nuclear factor-kB PI3K/Akt and protein kinase C pathway [84 - 86]. Flavonoids on binding to receptors might either inhibit or excite receptors and thus, they mediate their own actions *via* phosphorylation or gene expression modulation. They modulate the neuronal plasticity, synaptic protein synthesis as well as morphological changes, which are accountable for cognition impairment and neurodegenerative disorders. Metabolites of flavonoids also interacts with MAPKs signalling pathways (MEK2 and MEK1 receptors) resulting in cAMP downstream activation, thereby leading to alterations in memory and synaptic plasticity [87]. Anthocyanins and flavanols rich blueberry supplementation had also been reported for enhancing cognitive performance in case of animals by CREB activation and BDNF level elevation in the hippocampus.

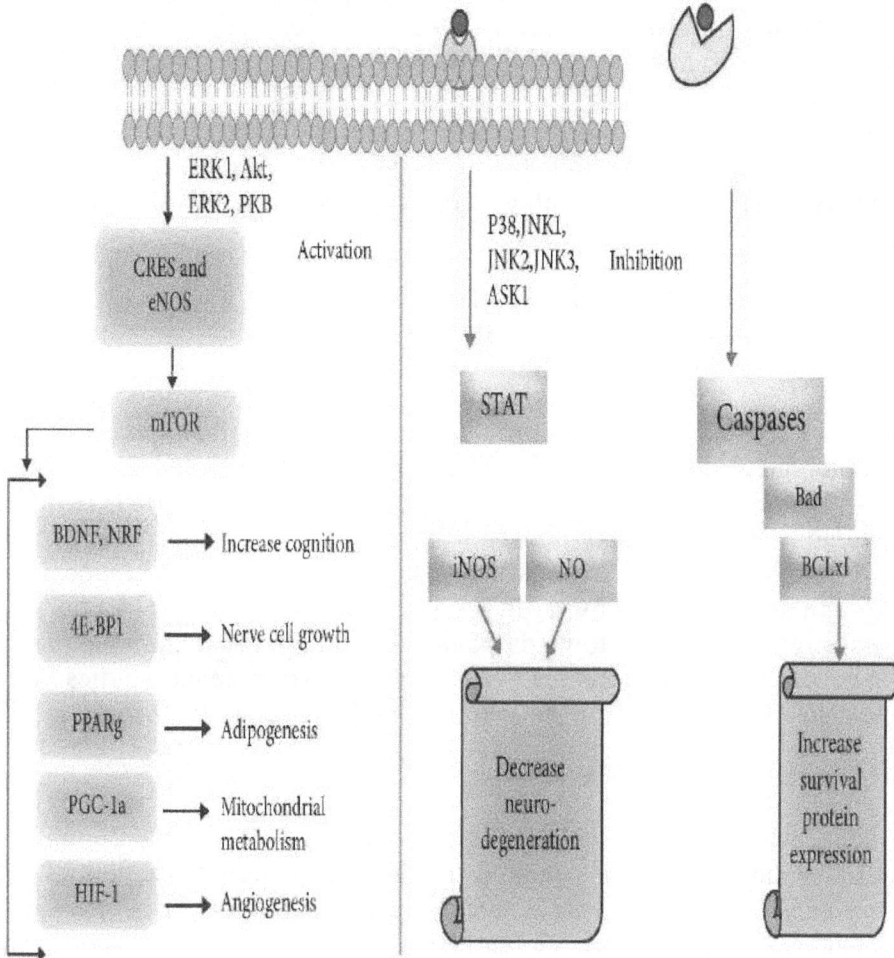

Fig. (5). Molecular binding of flavonoids which act on activation and inhibition.

Green tea catechins chronic administration could reduce $A\beta 1$–42 oligomers levels as well as up-regulates protein related synaptic plasticity action in hippocampus and elevates cAMP/ kinase A-response element binding protein (PKA/CREB) pathway [88]. Flavonoids activate peroxisome proliferator-activated receptor-g coactivator-1 (PGC-1a) pathway, stabilizing Nrf2 transcription factors and hypoxia inducible factor-1 (HIF-1) and acting as peroxisome proliferator-activated receptor gamma (PPAR-ɤ) modulators [89]. All the above flavonoid based molecular changes might recover AD pathophysiology as they protect neurons against reduced insulin resistance, oxidative stress, attenuates mitochondrial dysfunction and thus enhance cognitive impairment. Flavonoids direct interaction with ATP binding site and possess PI3-kinase modulating potentials [90]. Metabolites of Quercetin inhibit PI3-kinase activity thus inhibits prosurvival Akt/PKB signalling pathways (Fig. **5**). Hesperidin on the contrary activates Akt/PKB signalling pathway and imparts prosurvival features in cortical neurons [16].

Pathways of Various Signaling Proteins

EG moreover had also been reported for modulating, neurotransmission, reliant raise of PI3K in CREB phosphorylation, plasticity regulation *via* extracellular signal regulated kinase (ERK) stimulation, as well as GluR2 levels in neuronal corticol upregulation [91]. In one of the studies, chronic blueberry ingestion was reported to enhance mammalian target of rapamycin (mTOR) receptor downstream activation, Akt phosphorylation as well as increase Arc/Arg3.1 (activity-regulated cytoskeletal associated protein) content in hippocampus. As BDNF regulates Arc and is vital in long term potentiation (LTP), thus all these changes might be centred towards cognition and spatial memory improvement [92]. The above has been also proved by many experimental studies which are related to flavonoids effect on neuronal morphologies changes [93].

Toxicological Aspects of Flavonoids

Flavonoids wider accessibility, as well as their increased human consumption, also created major questions related to dietary components potential toxicity. Most of the natural products are better tolerated; but flavonoids as well as related phytochemicals exhibit neurobehavioral along with endocrine disrupting effects [94]. Flavonoids toxicity lies in the minimum range in case of animals, such as in rats, the LD50 found as 2–10 g/kg. Similar doses in humans are quite impracticable. Thus, as a preventive measure, doses less than 1 mg/adult/day were commended for humans [9]. In one study, quercetin, when administered as dietary supplement in both male and female albino rat in 27.8 mmol of concentration as daily dose, possesses carcinogenicity property. However, the exact mechanism of quercetin carcinogenicity is not specified. But these studies established that quercetin does not directly induce mutagenicity but indirectly activates mixed glucosidases [95]. Human cytochrome P450 (CYPs) could be either induced or inhibited by flavonoids depending upon their concentrations and structures. Flavonoids interacts with CYP3A4 is region of interest. Administering clinically used drugs and flavonoids might cause flavonoid–drug interactions as they modulate certain drug pharmacokinetics [9, 96].

CONCLUSION

Flavonoid-rich foodstuff's dietary usage may restore memory functions and possess the tendency of slowing down age-related decline in cognition as well as attenuate for the development of dementia conditions. The natural products' therapeutic importance in neurodegeneration attributes to modulatory neuropharmacological features. There are many further studies that need especially properly designed clinical trials for endorsing the flavonoids' clinical effectiveness with more prominent examples in clinical symptoms and signs of neurodegeneration. Several *In vivo* studies must be designed for obtaining a better insight related to efficacy of flavonoids related to their toxicities, bioavailability as well as accumulation in aging brain at targeted sites. By connecting a link among behavioural responses in test humans/ animals to hippocampal and cortical area changes, primary molecular events which are connected to neuronal stem cells, synaptic plasticity proliferation effects and cerebral blood flow changes would provide guidelines for dietary uses of flavonoids along with subsequent clinical endorsements in various neurological disorders. Employing spectroscopic and imaging techniques like NMR and MRI could provide a good idea of flavonoids attenuated changes in blood flow to cerebral, and electrophysiological changes as well as quantitative alterations in progenitor cells, grey matter density and neuronal stem cells. Coming to dementia and AD, it is vital to explore flavonoid anti-amyloid as well as tau modification properties both in *in vivo* and *in vitro* models. Considering the above, flavonoid tau modifying potential was investigated at a preliminary level, but there exist many detailed protocols on destabilization effects of tau proteins, β-amyloid and microglial activation effects which need to be explored. Further, endorsement related to the dose/daily intake and as well as duration of therapy should be given for efficacious and safe results. Molecular improvement CREB function reported for consolidating memory as they promote gene expression responsible for long term memory and synaptic morphology. Though there is a significant understanding of the biology of flavonoids, most clinicians consider them mistakenly as simple antioxidants, thus that remains barrier in the bioactive flavonoids development in preclinical studies. Presently it has been found that flavonoids by molecular brain and modulating cellular functions prevent both normal as well as disease-related deterioration in cognitive functions.

Therefore, flavonoids represent vital precursor molecules group in the quest for discovering newer memory enhancing agents that might be proven beneficial for counteracting and perhaps even suppressing decline in age-related cognitive functions.

CONSENT FOR PUBLICATION

Not applicable.

CONFLICT OF INTEREST

The authors declare no conflict of interest, financial or otherwise.

ACKNOWLEDGEMENTS

The authors acknowledge Department of Pharmaceuticals, Ministry of Chemical and Fertilizers, GOI, India.

REFERENCES

[1]   Havsteen BH. The biochemistry and medical significance of the flavonoids. Pharmacol Ther 2002; 96(2-3): 67-202.
        [http://dx.doi.org/10.1016/S0163-7258(02)00298-X] [PMID: 12453566]

[2]   Rice-Evans C, Packer L. Flavonoids. Flavonoids in Health and Disease 2003.

[3]   Havsteen B. Flavonoids, a class of natural products of high pharmacological potency. Biochem Pharmacol 1983; 32(7): 1141-8.
        [http://dx.doi.org/10.1016/0006-2952(83)90262-9] [PMID: 6342623]

[4]   Shukla R, Kakade S, Handa M, Kohli K. Emergence of Nanophytomedicine in Health Care Setting.Nanophytomedicine.   Singapore: Springer   Singapore   2020;   pp. 33-53.http://link.springer.com/10.1007/978-981-15-4909-0_3 Internet
        [http://dx.doi.org/10.1007/978-981-15-4909-0_3]

[5]   Robak J, Gryglewski RJ. Flavonoids are scavengers of superoxide anions. Biochem Pharmacol 1988; 37(5): 837-41.
        [http://dx.doi.org/10.1016/0006-2952(88)90169-4] [PMID: 2830882]

[6]   Cushnie TPT, Lamb AJ. Antimicrobial activity of flavonoids. Int J Antimicrob Agents 2005; 26(5): 343-56.
        [http://dx.doi.org/10.1016/j.ijantimicag.2005.09.002] [PMID: 16323269]

[7]   Middleton E Jr, Kandaswami C, Theoharides TC. The effects of plant flavonoids on mammalian cells: implications for inflammation, heart disease, and cancer. Pharmacol Rev 2000; 52(4): 673-751.
        [PMID: 11121513]

[8]   Marder M, Paladini A. GABA(A)-receptor ligands of flavonoid structure. Curr Top Med Chem 2002; 2(8): 853-67.
        [http://dx.doi.org/10.2174/1568026023393462] [PMID: 12171576]

[9]   Galati G, O'Brien PJ. Potential toxicity of flavonoids and other dietary phenolics: significance for their chemopreventive and anticancer properties. Free Radic Biol Med 2004; 37(3): 287-303.
        [http://dx.doi.org/10.1016/j.freeradbiomed.2004.04.034] [PMID: 15223063]

[10]   Handa M, Sharma A, Verma RK, Shukla R. Polycaprolactone based nano-carrier for co-administration

of moxifloxacin and rutin and its *In-vitro* evaluation for sepsis. J Drug Deliv Sci Technol 2019; 54(June): 101286.
[http://dx.doi.org/10.1016/j.jddst.2019.101286]

[11]   Macready AL, Kennedy OB, Ellis JA, Williams CM, Spencer JPE, Butler LT. Flavonoids and cognitive function: a review of human randomized controlled trial studies and recommendations for future studies. Genes Nutr 2009; 4(4): 227-42.
[http://dx.doi.org/10.1007/s12263-009-0135-4] [PMID: 19680703]

[12]   Spencer JPE. The impact of fruit flavonoids on memory and cognition. Br J Nutr 2010; 104(S3) (Suppl. 3): S40-7.
[http://dx.doi.org/10.1017/S0007114510003934] [PMID: 20955649]

[13]   Bakoyiannis I, Daskalopoulou A, Pergialiotis V, Perrea D. Phytochemicals and cognitive health: Are flavonoids doing the trick? Biomed Pharmacother 2019; 109: 1488-97.
[http://dx.doi.org/10.1016/j.biopha.2018.10.086] [PMID: 30551400]

[14]   Yevchak AM, Loeb SJ, Fick DM. Promoting Cognitive Health and Implications. Geriatr Nurs (Minneap) 2008; 29(5): 302-10.
[http://dx.doi.org/10.1016/j.gerinurse.2007.10.017] [PMID: 18929179]

[15]   Schroeter H, Boyd C, Spencer J, Williams R, Cadenas E, Riceevans C. MAPK signaling in neurodegeneration: influences of flavonoids and of nitric oxide. Neurobiol Aging 2002; 23(5): 861-80.
[http://dx.doi.org/10.1016/S0197-4580(02)00075-1] [PMID: 12392791]

[16]   Vauzour D, Vafeiadou K, Rice-Evans C, Williams RJ, Spencer JPE. Activation of pro-survival Akt and ERK1/2 signalling pathways underlie the anti-apoptotic effects of flavanones in cortical neurons. J Neurochem 2007; 103(4): 1355-67.
[http://dx.doi.org/10.1111/j.1471-4159.2007.04841.x] [PMID: 17961201]

[17]   Spencer JPE. Flavonoids: modulators of brain function? Br J Nutr 2008; 99(E-S1) (Suppl. 1): ES60-77.
[http://dx.doi.org/10.1017/S0007114508965776] [PMID: 18503736]

[18]   Lokesh BS, Kumar D, Handa M, Shukla R. History of Flavors Associated with Functional Foods and Nutraceuticals. 2019.
[http://dx.doi.org/10.1201/9780429470592-1]

[19]   Williams RJ, Spencer JPE. Flavonoids, cognition, and dementia: Actions, mechanisms, and potential therapeutic utility for Alzheimer disease. Free Radic Biol Med 2012; 52(1): 35-45.
[http://dx.doi.org/10.1016/j.freeradbiomed.2011.09.010] [PMID: 21982844]

[20]   Shukla R, Handa M, Pardhi VP. Introduction to Pharmaceutical Product Development 2020.https://www.taylorfrancis.com/books/9781000731323/chapters/10.1201/9780367821678-1
[http://dx.doi.org/10.1201/9780367821678-1]

[21]   Manach C, Scalbert A, Morand C, Rémésy C, Jiménez L. Polyphenols: food sources and bioavailability. Am J Clin Nutr 2004; 79(5): 727-47.
[http://dx.doi.org/10.1093/ajcn/79.5.727] [PMID: 15113710]

[22]   Manach C, Mazur A, Scalbert A. Polyphenols and prevention of cardiovascular diseases. Curr Opin Lipidol 2005; 16(1): 77-84.
[http://dx.doi.org/10.1097/00041433-200502000-00013] [PMID: 15650567]

[23]   Wang H, Murphy PA. Isoflavone Content in Commercial Soybean Foods. J Agric Food Chem 1994; 42(8): 1666-73.
[http://dx.doi.org/10.1021/jf00044a016]

[24]   Ding K, Wang S. Efficient synthesis of isoflavone analogues *via* a Suzuki coupling reaction. Tetrahedron Lett 2005; 46(21): 3707-9.
[http://dx.doi.org/10.1016/j.tetlet.2005.03.143]

[25]   Hoshino Y, Miyaura N, Suzuki A. Novel synthesis of isoflavones. Bull Chem Soc Jpn 1988; 61(8):

3008-10.
[http://dx.doi.org/10.1246/bcsj.61.3008]

[26]   Kochs G, Grisebach H. Enzymic synthesis of isoflavones. Eur J Biochem 1986; 155(2): 311-8.
[http://dx.doi.org/10.1111/j.1432-1033.1986.tb09492.x] [PMID: 3956488]

[27]   Donnelly DMX, Boland GM. Isoflavonoids and neoflavonoids: naturally occurring O-heterocycles.
Nat Prod Rep 1995; 12(3): 321-38.
[http://dx.doi.org/10.1039/np9951200321]

[28]   Chan SC, Chang YS, Kuo SC. Neoflavonoids from Dalbergia odorifera. Phytochemistry 1997; 46(5):
947-9.
[http://dx.doi.org/10.1016/S0031-9422(97)00365-8]

[29]   Singh RP, Pandey VB. Nivetin, a neoflavonoid from Echinops niveus. Phytochemistry 1990; 29(2):
680-1.
[http://dx.doi.org/10.1016/0031-9422(90)85148-9]

[30]   Sun X, Sneden A. Neoflavonoids from *Polygonum perfoliatum*. Planta Med 1999; 65(7): 671-3.
[http://dx.doi.org/10.1055/s-2006-960846] [PMID: 17260292]

[31]   Awale S, Shrestha SP, Tezuka Y, Ueda J, Matsushige K, Kadota S. Neoflavonoids and related
constituents from Nepalese propolis and their nitric oxide production inhibitory activity. J Nat Prod
2005; 68(6): 858-64.
[http://dx.doi.org/10.1021/np050009k] [PMID: 15974608]

[32]   Fukui K, Matsumoto T, Nakamura S, Nakayama M, Horie T. Synthetic Studies of the Flavone
Derivatives. VII. The Synthesis of Jaceidin. Bull Chem Soc Jpn 1968; 41(6): 1413-7.
[http://dx.doi.org/10.1246/bcsj.41.1413]

[33]   Bachman DL, Wolf PA, Linn R, *et al.* Prevalence of dementia and probable senile dementia of the
Alzheimer type in the Framingham Study. Neurology 1992; 42(1): 115-9.
[http://dx.doi.org/10.1212/WNL.42.1.115] [PMID: 1734291]

[34]   Atta-Ur-Rahman A, Nasim S, Baig I, *et al.* Two new isoflavanoids from the rhizomes of Iris soforana.
Nat Prod Res 2004; 18(5): 465-71.
[http://dx.doi.org/10.1080/14786410310001608136] [PMID: 15248616]

[35]   Orhan I, Kartal M, Tosun F, Şener B. Screening of various phenolic acids and flavonoid derivatives
for their anticholinesterase potential. Z Naturforsch C J Biosci 2007; 62(11-12): 829-32.
[http://dx.doi.org/10.1515/znc-2007-11-1210] [PMID: 18274286]

[36]   Lovell MA, Markesbery WR. Oxidative DNA damage in mild cognitive impairment and late-stage
Alzheimer's disease. Nucleic Acids Res 2007; 35(22): 7497-504.
[http://dx.doi.org/10.1093/nar/gkm821] [PMID: 17947327]

[37]   Mecocci P, Polidori MC, Cherubini A, *et al.* Lymphocyte oxidative DNA damage and plasma
antioxidants in Alzheimer disease. Arch Neurol 2002; 59(5): 794-8.
[http://dx.doi.org/10.1001/archneur.59.5.794] [PMID: 12020262]

[38]   Resende R, Ferreiro E, Pereira C, Resende de Oliveira C. Neurotoxic effect of oligomeric and fibrillar
species of amyloid-beta peptide 1-42: Involvement of endoplasmic reticulum calcium release in
oligomer-induced cell death. Neuroscience 2008; 155(3): 725-37.
[http://dx.doi.org/10.1016/j.neuroscience.2008.06.036] [PMID: 18621106]

[39]   Dumont M, Beal MF. Neuroprotective strategies involving ROS in Alzheimer disease. Free Radic Biol
Med 2011; 51(5): 1014-26.
[http://dx.doi.org/10.1016/j.freeradbiomed.2010.11.026] [PMID: 21130159]

[40]   Kowaltowski AJ, de Souza-Pinto NC, Castilho RF, Vercesi AE. Mitochondria and reactive oxygen
species. Free Radic Biol Med 2009; 47(4): 333-43.
[http://dx.doi.org/10.1016/j.freeradbiomed.2009.05.004] [PMID: 19427899]

[41]   Müller WE, Eckert A, Kurz C, Eckert GP, Leuner K. Mitochondrial dysfunction: Common final pathway in brain aging and alzheimer's disease-therapeutic aspects. Molecular Neurobiology. 2010; pp. 159-71.

[42]   Butterfield DA, Reed T, Newman SF, Sultana R. Roles of amyloid β-peptide-associated oxidative stress and brain protein modifications in the pathogenesis of Alzheimer's disease and mild cognitive impairment. Free Radic Biol Med 2007; 43(5): 658-77.
[http://dx.doi.org/10.1016/j.freeradbiomed.2007.05.037] [PMID: 17664130]

[43]   Craft JM, Watterson DM, Van Eldik LJ. Neuroinflammation: A potential therapeutic target. 2005.

[44]   Balducci C, Forloni G. Novel targets in Alzheimer's disease: A special focus on microglia. Pharmacol Res 2018; 130: 402-13.
[http://dx.doi.org/10.1016/j.phrs.2018.01.017] [PMID: 29391235]

[45]   Park L, Zhou P, Pitstick R, *et al.* Nox2-derived radicals contribute to neurovascular and behavioral dysfunction in mice overexpressing the amyloid precursor protein. Proc Natl Acad Sci USA 2008; 105(4): 1347-52.
[http://dx.doi.org/10.1073/pnas.0711568105] [PMID: 18202172]

[46]   Singh K, Rani A, Kumar S, *et al.* An early gene of the flavonoid pathway, flavanone 3-hydroxylase, exhibits a positive relationship with the concentration of catechins in tea (*Camellia sinensis*). Tree Physiol 2008; 28(9): 1349-56.
[http://dx.doi.org/10.1093/treephys/28.9.1349] [PMID: 18595847]

[47]   Mandel SA, Amit T, Kalfon L, Reznichenko L, Weinreb O, Youdim MBH. Cell signaling pathways and iron chelation in the neurorestorative activity of green tea polyphenols: special reference to epigallocatechin gallate (EGCG). J Alzheimers Dis 2008; 15(2): 211-22.
[http://dx.doi.org/10.3233/JAD-2008-15207] [PMID: 18953110]

[48]   Lee JW, Lee YK, Ban JO, *et al.* Green tea (-)-epigallocatechin-3-gallate inhibits beta-amyloid-induced cognitive dysfunction through modification of secretase activity *via* inhibition of ERK and NF-kappaB pathways in mice. J Nutr 2009; 139(10): 1987-93.
[http://dx.doi.org/10.3945/jn.109.109785] [PMID: 19656855]

[49]   Choi YT, Jung CH, Lee SR, *et al.* The green tea polyphenol (−)-epigallocatechin gallate attenuates β-amyloid-induced neurotoxicity in cultured hippocampal neurons. Life Sci 2001; 70(5): 603-14.
[http://dx.doi.org/10.1016/S0024-3205(01)01438-2] [PMID: 11811904]

[50]   Vepsäläinen S, Koivisto H, Pekkarinen E, *et al.* Anthocyanin-enriched bilberry and blackcurrant extracts modulate amyloid precursor protein processing and alleviate behavioral abnormalities in the APP/PS1 mouse model of Alzheimer's disease. J Nutr Biochem 2013; 24(1): 360-70.
[http://dx.doi.org/10.1016/j.jnutbio.2012.07.006] [PMID: 22995388]

[51]   Onozuka H, Nakajima A, Matsuzaki K, *et al.* Nobiletin, a citrus flavonoid, improves memory impairment and Abeta pathology in a transgenic mouse model of Alzheimer's disease. J Pharmacol Exp Ther 2008; 326(3): 739-44.
[http://dx.doi.org/10.1124/jpet.108.140293] [PMID: 18544674]

[52]   Wang SY, Bowman L, Ding M. Methyl jasmonate enhances antioxidant Food Chem 2008; 107(3): 1261-9.

[53]   Rezai-Zadeh K, Douglas Shytle R, Bai Y, *et al.* Flavonoid-mediated presenilin-1 phosphorylation reduces Alzheimer's disease β-amyloid production. J Cell Mol Med 2009; 13(3): 574-88.
[http://dx.doi.org/10.1111/j.1582-4934.2008.00344.x] [PMID: 18410522]

[54]   Rezai-Zadeh K, Shytle D, Sun N, *et al.* Green tea epigallocatechin-3-gallate (EGCG) modulates amyloid precursor protein cleavage and reduces cerebral amyloidosis in Alzheimer transgenic mice. J Neurosci 2005; 25(38): 8807-14.
[http://dx.doi.org/10.1523/JNEUROSCI.1521-05.2005] [PMID: 16177050]

[55]   Rezai-Zadeh K, Arendash GW, Hou H, *et al.* Green tea epigallocatechin-3-gallate (EGCG) reduces β-

amyloid mediated cognitive impairment and modulates tau pathology in Alzheimer transgenic mice. Brain Res 2008; 1214: 177-87.
[http://dx.doi.org/10.1016/j.brainres.2008.02.107] [PMID: 18457818]

[56]   Shimmyo Y, Kihara T, Akaike A, Niidome T, Sugimoto H. Epigallocatechin-3-gallate and curcumin suppress amyloid beta-induced beta-site APP cleaving enzyme-1 upregulation. Neuroreport 2008; 19(13): 1329-33.
[http://dx.doi.org/10.1097/WNR.0b013e32830b8ae1] [PMID: 18695518]

[57]   Asha D, Sumathi T. Nootropic activity of isorhamnetin in amyloid beta 25-35 induced cognitive dysfunction and its related MRNA expressions in Alzheimer's Int J Pharm Sci Res 2016; 7(8)

[58]   Ishola IO, Jacinta AA, Adeyemi OO. Cortico-hippocampal memory enhancing activity of hesperetin on scopolamine-induced amnesia in mice: role of antioxidant defense system, cholinergic neurotransmission and expression of BDNF. Metab Brain Dis 2019; 34(4): 979-89.
[http://dx.doi.org/10.1007/s11011-019-00409-0] [PMID: 30949953]

[59]   Babaei P, Kouhestani S, Jafari A. Kaempferol attenuates cognitive deficit *via* regulating oxidative stress and neuroinflammation in an ovariectomized rat model of sporadic dementia. Neural Regen Res 2018; 13(10): 1827-32.
[http://dx.doi.org/10.4103/1673-5374.238714] [PMID: 30136699]

[60]   Darbandi N, Ramezani M, Khodagholi F, Noori M. Kaempferol Biologija (Vilnius) 2016; 62(3)

[61]   Wang X, Ouyang YY, Liu J, Zhao G. Flavonoid intake and risk of CVD: a systematic review and meta-analysis of prospective cohort studies. Br J Nutr 2014; 111(1): 1-11.
[http://dx.doi.org/10.1017/S000711451300278X] [PMID: 23953879]

[62]   Fernandez JW, Rezai-Zadeh K, Obregon D, Tan J. EGCG functions through estrogen receptor-mediated activation of ADAM10 in the promotion of non-amyloidogenic processing of APP. FEBS Lett 2010; 584(19): 4259-67.
[http://dx.doi.org/10.1016/j.febslet.2010.09.022] [PMID: 20849853]

[63]   Ehrnhoefer DE, Bieschke J, Boeddrich A, *et al.* EGCG redirects amyloidogenic polypeptides into unstructured, off-pathway oligomers. Nat Struct Mol Biol 2008; 15(6): 558-66.
[http://dx.doi.org/10.1038/nsmb.1437] [PMID: 18511942]

[64]   Bieschke J, Russ J, Friedrich RP, *et al.* EGCG remodels mature α-synuclein and amyloid-β fibrils and reduces cellular toxicity. Proc Natl Acad Sci USA 2010; 107(17): 7710-5.
[http://dx.doi.org/10.1073/pnas.0910723107] [PMID: 20385841]

[65]   Hirohata M, Hasegawa K, Tsutsumi-Yasuhara S, *et al.* The anti-amyloidogenic effect is exerted against Alzheimer's beta-amyloid fibrils in vitro by preferential and reversible binding of flavonoids to the amyloid fibril structure. Biochemistry 2007; 46(7): 1888-99.
[http://dx.doi.org/10.1021/bi061540x] [PMID: 17253770]

[66]   Ono K, Yoshiike Y, Takashima A, Hasegawa K, Naiki H, Yamada M. Potent anti-amyloidogenic and fibril-destabilizing effects of polyphenols *in vitro*: implications for the prevention and therapeutics of Alzheimer's disease. J Neurochem 2003; 87(1): 172-81.
[http://dx.doi.org/10.1046/j.1471-4159.2003.01976.x] [PMID: 12969264]

[67]   Baptista R, Madureira AM, Jorge R, Adão R, Duarte A, Duarte N, *et al.* Antioxidant and antimycotic activities of two native Lavandula species from Portugal. Evidence-based Complement Altern Med 2015.

[68]   Calcul L, Zhang B, Jinwal UK, Dickey CA, Baker BJ. Natural products as a rich source of tau-targeting drugs for Alzheimer's disease. Future Med Chem 2012; 4(13): 1751-61.
[http://dx.doi.org/10.4155/fmc.12.124] [PMID: 22924511]

[69]   Taniguchi S, Suzuki N, Masuda M, *et al.* Inhibition of heparin-induced tau filament formation by phenothiazines, polyphenols, and porphyrins. J Biol Chem 2005; 280(9): 7614-23.
[http://dx.doi.org/10.1074/jbc.M408714200] [PMID: 15611092]

[70]   Rezai-Zadeh K, Ehrhart J, Bai Y, *et al.* Apigenin and luteolin modulate microglial activation *via* inhibition of STAT1-induced CD40 expression. J Neuroinflammation 2008; 5(1): 41.
[http://dx.doi.org/10.1186/1742-2094-5-41] [PMID: 18817573]

[71]   Pasinetti G, Ho L. Role of grape seed polyphenols in Alzheimer's disease neuropathology. Nutr Diet Suppl 2010; 2010(2): 97-103.
[http://dx.doi.org/10.2147/NDS.S6898] [PMID: 23730149]

[72]   Gong EJ, Park HR, Kim ME, *et al.* Morin attenuates tau hyperphosphorylation by inhibiting GSK3β. Neurobiol Dis 2011; 44(2): 223-30.
[http://dx.doi.org/10.1016/j.nbd.2011.07.005] [PMID: 21782947]

[73]   Qin P, Wu L, Yao Y, Ren G. Changes in phytochemical compositions, antioxidant and α-glucosidase inhibitory activities during the processing of tartary buckwheat tea. Food Res Int 2013; 50(2): 562-7.
[http://dx.doi.org/10.1016/j.foodres.2011.03.028]

[74]   Jellinger KA, Paulus W, Wrocklage C, Litvan I. Traumatic brain injury as a risk factor for Alzheimer disease. Comparison of two retrospective autopsy cohorts with evaluation of ApoE genotype. BMC Neurol 2001; 1(1): 3.
[http://dx.doi.org/10.1186/1471-2377-1-3] [PMID: 11504565]

[75]   Mandel S, Youdim MBH. Catechin polyphenols: neurodegeneration and neuroprotection in neurodegenerative diseases. Free Radic Biol Med 2004; 37(3): 304-17.
[http://dx.doi.org/10.1016/j.freeradbiomed.2004.04.012] [PMID: 15223064]

[76]   Mandel SA, Avramovich-Tirosh Y, Reznichenko L, *et al.* Multifunctional activities of green tea catechins in neuroprotection. Modulation of cell survival genes, iron-dependent oxidative stress and PKC signaling pathway. Neurosignals 2005; 14(1-2): 46-60.
[http://dx.doi.org/10.1159/000085385] [PMID: 15956814]

[77]   Weinreb O, Amit T, Mandel S, Youdim MBH. Neuroprotective molecular mechanisms of (−)-epigallocatechin-3-gallate: a reflective outcome of its antioxidant, iron chelating and neuritogenic properties. Genes Nutr 2009; 4(4): 283-96.
[http://dx.doi.org/10.1007/s12263-009-0143-4] [PMID: 19756809]

[78]   Lau FC, Shukitt-Hale B, Joseph JA. Nutritional intervention in brain aging: reducing the effects of inflammation and oxidative stress. Subcell Biochem 2007; 42: 299-318.
[http://dx.doi.org/10.1007/1-4020-5688-5_14] [PMID: 17612057]

[79]   Chen D, Daniel KG, Chen MS, Kuhn DJ, Landis-Piwowar KR, Dou QP. Dietary flavonoids as proteasome inhibitors and apoptosis inducers in human leukemia cells. Biochem Pharmacol 2005; 69(10): 1421-32.
[http://dx.doi.org/10.1016/j.bcp.2005.02.022] [PMID: 15857606]

[80]   Lee H, Kim YO, Kim H, *et al.* Flavonoid wogonin from medicinal herb is neuroprotective by inhibiting inflammatory activation of microglia. FASEB J 2003; 17(13): 1-21.
[http://dx.doi.org/10.1096/fj.03-0057fje] [PMID: 12897065]

[81]   Zheng Y, Valdez PA, Danilenko DM, *et al.* Interleukin-22 mediates early host defense against attaching and effacing bacterial pathogens. Nat Med 2008; 14(3): 282-9.
[http://dx.doi.org/10.1038/nm1720] [PMID: 18264109]

[82]   Hernandez-Montes E, Pollard SE, Vauzour D, *et al.* Activation of glutathione peroxidase *via* Nrf1 mediates genistein's protection against oxidative endothelial cell injury. Biochem Biophys Res Commun 2006; 346(3): 851-9.
[http://dx.doi.org/10.1016/j.bbrc.2006.05.197] [PMID: 16780800]

[83]   Katavic PL, Lamb K, Navarro H, Prisinzano TE. Flavonoids as opioid receptor ligands: identification and preliminary structure-activity relationships. J Nat Prod 2007; 70(8): 1278-82.
[http://dx.doi.org/10.1021/np070194x] [PMID: 17685652]

[84]   Incani A, Deiana M, Corona G, *et al.* Involvement of ERK, Akt and JNK signalling in H2O2-induced

cell injury and protection by hydroxytyrosol and its metabolite homovanillic alcohol. Mol Nutr Food Res 2010; 54(6): 788-96.
[http://dx.doi.org/10.1002/mnfr.200900098] [PMID: 20024934]

[85]   Schroeter H, Spencer JPE, Rice-Evans C, Williams RJ. Flavonoids protect neurons from oxidized low-density-lipoprotein-induced apoptosis involving c-Jun N-terminal kinase (JNK), c-Jun and caspase-3. Biochem J 2001; 358(3): 547-57.
[http://dx.doi.org/10.1042/bj3580547] [PMID: 11535118]

[86]   Gamet-Payrastre L, Manenti S, Gratacap MP, Tulliez J, Chap H, Payrastre B. Flavonoids and the inhibition of PKC and PI 3-kinase. Gen Pharmacol 1999; 32(3): 279-86.
[http://dx.doi.org/10.1016/S0306-3623(98)00220-1] [PMID: 10211581]

[87]   Impey S, Obrietan K, Storm DR. Making new connections: role of ERK/MAP kinase signaling in neuronal plasticity. Neuron 1999; 23(1): 11-4.
[http://dx.doi.org/10.1016/S0896-6273(00)80747-3] [PMID: 10402188]

[88]   Li LL, McCorkle SR, Monchy S, Taghavi S, van der Lelie D. Bioprospecting metagenomes: glycosyl hydrolases for converting biomass. Biotechnol Biofuels 2009; 2(1): 10.
[http://dx.doi.org/10.1186/1754-6834-2-10] [PMID: 19450243]

[89]   Feng Y, Lin W, Li W, Wang Q. Equations of state and diagrams of two-dimensional liquid dusty plasmas. Phys Plasmas 2016; 23(9): 093705.
[http://dx.doi.org/10.1063/1.4962685]

[90]   Vlahos NJ, Khattak A, Manheim ML, Kanafani A. The role of teamwork in a planning methodology for intelligent urban transportation systems. Transp Res, Part C Emerg Technol 1994; 2(4): 217-29.
[http://dx.doi.org/10.1016/0968-090X(94)90011-6]

[91]   Schroeter C, House L, Lorence A. Fruit and vegetable consumption among college students in Arkansas and Florida: Food culture vs. health knowledge. Int Food Agribus Manag Rev 2007; 10(3): 63-89.

[92]   Waltereit P, Brandt O, Ramsteiner M, *et al.* M-plane GaN grown on γ-LiAlO2(100): nitride semiconductors free of internal electrostatic fields. J Cryst Growth 2001; 227-228: 437-41.
[http://dx.doi.org/10.1016/S0022-0248(01)00739-4]

[93]   van Praag H, Lucero MJ, Yeo GW, *et al.* Plant-derived flavanol (-)epicatechin enhances angiogenesis and retention of spatial memory in mice. J Neurosci 2007; 27(22): 5869-78.
[http://dx.doi.org/10.1523/JNEUROSCI.0914-07.2007] [PMID: 17537957]

[94]   Bügel SG, Hertwig J, Kahl J, Lairon D, Paoletti F, Strassner C. The New Nordic Diet as a prototype for regional sustainable diets. Sustain Value Chain Sustain. Food Syst 2016; 2016: 109-6.

[95]   Dunnick J, Hailey JR. Toxicity and carcinogenicity studies of quercetin, a natural component of foods. Fundam Appl Toxicol 1992; 19(3): 423-31.
[http://dx.doi.org/10.1016/0272-0590(92)90181-G] [PMID: 1459373]

[96]   Hodek P, Trefil P, Stiborová M. Flavonoids-potent and versatile biologically active compounds interacting with cytochromes P450. Chem Biol Interact 2002; 139(1): 1-21.
[http://dx.doi.org/10.1016/S0009-2797(01)00285-X] [PMID: 11803026]

[97]   Uriarte-Pueyo I, Calvo MI. Flavonoids as acetylcholinesterase inhibitors. Curr Med Chem 2011; 18(34): 5289-302.
[http://dx.doi.org/10.2174/092986711798184325] [PMID: 22087826]

CHAPTER 2

Potential Uses of Plant and Marine Derived Bioactive Compounds for Cancer Theragnostic

Neha Jain[1], Mukesh Kumar Sharma[2,*], Yoshihisa Matsumoto[3] and Pallavi Kaushik[1]

[1] *Department of Zoology, University of Rajasthan, Jaipur-302004, India*

[2] *Department of Zoology, SPC Government College, Ajmer-305001, India*

[3] *Institute of Innovative Research, Tokyo Institute of Technology, Tokyo, Japan*

Abstract: The evolution of novel strategies for application in all facets of cancer theragnostic has shown great progress in the past several decades. Bioactive compounds collected from plants and marine natural provenances have now been accredited as the crucial stepping stone to endow with fortification approach against several relentless ailments counting cancer. As per sundry investigations reports, the naturally occurring bioactive compounds possess an unprecedented molecular diversity with the potential to modulate several metabolic processes with high priority objectives such as low toxicity, targeting multiple drug resistance and heterogeneity of the tumor cells. These attributes with bioactive compounds can provide safe and high quality of healthy life achievable with easily available low-cost alternatives and nominal or no side effects. In topical quondam, numerous potent phytochemicals and marine molecules have been isolated, exemplified, identified, and are under disparate phases of clinical trials for human welfare. In this context, the chapter addresses recently discovered plant and marine originated natural compounds for cancer therapeutics concerning with more targeted and innoxious approach with future outlook. Moreover, an attempt to consolidate data on various bioactive compounds has been made which herald to aid in unrelenting research into potential use either solely or in combination with other widely employed therapies.

Keywords: Anticancer therapeutics, Bioactive compounds, Cytotoxic, Phytochemicals, Tumorigenesis.

INTRODUCTION

CANCER is the second significant leading cause of mortality worldwide giving rise to an immense burden on communal health and is reflected to be one of the

* **Corresponding author Mukesh Kumar Sharma:** Department of Zoology, SPC Government College, Ajmer-305001, India; Tel: +91-98291 99444; E-mail: mkshrma@hotmail.com

major challenges of the century, allied with severe medical connotation in concert with social and economic impacts [1 - 6]. World Health Organization projects 100 million cancer cases per year, causing 6 million deaths all around the world. According to them, if the trend continues, there will be a high probability of a boost in cancer cases (up to 60%) in the coming two decades.

Cancer is an uncontrolled proliferation of cells which invade other parts of the body causing acute damage at the molecular and cellular levels [3]. Moreover, it also stimulates chronic inflammation which accelerates consequences like apoptosis evasion, metastasis, angiogenesis and DNA damage [8 - 10]. The standard therapies used for cancer treatment confer lifelong morbidities along with other issues like bystander effects, multi-drug resistance, untimely relapses, low efficacy, are expensive and have several other lethal side effects [1, 2, 9, 11 - 14].

Therefore, there is an imperative need for devising castigating therapeutic interventions with broad exploration and novel health promising strategies comprising of naturally occurring bioactive compounds.

Biologically active natural compounds are used in about 80% of licensed chemotherapeutic drugs and more than half of all primary drugs. These are also responsible for curing 87% of human illnesses, including various types of malignancies [15, 16]. Natural products and their derivatives act on the life-threatening disease by interfering with the mechanism of carcinogenesis and its multistep progression, preventing proliferation by one or more pathways. The prime mechanisms of anticancer properties of bioactive compounds include; arresting cell cycle modulating processes, inhibiting metastasis [15, 16], inducing apoptosis, cleaving DNA [17, 18], permeabilizing mitochondrial membrane [11] and inhibiting angiogenesis [15], *etc.*

Many natural bioactive products derived from plant, marine and microbial sources have the potentiality to serve as chemotherapeutic as well as chemo-preventive agents [6, 10]. The phytochemicals from therapeutic plants have been employed in traditional medicines for centuries and have been the subject of scientific drug discovery even in present times. Although, the bioactives from marine sources seem as a newer dimension of study, being exploited since 1970s, but hold auspicious sources, as their chemical ingenuity and diversity outweigh terrestrial founts [17]. These pharmacologically active bioactive compounds are either refined into medicament directly or serve as "pharmacophores" for the chemical production of cognates with enhanced potencies and physicochemical attributes [19].

Plants Derived Bioactive Compounds

Among enormous miscellany of functional bioactive compounds or phytochemicals have engrossed broad recognition for their extensive anticancer bioactivities linked with antioxidant and immune-stimulating applications impacting health and wellness. Major therapeutic properties of bioactive compounds are demonstrated in Fig. (**4**). Numerous findings have highlighted that therapeutic plant derived compounds can augment the effectiveness of various cancer remedial treatments and in some cases, alleviate many of the detrimental concomitants of chemotherapeutic agents. Some of the significant bioactive compounds with prospective use in malignant therapeutics are described in the following text.

Curcumin

A polyphenolic metabolite (Fig. **1**) isolated from the rhizome of *Curcuma longa*, *C. zedoaria* and *Acorus calamus L.*(Zingiberaceae) which is accredited to broad spectrum of pharmacological activities such as antioxidant, chemotherapeutic, chemopreventive, and chemo-sensitizing pursuits [5, 20 - 25]. Antiproliferative properties of Curcumin have been demonstrated in *in vivo* and *in vitro* models against breast, pancreatic, prostate, colorectal, ovarian, skin and blood cancer, hematological malignancies and esophageal squamous cell carcinoma (EC1, KYSE450, EC9706, TE13cell lines) [5, 20, 25]. It pertains various anti-cancer attributes like: inhibiting associated enzymes such as Cyclooxygenase (COX)-2, 5-LOX and iNOS. Other anti-cancer mechanisms include caspase activation, cytochrome P450 enzymes modulation, upregulation of CDKIs, cell cycle arrest at G1, S-phase and G2/M phase check points, inhibition of NF-κB transcription factor and down-regulation of vascular endothelial growth factor's expressions, platelet- derived growth factor and fibroblast growth factors [23, 24]. Although, Curcumin plays an important role as chemo-sensitizer with some anti-tumor drugs like 5-fluorouracil, gemcitabine, paclitaxel, doxorubicin and also work as synergist with natural drugs like honokiol, resveratrol, epigallocatechin-3-gallate, omega-3 and licochalcone but the studied metabolite has exceptionally low absorptivity, demonstrates meager systemic bioavailability and is indecently metabolized [23].

Camptothecin

Quinolone alkaloids (Fig. **1**) are extracted from *Camptotheca acuminata*, a Chinese ornamental plant. The complex and its derivatives possess antineoplastic properties [1, 5, 26] linking with DNA topoisomerase 1 and inhibiting DNA's relegation and cleavage, thus leading to DNA sever and cytotoxicity [5, 26]. At present, topotecan and irinotecan, the two well-known derivatives of camptothecin which are the semi-synthetic in nature, are clinically approved for the treatment of recurring ovarian cancer, cervical cancer, small cell lung cancer; and rectum and large intestine cancers, respectively with a reduced amount of toxicity than the parent compound [1, 5, 26].

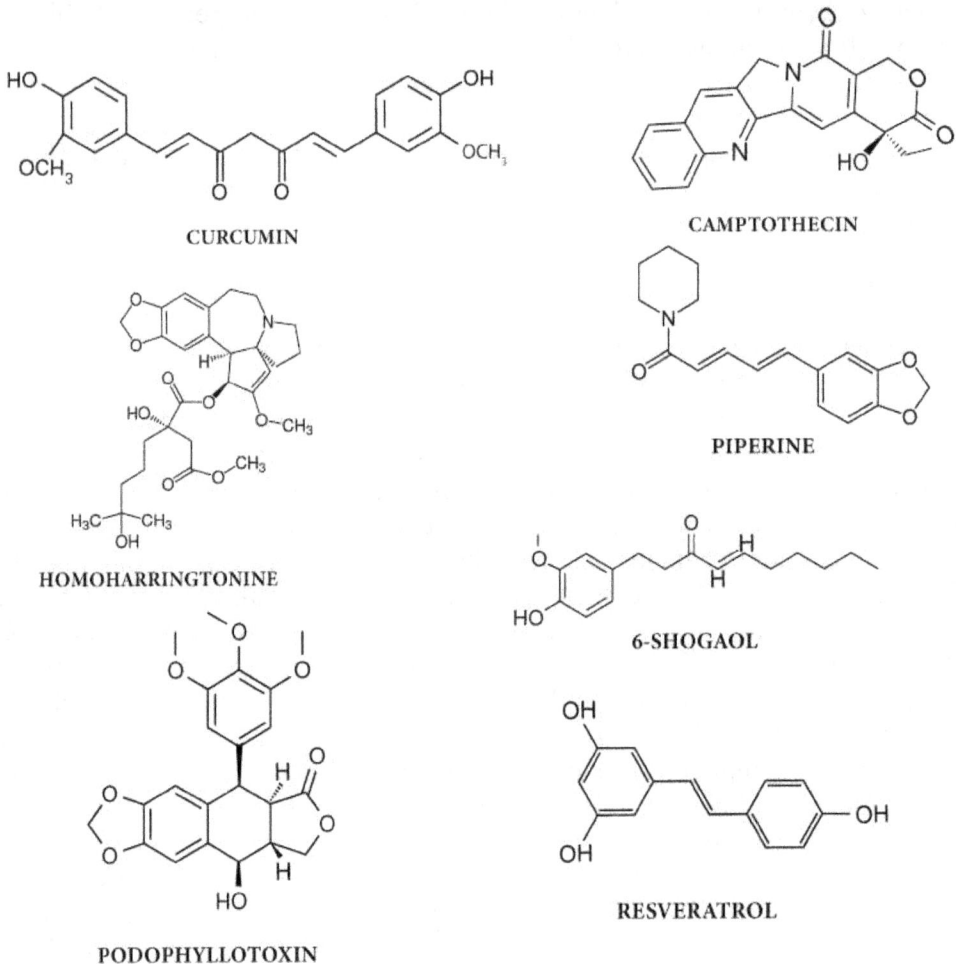

CURCUMIN

CAMPTOTHECIN

HOMOHARRINGTONINE

PIPERINE

6-SHOGAOL

RESVERATROL

PODOPHYLLOTOXIN

Fig. (1). Structures of various plant derived bioactive compounds.

Homoharringtonine

Cephalotaxine's esters (Fig. **1**) isolated from *Cephalotaxus harringtonia* are acknowledged to operate against breast cancer [26] and chronic myeloid leukemia [1, 5, 26]. In addition, the compound has been investigated to deliver absolute hematologic diminution in patients anguishing from late-stage chronic myelogenous leukemia [1]. Mechanistically, it induces apoptosis and trusses the A-site cleft of the large ribosomal subunit, thus blocking the admittance of charged tRNA thereby eventually inhibiting course of action of translation [5, 23, 25]. Furthermore, one of the prominent therapeutic semi-synthetic derivatives of homoharringtonine *i.e.* omacetaxine mepesuccinate has been proved to be effective for treating myelodysplastic syndromes and chronic myelomonocytic leukemia in patients suffering from aversion and resistance to hypomethylating agents [5].

Piperine (1-piperoyl piperidine)

An alkaloid (Fig. **1**), isolated from *Piper nigrum* [20, 27] and *Piper longum* [27] that has been recognized for numerous anti- malignant characteristics for example, decreased metastasis and neo-angiogenesis; lowering of polyamine synthesis, cytokines reduction, tempering of lipid peroxidation, and alterations of many pathways to perform in opposition to melanoma, sarcoma, lung cancer, and colon cancer and thereby performing a promising anti- tumorigenic bioactive source [20, 27]. Moreover, it is investigated that the compound has the capability to activate caspase- 3 in ovarian and melanoma cancer cell lines; activate procaspase-3, 7 and inhibit the expression of survivin gene whose major function is to inhibit caspase activation expression in colon cancer cells and also in murine breast cancer cells. It also has the competence of inhibiting phosphorylation of **Survivin's** transcription factor [p65] leading to the process of **Survivin** inhibition [27]. Additionally, when employed in combination with other metabolites, piperine not only augments their bioactivity, but also amplifies their effectiveness. For case, a combination of piperine and curcumin in a study dramatically abridged the amount of DNA damage and 8-oxo-dG concentration in BP- persuaded DNA break in lungs, livers, and colon in *in vivo* model, signifying a superior geno-protective competence in contrast to curcumin exclusively [20].

Podophyllotoxin

A natural therapeutic agent known for its latent anti- neoplastic potency to medicate skin cancer, which is isolated from *Podophyllum emodi* and *Podophyllum peltatum* (Fig. **1**) [1, 5, 26].The compound tends to bind with tubulin so as to suppress its activity in a reversible manner and thus interrupting the karyokinetic spindle organization [5, 26]. Further, by means of their encounters with DNA topoisomerase II, the podophyllotoxins cause cell cycle arrest in G2 phase by inducing single and double stranded DNA breaks. Some of the major semi-synthetic derivatives of the compound namely, etopophos, teniposide, etoposide, azatoxin, tafluposide, GL33, NK61, and TOP-53, also bear anti-tumor proficiency by distressing the metaphase of cell cycle, thus paving the way to apoptosis [26]. Furthermore, these compounds also exhibit anti-multidrug resistance in several cancer cells. For instance, by controlling topoisomerase- IIa activity, CIP-36, a derivative of podophyllotoxin, has been evaluated to resolve the multidrug resistance in adriamycin-resistant human leukemia (K562/ADR) cell line [5]. Podophyllotoxin with its derivatives has been effectively explored its anticancer properties against lymphomas, neuroblastomas, sarcomas, gliomas, carcinomas, cervical, testicular, ovarian, colon, lung, breast, prostate, gastrointestinal and brain cancers [26].

Resveratrol (trans-3,5,4'-trihydroxystilbene)

A natural polyphenol (Fig. **1**) that belongs to a stillbenoid composition and primarily isolated from red grapes, peanuts, blueberry mulberry, cranberries, *etc* [5, 24, 25]. The compound possesses various beneficial aspects comprising anti-estrogenic, anti-oxidative activities [24] and anti-tumourigenesis which has been reported in esophageal, prostate, pancreatic, gastric, ovarian, melanoma, endometrial, thyroid, lung, colon, liver, head and neck cancers as well as colon cancer cell line (Caco-2, HCT 116 and HT29). Resveratrol's inhibitory functions have been demonstrated to be indispensable in order to amend a diverse spectrum of cellular components and proliferation causative pathways. In addition, LOX, iNOS, COX2 and other inflammation molecules are also known to be suppressed by the therapeutic agent [20]. The phytochemical has twofold role on cells *i.e.* it can either cause or inhibit angiogenic effects, revealing its salutary action in separate tumor cells based on their environmental conditions [24].

Vinca Alkaloids (Catharanthus Alkaloids)

Compounds (Fig. **2**) derived from the *Catharanthus roseus*, are the first known agents to be introduced in the health sector. It comprises 130 terpenoid indole alkaloids out of which Vinblastine is the foremost to be extracted from the beneficial plant [19, 26, 28]. Vinblastine, vincristine and anhydrovinblastine are the major known alkaloids and vinflunine, vindesine and vinorelbine conclude some of the chief semi-synthetic derivatives of the phytochemical [1, 5, 23, 26] as mentioned in Fig. (**2**). *Catharanthus* alkaloids exhibit cytotoxic effects on cancerous cells by targeting microtubules and binding to their tubulin subunits. Apparently, based on their concentration, the agents illustrate diverse action mechanisms. At low concentrations [<1 μmol], these are capable of maintaining and suppressing the dynamics of the microtubules, whereas at high concentrations [>1–2 μmol], these have the caliber to induce the direct collapse of the microtubules and disruption the mitotic spindle, contributing to mitosis inhibition and apoptosis [5, 26]. To treat non-small cell lung, renal, bladder, ovarian, breast cancer, Kaposi's sarcoma and soft tissue sarcoma, the alkaloids are employed in chemotherapy. These are also acknowledged to cure idiopathic thrombocytopenic purpura, malignant lymphomas, acute lymphocytic leukemia, and various solid tumors namely Ewing's sarcoma, Wilms' tumor, neuroectodermal tumors and retinoblastoma [1, 5, 26]. More than 160 of over 2069 therapeutic investigations identified by National Cancer Institute for drug formulations are employing vinca alkaloids as mediators countering a wide range of malignancies [1].

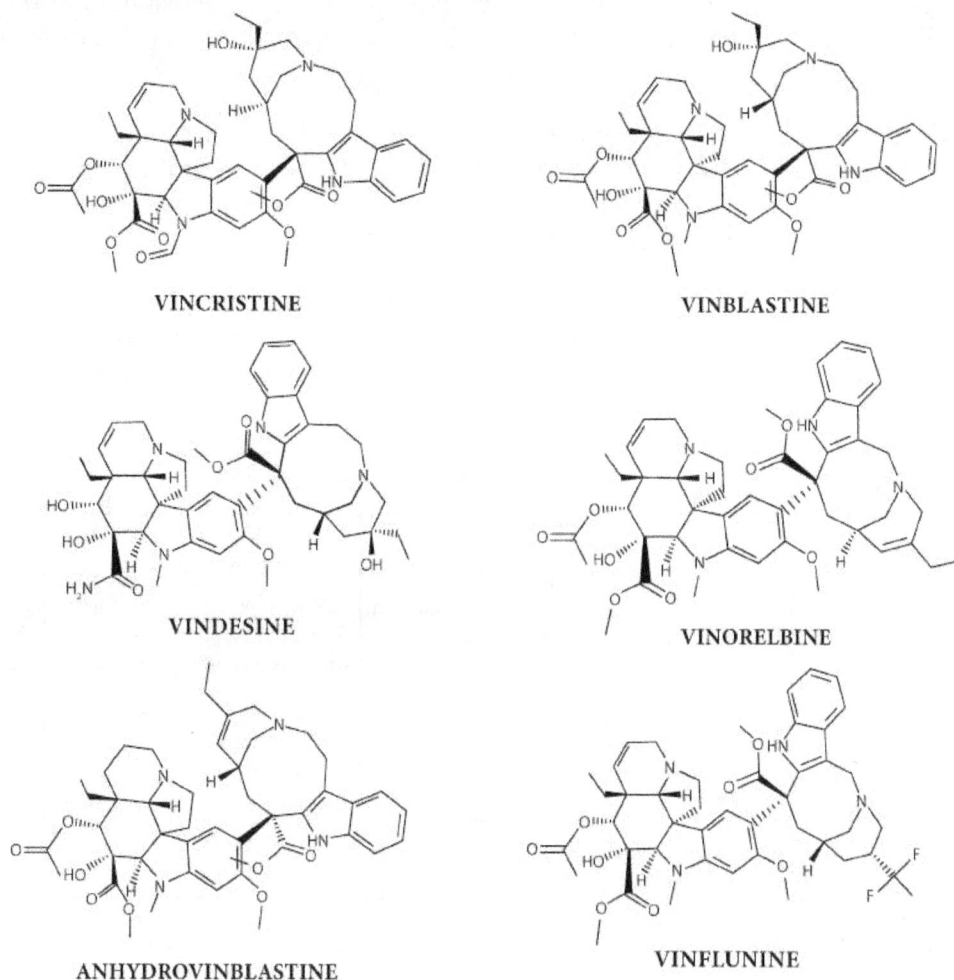

VINCRISTINE

VINBLASTINE

VINDESINE

VINORELBINE

ANHYDROVINBLASTINE

VINFLUNINE

Fig. (2). Structures of various vinca alkaloids (*Catharanthus* alkaloids).

6-Shogaol

A potent bioactive compound (Fig. **1**), isolated from dried ginger (*Zingiber officinale* Roscoe), that have the capacity to meddle with the carcinogenic processes of pancreatic [29] colorectal, lung, liver and prostate cancer, in *in vitro*

(LNCaP, DU145, and PC3) as well as *in vivo* mouse (HMVP2) prostate cancer cells [30] by the means of caspase-independent cell death and relative oxygen species generation, devoid of any stern adverse outcomes [29]. Mechanistically, the compound inhibits NF-kB, STAT3 and other signaling induced by interleukin (IL-6) thereby decreasing the protein level targeted genes such as survivin, cyclin D1, and cMyc. The study demonstrates that the compound restrains constitutive (DU145 and HMVP2) as well as IL-6–induced (LNCaP) phosphorylation of STAT3^{Tyr705} in prostate cancer by not allowing its nuclear translocation and binding on the specific nuclear target genes.

Furthermore, it has the competence to alter mRNA levels of cytokine, cyclooxygenase-1 (COX-1), glutathione-S-transferase, multidrug resistance associated protein 1 (MRP1), chemokine apoptosis and cell cycle regulatory genes (CCL5, IL-7, BAX, p21, BCL2 and p27) [30].

Other important bioactive compounds that retain inherent characteristics to act in opposition to assorted cancers are lycopenes, honokiol, anthocyanins, apigenins, quercetin, isothyocyanates, withaferin-A, *etc.* from the explicit medicinal plants are mentioned in Table **1**.

Table 1. Phytochemicals with their mechanism of action against various cancers.

Name	Source	Therapeutic Applications	Biological Effect And/Or Action Mechanism	Refs.
Epigallocatechin gallate (EGCG)	White, green and black tea.	Epidermoid carcinoma, oral cancer, ovarian carcinoma, colon and rectal cancer	Conceal proliferation, induce apoptosis, promote tumor suppressors and inhibit group of cytokines	[1, 9, 13, 24, 25, 31]
Lycopene	Carotenoids family belonging fruits and vegetables like tomato, apricot, guava, watermelon, pink grapefruit.	Prostate and colon cancer	Anti-oxidant, decrease malignancy, anti-inflammatory and immune suppression	[5, 9, 13, 22, 32, 33]
Anthocyanins	Black currant skin, berries, black rice, black soyabean etc	Lung cancer	Down regulation of protein oxidation, iNOS NF-KB, COX-2, 3-NT	[9, 13]
Genistein (GEN)	*Genista tinctoria*	Bladder cancer	Induce AKT controlled apoptosis, inhibit proliferation	[9, 13, 24]
Apigenin	*Matricaria chamomillla, Petroselinium crispum, Apium graveolens*	Prostate cancer	Antioxidant, anti- mutagenic, anti-proliferative and anti-inflammatory	[9, 13]

(Table 1) cont.....

Quercetin (flavonoid)	Apples, berries, grapes, onions, Brassica vegetables, seeds, bark, leaves	Prostate, cervical, lung, breast and colon cancer.	Antioxidant	[9, 13, 24]
Isothyocyanate	Cruciferous vegetables	Prostate cancer	Detoxification of carcinogens.	[9, 13]
Ursolic acid	Medicinal plants, apple peel	Lungs, uterus, ovary, liver, stomach, rectum, colon and brain cancer	Antioxidant	[22, 25, 33, 34]
Taxanes, Taxol (paclitaxel)	*Taxus brevifolia*	Breast, pancreas, ovarian, lung, Kaposi sarcoma, head and neck carcinoma and prostate cancer	Antiproliferative, inhibit microtubule depolymerisation, enhance and tubulin polymerization	[1, 11, 19, 23, 26, 28]
Napthoquinone (shikonin pigment)	*Lithospermum erythrorhizon*	Lung, colon, and breast cancer	Induce apoptosis, necrosis, autophagy, cell cycle arrest, inhibit cell proliferation and metastasis	[11, 19, 25]
Oleanolic Acid	Olive oil, garlic	Ovary, breast, oral and colon cancer	DNA fragmentation, inhibition of MMPs	[20]
Lupeol (Fagarsterol)	Strawberry, olive, white cabbage, mangoes, green pepper, grapes, figs	Breast, ovarian, pancreatic, colon, stomach, colon, renal and bladder cancer	Inhibit inflammation	[20]
Withaferin-A	*Withania somnifera*	Cervical cancer	Reduce tumor	[1, 22]
Honokiol	*Magnolia sp.*	Bone, pancreatic, lung, cervix, fibroblast, brain, bladder, colon, breast and blood cancer	Arrest G0/G1 and G2/M cell cycle, inhibit epithelial-mesenchymal transition and metastasis, induce anti-angiogenesis activity	[7]
Myricetin	*Myrica nagi Thunb,* Tea, berries, red wine and medicinal plants.	ovarian, liver, colon, skin, bladder and breast cancers	Cell cycle arrest at the G2/M phase by down regulating cyclin-dependent kinase and cdc2- cyclin B1	[6]
Gymnemagenol gymnemagenin, gymnemic acids, gymnemanol, and β-amyrin-related glycosides	*Gymnema sylvestre*	Human lung adenocarcinoma cell lines (A549) and human breast carcinoma cell on HeLa cancer lines (MCF7)	Cytotoxic, antioxidant	[35]

Bioactives Obtained from Marine Organisms

Marine acquired natural products have, as of now, been accredited as one of the outstanding sources of bioactive substances exerting vast pharmacological activities exhibiting an alternative fount of secure, valuable, and economical medications. Therapeutic metabolites generally belong to peptides, phenols, sulfated polysaccharides, carotenoids, and their derivatives *etc.* demonstrating anti-tumor capacity *viz* impending migration, growth and development of cancer cells. The most promising anticancer marine compounds that have been explored in cancer models are illustrated subsequently: -

Trabectedin (Ecteinascidin-743 or ET-743)

A chemopreventive bioactive compound which is extracted from ascidian *Ecteinascidia turbinate* possesses immense anticancer effect [28, 36 - 38, 42]. The alkaloid (Fig. **3**) was the first known marine source to get European Union's approval to treat reverted sarcoma and ovarian cancer in the year 2007 and in 2015 by FDA [37], and has been commercialized in the name of Yondelis® (PharmaMar SA) [36]. Trabectedin's cytotoxic activity is attributed to bind minor groove of DNA, blocking transcription by inhibiting the transcription factors. Furthermore, it competes primarily with RNA polymerase II enzyme. It is deliberated to alter the tumor micromilieu by regulating the development of tumor linked macrophages thereby controlling the production of cytokines and related angiogenic factors [37].

Dolastatins 10

A cytotoxic compound (Fig. **3**) isolated from opisthobranch gastropod, Mollusca *Dolabella auricularia* and cyanobacteria *Symploca* and *Lyngbya* sp [17, 26, 36, 37, 39 - 41]. The metabolite has been investigated its promising anti- tumor prospective against murine leukemia (P338), melanoma (SK-MEL-5), ovarian (OVCAR-3), colon (KM20L2), lung (NCI-H460), glioma (SF-295) and kidney (A498) colon adenocarcinoma (LoVo) and the HeLa-derived (KB) cell lines [26, 36]. Mode of action of Dolastatin 10 comprises its anti-mitotic and anti-microbial maneuver that leads to impediment of tubulin polymerization, guanosine triphosphate hydrolysis, nucleotide exchange and apoptotic activity [17, 36, 37, 41]. Although having numerous beneficial aspects, the compound could not successfully complete the clinical trial [36, 39]. Therefore, its derivatives like auristatin PE, soblidotin and tetrapeptide TZT-1027 are designed to maintain anti-proliferative potential with reduced toxicity in (M5076) sarcoma, colon 26 adenocarcinoma, murine (P338) leukemia and (B16) melanoma *in vivo* models [26, 36, 37, 42].

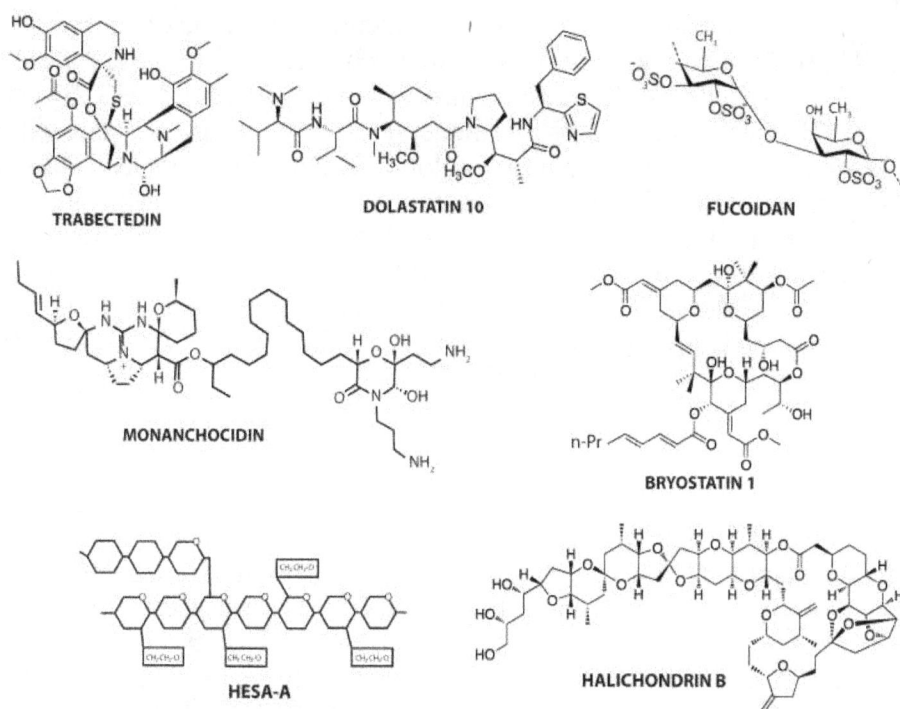

Fig. (3). Structures of various marine organisms derived bioactive compounds.

Monanchocidin

A polycyclic guanidine alkaloid (Fig. **3**), generally extracted from marine sponge *Monanchora pulchra* found cytotoxic against human acute monocytic leukemia cell line (THP-1), mouse epidermal cell line (JB6 Cl41), human cervix epithelioid carcinoma HeLa cell line, prostate cancer cell line (PC-3M) and human metastatic breast, cancer cell line (MDA-MB-231) [16, 43, 44]. At higher concentrations, the alkaloids have the efficacy to treat genito-urinary and bladder cancer cell lines by the means of induction of autophagy [42 - 44]. Monanchocidin A, monanchocidin B, monanchomycalin C, urupocidin A, pulchranin A, ptilomycalin A, monanchomycalin B and normonanchocidin D, are the major representatives of the monanchocidin family and are known to be effectual in inducing apoptosis and cell cycle arrest in JB6 P+ Cl41, HeLa cancerous cell lines. Moreover, EGF-induced neoplastic transformation of JB6 P+ Cl41 cells was also reported to be subdued by the remedial compounds [42, 44, 45].

Fucoidan

A sulphated polysaccharide (Fig. **3**) extracted from cell wall of brown macroalgae *Undaria pinnatifida* that has been evaluated to cure wide range of cancers [16, 28, 36, 37, 41] in *in vitro* and in *in vivo* studies, comprising of breast cancer, lung cancer, head and neck cancer [36]and also in human lymphoma HS- Sultan cell line [16, 17]. Furthermore, anti-carcinogenic ability of the fucoidan extracted from *Ascophyllum nodosum* has been explored in sigmoid colon adenocarcinoma cells (COLO 320 DM) [17, 41]. The compound has been actively employed for cancer chemotherapy's efficacy as well as in opposition to its after effects [36]. In broad spectrum, the agent functions to modulate angiogenesis, atherosclerosis, and metastasis in the malignant cells. At molecular level, it is known to down regulate kinase pathway by initiating the caspase-3 activity [17]. Additionally, it also has the competence to stall PI3K/AKT and p38 MAPK signaling pathways for which, the compound has been undergoing therapeutic evaluation in phase II [28].

Bryostatin 1

Macrocyclic lactones (Fig. **3**) procured from the marine based bryozoan *i.e.* *Bugula neritina* (Bugulidae) have been known for their great anti-neoplastic properties [16, 17, 28, 36, 37]. Its anti-carcinogenic activity has been explored in the murine leukemia cell line P338 and colorectal cancer [36] *via* the process of protein kinase C (PKC) downregulation, apoptosis and modulation of cancer cell differentiation [36, 37]. It also demonstrates cytokine release activation, immune-modulation and tumor-specific lymphocyte community growth in the cells [37, 41]. Additionally, analogs of Bryostatin 1, that is Bryostatin 8 and Bryostatin 5 have been investigated and revealed to have anti-proliferative efficacy in melanoma K1735-M2 allografts *in vivo* but these tend to display lower loss in body's weight [36, 42].

HESA-A

A herbal-marine compound sequestered from some microalgae [16], *Penaeus latisculatus* [king prawn] and also seen in *Carum carvi* [Persian cumin], *Apium graveolens* (celery) [45, 46]. The biological agent (Fig. **3**) has been reported as a convincing chemoprotective contender in opposition to breast [16, 47] colon [46] and MDA-MB-46, Hela and Hep-2 cancer cell lines [48]. Apart from being an affluent mineral [50%], organic [45%] and aqueous elements [5%] source [16, 47], HESA-A comprehends rich amount of necessitated trace elements such as Vanadium, Nickel, Titanium, Selenium, Zinc, Cobalt which plays the major antioxidant role against the malignant cells. Although, the mechanism of action of the compound is yet unknown, it certainly appears to exert several pharmacological effects on the tumor cells making it a non-toxic, effective, selective and safe, chemotherapeutic agent [16, 46 - 48].

Halichondrin B

A polyether macrolide compound (Fig. **3**) obtained from marine sponges *Halichondria okadai* [28, 36, 37, 42, 43], *Lissodendoryx* [28, 37], *Axinella* and *Phakellia* [28]. The biological product has been found cytotoxic to various cancers including melanoma cell line B16 and its allograft as well as Murine leukemia cell lines L-1210, P338 and allografts where the major action of molecule resides in its macrocyclic C1-C38 moiety [36]. Due to lack of Halichondrin's sustainable supply, its truncated synthetic analogue Eribulin mesylate (Halaven®) has been developed as clinical potent polyketides nontaxane derivative [17, 28, 36, 37, 42, 43]. It has the capacity to destabilize microtubules by firmly inhibiting the dynamics of microtubule polymerization at elevated concentrations [28, 42]. Mechanistically, it irreversibly binds the positive ends of protofilament resulting in cell cycle arrest at G2/M phase [17, 28, 36, 37, 43]. Moreover, the agent has been successfully investigated in metastatic breast cancer and led to the EMA and FDA approval in 2010 [17, 36, 43].

Other major bioactive compounds obtained from marine sources are used against various types of cancers as mentioned in Table **2**.

Table 2. Marine bioactive compounds with their mechanism of action against various cancers.

Name	Source	Therapeutic Applications	Biological Effect And/Or Action Mechanism	Refs.
Non-cembranoidal diterpene 5-episinuleptolide acetate	*Sinularia sp.*	Human leukemia K562 and HL 60 and lymphoblastic leukemia MOLT-4 cell line	Apoptosis	[16]
Carrageenans	*Chondrus, Gigartina, Hypnea,* and *Eucheuma,*	Cervical cancer	Primarily act on human papilloma virus *In-vitro*	[16, 28, 49]
Renieramycin M	Sponges	Lung carcinomas	Apoptosis	[16, 39]

(Table 2) cont.....

Heteronemin	*Hippospongia sp.*	Chronic myelogenous leukemia	Induce apoptosis, cell cycle arrest, control mitogen-initiated protein kinases pathway and the nuclear factor kappa B signaling cascade	[16]
Scopararane I	*Eutypella sp.*	Breast MCF-7, non small cell lung NCI-H460 and glioblastoma SF-268 tumour cell line	Apoptosis	[16]
Frondoside A	*Cucumaria Frondosa japonica, Cucumaria okhotensis*	Prostate and lung cancer	Inhibits cell proliferation, induce cell cycle arrest and apoptosis	[42, 44]
Cucumarioside A2-2	*Cucumaria Frondosa japonica*	Human cervix carcinoma HeLa cells, mouse Ehrlich carcinoma cells and mouse epidermal JB6 Cl41 P+ cells,	Block the membrane transporter by P-glycoprotein, and suppress colony formation and proliferation of tumor cells	[42, 44]
Pyrroloformamide	*Streptomyces sp.* symbiotic with the ascidian *Eudistoma vannamei.*	Prostate cancer cell line PC3M	Anti-proliferative activity	[44]
Urukthapelstatin A	Actinobacteria *Mechercharimyces asporophorigenens*	Human lung cancer lines A549, DMS114, and NCIH460; human ovarian cancer cell lines OVCAR-3, OVCAR-4, OVCAR-5, OVCAR-8, and SK-OV3; human breast cancer cell line MCF-7 and; human colon cancer cell line HCT-116	Apoptotic and anti-proliferative effect	[44, 50]
Ketosteroids	*Acanthophora spicifera*	Human cancer lines Bel-7402, HCT-8, A549, BGC-823 and HeLa	Relapse viable cell count and tumour volume	[37, 51]

(Table 2) cont.....

Thicoraline	*Micromonospora marina*	Human colon cancer cell lines LOVO and SW620	Arrest cell cycle in G1 phase and a decrease in the rate of S phase progression towards G2/M phase	[17, 50]

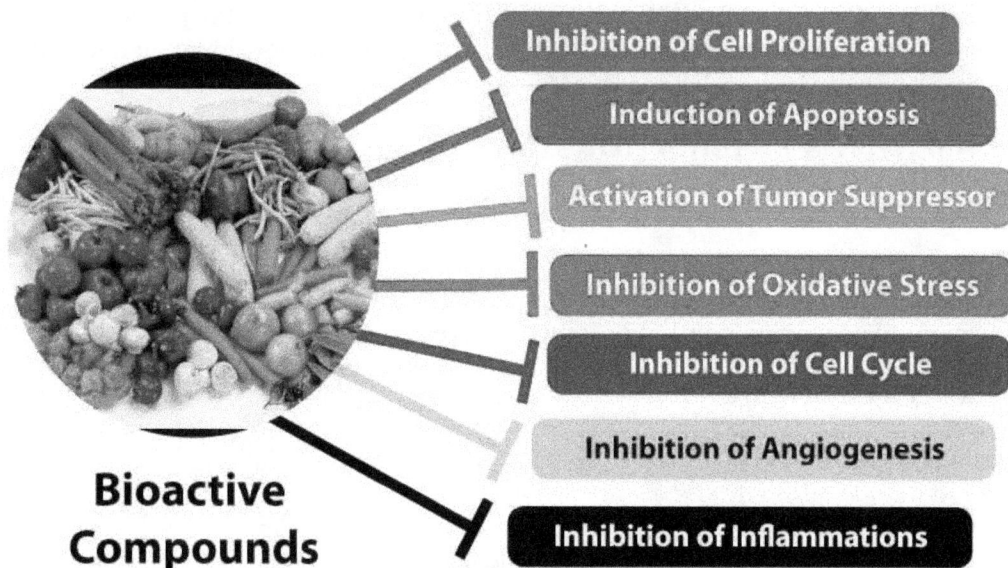

Fig. (4). Schematic illustration of various modes involved in anticancerous potentialities of bioactive compounds.

CONCLUSION AND FUTURE PROSPECTIVES

Cancer has now become a high-profile disease with a booming number of cases in both developed and developing nations, and its treatment is a huge concern across the world. Drugs that are synthesized and used in conventional therapies, on the other hand, have significant flaws due to their toxic effects on non-targeted cells, culminating in a range of health problems. As a result, demand for alternatives, such as naturally occurring substances, has intensified as these have novel chemical signatures that are quite productive and pharmacologically active providing vast opportunities for future of new anti-cancer agents. In sum, we discussed the use of natural organic ingredients in the therapeutic intervention in tumor genesis and its effects, with particular emphasis on bioactive compounds and their derivatives ubiquitously expressed in some medicinal plants and marine sources. The impact of a specific biologically active compound is evaluated by their interaction with number of pro-oncogenic or anti- oncogenic intermediaries as well as their aptitude to regulate the specific targets. However, one of the major setbacks of these active compounds is their low bio-availability because of probable dilapidation under rigorous gastro- intestinal environment, diffusion, absorption or interaction with other nutrients could impede research progress in drug formulations and their targeted delivery. Nevertheless, standard delivery system such as nanoparticles, liposomes, micelles, antibody-drug conjugates [ADCs] generation, *etc.* could enhance the targeted approach. Further development in the regarding field is required to make natural products as an essential asset for better perspective towards research and development and future success of pharmaceuticals industries.

CONSENT FOR PUBLICATION

Not applicable.

CONFLICT OF INTEREST

The authors declare no conflict of interest, financial or otherwise.

ACKNOWLEDGEMENTS

Declared none.

REFERENCES

[1]   Prakash O, Kumar A, Kumar P, Ajeet A. Anticancer Potential of Plants and Natural Products: A Review. Am J Pharmacol Sci 2013; 1(6): 104-15.
        [http://dx.doi.org/10.12691/ajps-1-6-1]

[2]   Block K, Gyllenhaal C, Lowe L, *et al.* A Broad-spectrum Integrative Prevention Design for Cancer Prevention and Therapy. Semin Cancer Biol 2015; 35 (Suppl.): S276-304.
        [http://dx.doi.org/10.1016/j.semcancer.2015.09.007] [PMID: 26590477]

[3]   Hassanpour SH, Dehghani M. Review of cancer from perspective of molecular. J Cancer Res Pract 2017; 4(4): 127-9.
        [http://dx.doi.org/10.1016/j.jcrpr.2017.07.001]

[4]   Alizadeh SA, Hashemi SM. Development and therapeutic potential of 2-aminothiazole derivatives in anticancer drug discovery. Medicinal Chemistry Research Springer US2021 2021; 30: 771-806.

[5]   Choudhari AS, Mandave PC, Deshpande M, Ranjekar P, Prakash O. Phytochemicals in Cancer Treatment: From Preclinical Studies to Clinical Practice. Front Pharmacol 2020; 10(January): 1614.
        [http://dx.doi.org/10.3389/fphar.2019.01614] [PMID: 32116665]

[6]   Subramaniam S, Selvaduray KR, Radhakrishnan AK. Bioactive Compounds : Natural Defense Against Cancer ? Biomolecules 2019; 9: 12 758.

[7]   Ong CP, Lee WL, Tang YQ, *et al.* Honokiol. J Cancer 2020; 12(1): 1-44.
        [PMID: 31892967]

[8]   Ohnishi S, Ma N, Thanan R, *et al.* DNA Damage in Inflammation-Related Carcinogenesis and Cancer Stem Cells. Oxid Med Cell Longev 2013; 2013: 387014.

[9]   Samadi AK, Bilsland A, Georgakilas AG, *et al.* A multi-targeted approach to suppress tumor-promoting inflammation. Semin Cancer Biol 2015; 35(May) (Suppl.): S151-84.
        [http://dx.doi.org/10.1016/j.semcancer.2015.03.006] [PMID: 25951989]

[10] Badraoui R, Rebai T, Elkahoui S, *et al. Allium subhirsutum* L. as a Potential Source of Antioxidant and Anticancer Bioactive Molecules: HR-LCMS Phytochemical Profiling, *In Vitro* and *In Vivo* Pharmacological Study. Antioxidants 2020; 9(10): E1003.
[http://dx.doi.org/10.3390/antiox9101003] [PMID: 33081189]

[11] Demain AL, Vaishnav P. Natural products for cancer chemotherapy. Microb Biotechnol 2011; 4(6): 687-99.
[http://dx.doi.org/10.1111/j.1751-7915.2010.00221.x] [PMID: 21375717]

[12] Badawy AA, El-Magd MA, AlSadrah SA. Therapeutic. Integr Cancer Ther 2018; 17(4): 1235-46.
[http://dx.doi.org/10.1177/1534735418786000] [PMID: 29986606]

[13] Feitelson MA, Arzumanyan A, Kulathinal RJ, *et al.* Sustained proliferation in cancer: Mechanisms and novel therapeutic targets. Semin Cancer Biol 2015; 35 (Suppl.): S25-54.
[http://dx.doi.org/10.1016/j.semcancer.2015.02.006] [PMID: 25892662]

[14] Deshmukh S, Gupta M, Prakash V, Reddy MS. Mangrove-Associated Fungi: A Novel Source of Potential Anticancer Compounds. J Fungi (Basel) 2018; 4(3): 101.
[http://dx.doi.org/10.3390/jof4030101] [PMID: 30149584]

[15] M HR. Suppression of VEGF-induced angiogenesis and tumor growth by Eugenia jambolana , Musa paradisiaca , and Coccinia indica extracts. Pharm Biol 2017; 2013: 12 758.

[16] Wali AF, Majid S, Rasool S, *et al.* Natural products against cancer: Review on phytochemicals from marine sources in preventing cancer. Saudi Pharm J 2019; 27(6): 767-77.
[http://dx.doi.org/10.1016/j.jsps.2019.04.013] [PMID: 31516319]

[17] Khalifa SAM, Elias N, Farag MA, *et al.* Marine natural products: A source of novel anticancer. Mar Drugs 2019; 17(9): 491.
[http://dx.doi.org/10.3390/md17090491] [PMID: 31443597]

[18] Le TN, Chiu C, Hsieh P. Bioactive Compounds and Bioactivities of *Brassica oleracea L. var.* Italica Sprouts and Microgreens : An Updated Overview from a Nutraceutical Perspective. Plant J 2020; 9: 8 946.

[19] Agarwal G, Carcache PJB, Addo EM, Kinghorn AD. Current status and contemporary approaches to the discovery of antitumor agents from higher plants. Biotechnol Adv 2020; 38: 107337.
[http://dx.doi.org/10.1016/j.biotechadv.2019.01.004] [PMID: 30633954]

[20] Madka V, Rao C. Anti-inflammatory phytochemicals for chemoprevention of colon cancer. Curr Cancer Drug Targets 2013; 13(5): 542-57.
[http://dx.doi.org/10.2174/15680096113139990036] [PMID: 23597198]

[21] Khan T, Ali M, Khan A, *et al.* Anticancer Plants: A Review of the Active Phytochemicals, Applications in Animal Models, and Regulatory Aspects. Biomolecules 2019; 10(1): 47.
[http://dx.doi.org/10.3390/biom10010047] [PMID: 31892257]

[22] Ashraf MA. Phytochemicals as Potential Anticancer Drugs : Time to Ponder Nature ' s Bounty. Biomed Res Int 2020; 2020

[23] Seca AML, Pinto DCGA. Plant Secondary Metabolites as Anticancer Agents : Successes in Clinical Trials and Therapeutic Application. Int J Mol Sci 2018; 19: 1 263. 1.

[24] Sun Q, Heilmann J, König B. Natural phenolic metabolites with anti-angiogenic properties – a review from the chemical point of view. Beilstein J Org Chem 2015; 11: 249-64.
[http://dx.doi.org/10.3762/bjoc.11.28] [PMID: 25815077]

[25] Luo H, Vong CT, Chen H, *et al.* Naturally occurring anti-cancer compounds: shining from Chinese herbal medicine. Chin Med 2019; 14(1): 48.
[http://dx.doi.org/10.1186/s13020-019-0270-9] [PMID: 31719837]

[26] Lichota A, Gwozdzinski K. Anticancer Activity of Natural Compounds from Plant and Marine Environment. Int J Mol Sci 2018; 19: 11 3533.

[http://dx.doi.org/10.3390/ijms19113533]

[27] Turrini E, Sestili P. Overview of the Anticancer Potential of the " King of Spices " Piper nigrum and Its Main. Toxins. 2020; 12,12 747.

[28] Barreca M, Span V, Montalbano A, *et al.* Marine Anticancer Agents : An Overview with a Particular Focus on Their Chemical Classes. Marine Drugs, volume no.2020; 18(12):619.

[29] Mao QQ, Xu XY, Cao SY, *et al.* Bioactive Compounds and Bioactivities of Ginger (*Zingiber officinale Roscoe*). Foods 2019; 8(6): 185.
[http://dx.doi.org/10.3390/foods8060185] [PMID: 31151279]

[30] Saha A, Blando J, Silver E, Beltran L, Sessler J, DiGiovanni J. 6-Shogaol from dried ginger inhibits growth of prostate cancer cells both *in vitro* and *in vivo* through inhibition of STAT3 and NF-κB signaling. Cancer Prev Res (Phila) 2014; 7(6): 627-38.
[http://dx.doi.org/10.1158/1940-6207.CAPR-13-0420] [PMID: 24691500]

[31] Ackova DG, Smilkov K, Bosnakovski D. Contemporary Formulations for Drug Delivery of Anticancer Bioactive Compounds. Recent Patents Anticancer Drug Discov 2019; 14(1): 19-31.
[http://dx.doi.org/10.2174/1574892814666190111104834] [PMID: 30636616]

[32] Pouchieu C, Galan P, Ducros V, Latino-Martel P, Hercberg S, Touvier M. Plasma carotenoids and retinol and overall and breast cancer risk: a nested case-control study. Nutr Cancer 2014; 66(6): 980-8.
[http://dx.doi.org/10.1080/01635581.2014.936952] [PMID: 25072980]

[33] Omara T, Kiprop AK, Ramkat RC, *et al.* Medicinal Plants Used in Traditional Management of Cancer in Uganda : A Review of Ethnobotanical Surveys, Phytochemistry, and Anticancer Studies. Evid Based Complement Alternat Med 2020; 3529081.

[34] Rajesh E, Sankari LS, Malathi L, Krupaa JR. Naturally occurring products in cancer therapy. J Pharm Bioallied Sci 2015; 7(April) (Suppl. 1): S181-3.
[PMID: 26015704]

[35] Arunachalam K, Arun LB, Annamalai SK, Arunachalam AM. Potential anticancer properties of bioactive compounds of Gymnema sylvestre and its biofunctionalized silver nanoparticles. Int J Nanomedicine 2014; 10: 31-41.
[http://dx.doi.org/10.2147/IJN.S71182] [PMID: 25565802]

[36] Wang E, Sorolla MA, Gopal Krishnan PD, Sorolla A. From Seabed to Bedside: A Review on Promising Marine Anticancer Compounds. Biomolecules 2020; 10(2): 248.
[http://dx.doi.org/10.3390/biom10020248] [PMID: 32041255]

[37] Nigam M, Suleria HAR, Farzaei MH, Mishra AP. Marine anticancer drugs and their relevant targets: a treasure from the ocean. Daru 2019; 27(1): 491-515.
[http://dx.doi.org/10.1007/s40199-019-00273-4] [PMID: 31165439]

[38] Avila C, Preckler CA. Bioactive Compounds from Marine Heterobranchs. Mar. Drugs. 2020; 18,12 657:19–29.
[http://dx.doi.org/10.3390/md18120657]

[39] Ciavatta ML, Lefranc F, Carbone M, *et al.* Marine Mollusk-Derived Agents with Antiproliferative Activity as Promising Anticancer Agents to Overcome Chemotherapy Resistance. Med Res Rev 2017; 37(4): 702-801.
[http://dx.doi.org/10.1002/med.21423] [PMID: 27925266]

[40] Pham JV, Yilma MA, Feliz A, *et al.* A Review of the Microbial Production of Bioactive Natural Products and Biologics. Front Microbiol 2019; 10(June): 1404.
[http://dx.doi.org/10.3389/fmicb.2019.01404] [PMID: 31281299]

[41] Mondal A, Bose S, Banerjee S, *et al.* Marine Cyanobacteria and Microalgae Metabolites — A Rich Source of Potential. Mar Drugs 2020; 18, 9: 476.

[42] Ruiz-Torres V, Encinar J, Herranz-López M, *et al.* An Updated Review on Marine Anticancer

Compounds: The Use of Virtual Screening for the Discovery of Small-Molecule Cancer Drugs. Molecules 2017; 22(7): 1037.
[http://dx.doi.org/10.3390/molecules22071037] [PMID: 28644406]

[43]   Gomes N, Dasari R, Chandra S, Kiss R, Kornienko A. Marine Invertebrate Metabolites with Anticancer Activities: Solutions to the "Supply Problem". Mar Drugs 2016; 14(5): 98.
[http://dx.doi.org/10.3390/md14050098] [PMID: 27213412]

[44]   Katanaev VL, Di Falco S, Khotimchenko Y. The anticancer. Mar Drugs 2019; 17(8): 474.
[http://dx.doi.org/10.3390/md17080474] [PMID: 31426365]

[45]   Schumacher M, Kelkel M, Dicato M, Diederich M. A survey of marine natural compounds and their derivatives with anti-cancer activity reported in 2010. Molecules 2011; 16(7): 5629-46.
[http://dx.doi.org/10.3390/molecules16075629] [PMID: 21993222]

[46]   Ahmadi A, Mohagheghi M, Karimi M, Naseri M. Anticancer effects of HESA-A in patients with metastatic colon cancer. Integr Cancer Ther 2009; 8(1): 71-4.
[http://dx.doi.org/10.1177/1534735408327995] [PMID: 19147644]

[47]   Ahmadi A, Mohagheghi MA, Fazeli MS, *et al.* HESA-A: new treatment for breast cancer and choroidal metastasis. Med Sci Monit 2005; 11(6): CR300-3.
[PMID: 15917722]

[48]   Ahmadi A, Mohagheghi M, Karimi M, *et al.* Therapeutic effects of HESA-A in patients with end-stage metastatic cancers. Integr Cancer Ther 2010; 9(1): 32-5.
[http://dx.doi.org/10.1177/1534735409357934] [PMID: 20150223]

[49]   Moghadamtousi SZ, Karimian H, Khanabdali R, *et al.* Anticancer and Antitumor Potential of Fucoidan and Fucoxanthin, Two Main Metabolites Isolated from Brown Algae. Sci World J 2014; 2014

[50]   Zhang JN, Xia YX, Zhang HJ. Natural Cyclopeptides as Anticancer Agents in the Last 20 Years. Int J Mol Sci 2021; 22(8): 3973.
[http://dx.doi.org/10.3390/ijms22083973] [PMID: 33921480]

[51]   Shi D, Guo S, Fan X. A new ketosteroid from red alga Acanthophora spicifera. Chin J Oceanology Limnol 2011; 29(3): 674-8.
[http://dx.doi.org/10.1007/s00343-011-0183-7]

CHAPTER 3

Natural Bio-actives Acting Against Clinically Important Bacterial Biofilms

Amrita C. Bhagwat[1], Amrita M. Patil[1] and Sunil D. Saroj[1,*]

[1] *Symbiosis School of Biological Sciences, Symbiosis International (Deemed University), Lavale, Pune, Maharashtra, India*

Abstract: Biofilm research is growing rapidly due to the widespread existence of biofilms in pathogens and their resistance to a variety of antimicrobial therapies. World Health Organization in 2017 categorised pathogens into three categories based on their AMR [Antimicrobial resistance] and severity of infection *viz.* critical, high and medium. *Acinetobacter baumannii, Pseudomonas aeruginosa* and organisms belonging to *Enterobacteriaceae* family are top priority pathogens- 'critical', amongst which the majority of them are reported to cause the infection due to biofilm formation. As antibiotic resistance has increased tremendously in the last few years, the current research is concentrated on the development of effective approaches to inhibit biofilm formation by bacteria. Anti-biofilm activity is mediated by a spectrum of molecules obtained from plants, mammals, fungi, microbes, and marine sponges. The chapter gives a comprehensive idea about natural bioactives from plant and other sources that act as anti-biofilm agents. Clinical validation of these bioactives will aid the medical field with alternate preventive and treatment methods against pathogenic biofilms.

Keywords: Anti-biofilm agents, Antibiotic resistance, *Acinetobacter baumannii*, Bioactives, *Enterobacteriaceae, Pseudomonas aeruginosa.*

INTRODUCTION

A product that exhibits biological activity is termed as bioactive. These active products exert either positive or negative biological effects based on the nature of the substance, the dosage or the bioavailability [1]. Bioactive compounds have the potential to affect metabolic processes and perform functions like receptor suppression, inhibition or enzyme activation, and also involved in gene induction and suppression [2]. Bioactive compounds are important for human well-being due to their various biochemical activities, involving antioxidant, anticarcinogenic, antimutagenic, antiallergenic, anti-inflammatory, and antimi-

* **Corresponding author Sunil D. Saroj:** Symbiosis School of Biological Sciences, Symbiosis International (Deemed University), Lavale, Pune, Maharashtra, India; Tel: +91 20 61936532; E-mail: sunil.saroj@ssbs.edu.in

Mukesh Kumar Sharma and Pallavi Kaushik (Eds.)

crobial activities, as well as the reduction in cardiovascular disease risk factors [3 - 5].

Solid-liquid extraction using organic solvents and other methods, such as supercritical fluid extraction, high-pressure procedures, microwave or ultrasound-aided extraction and subcritical water extraction, are some commonly used methods for extracting bioactive compounds from their natural sources [4, 6 - 9]. There can be multiple sources of bioactives like plants, animal, bacteria, marine sponges, algae, fungi, *etc.* of which plants are most commonly and widely explored for their bioactives due to their strong phytochemical profile. There is a wide range of bioactive applications. However, their potential in eradicating biofilms of clinically challenging pathogens is currently under investigation.

By carrying the microscopic analysis of mucus and lung tissue in chronically compromised cystic fibrosis patients, Hoiby discovered aggregates of *Pseudomonas aeruginosa* cells and termed it as "biofilm infection." Nickel *et al.* introduced the word "biofilm" to medicine and medical microbiology in 1985. Microbial biofilms were described by Niels Hoiby as "a clump or cluster of microbes which is surrounded by an extracellular self-generated polymer matrix" [10]. The persistence of these microbial biofilms has caused severe damages to food processing industries and is considered as major obstacle in clinical treatments of chronic infections.

Biofilms are microbes extracellular secretions made up mostly of polymeric substances such as polysaccharides, proteins, and DNA. The organisms in the core of these biofilms decrease their metabolic activities acquiring a dormant state, making them more tolerant to antibiotics. Bacteria within biofilms gain resistance to antibiotics by a variety of mechanisms, including synthesis β lactamase, upregulating efflux pumps, and by modifying antibiotic target in bacteria [11]. The ECM (extracellular matrix) is a stubborn source of defence for bacteria against stress conditions *e.g.* physical, environmental, chemical and biological [12]. Increasing antibiotic resistance among microorganisms is currently one of the most serious threats to the health sector around the world [13]. These biofilms are also tolerant towards disinfectant chemicals as well as resistant to the body's defence system. Bacteria within biofilms are relatively more resistant than outside biofilm. Biofilms are found to be resistant to carbapenems and third-generation cephalosporins, which are known to be the best antibiotics currently available for treating multidrug-resistant bacteria. Based on the above characteristics, biofilm plays a vital role in human infections and exhibits important adaptive mechanisms making their eradication a challenging task.

In 2017, WHO categorised these pathogens according to their infection severity into three priority tiers: critical, high and medium. The critical group includes *Acinetobacter baumannii*, *Pseudomonas aeruginosa*, Enterobacteriaceae and effective therapies targeted towards their biofilms that need to be developed immediately [14]. Moreover, a recent review anticipated 10 million deaths per annum by 2050 due to antimicrobial resistance [15]. Since July 2020, the CDC (Centers for Disease Control and Prevention) has issued eight complaints of infections caused by *P. aeruginosa* in patients who had surgery or other invasive procedures in Mexico. Six of these occurred in patients undergoing surgical treatments [bariatric surgery, cosmetic surgery, cholecystectomy, and cancer treatment] at various healthcare facilities in Tijuana, Baja California, Mexico (CDC site: Health associated infections). *A. baumannii* is a bacteria that cause healthcare-associated infections (HAIs). An outbreak of *A. baumannii* infection was observed in the University Hospital of Angers in France and in that nearly 49 patients were infected with drug-resistant *A. baumannii* [16]. Antibiotic resistance in biofilm-forming organisms is usually associated with considerably higher mortality, morbidity, and economic burden [17]. As a result, antibiotic resistance and the potential to form single-species and polymicrobial biofilms limit the effectiveness of existing therapies, putting a financial strain on the healthcare system [18]. This creates an urge to discover either biofilm inhibiting or biofilm eradicating agents.

Some of the strategies currently being used to treat biofilms are enzymes that impair the biofilm matrix or compounds that inhibit bacterial communication, thereby increasing sensitivity to antibiotics, phage therapy, *etc.* While a few synthetic compounds demonstrated promise as anti-biofilm agents, but the natural compound drugs are preferable in terms of processing costs and success rates [19]. Thus, considering the advantages offered by the natural sources, they are being explored for anti-biofilm bioactives.

This chapter gives an insight into different natural bioactives (plants, animal, bacteria, fungi or marine organisms) that are reported to inhibit biofilms formation in critical priority pathogens (*Acinetobacter baumannii*, *Pseudomonas aeruginosa* and Enterobacteriaceae) listed by WHO. The chapter also discusses how the lack of clinical trials and other research gaps in the discovery and applications of natural bioactives as anti-biofilm agents has narrowed its usage while emphasizing the importance of *in vivo* and translational research.

Natural Bioactives against *Acinetobacter baumannii* Biofilms

A. baumannii is a major etiological agent of nosocomial infection. It possesses an ability to form a biofilm which aggravates its virulence and antibiotic resistance, thereby, causing a great challenge to global health. The chapter includes an elucidatory Table **1** that gives brief description regarding the source of bioactive and its action against particular pathogen.

Table 1. Natural bioactives against *Acinetobacter baumannii*, *Pseudomonas aeruginosa*, Enterobacteriaceae (*e.g. Shigella* spp., *E. coli*, *Klebsiella pneumoniae* and *Salmonella* spp.).

Pathogen	Source of Bioactives	Bioactive	Anti-biofilm Activity (*In vitro/in vivo*, Polymicrobial/Monomicrobial, Effective Concentration/ Percent Inhibition)	Additional Activities	Refs.
Acinetobacter baumannii	Plant	Propolin- D from fruits of *Macaranga tanarius* (L.)	*In vitro*, monomicrobial biofilm	Minimal toxicity in Caenorhabditis elegans model	[26]
		Sanquinarine and hydroxyflavone from kiwi (*Actinidia deliciosa*)	*In vitro*, monomicrobial biofilm	-	[20]
		Thymol (40%), Y-terpinene (36%) and pcymene (21%) from *Carum copticum*	*In vitro*, monomicrobial biofilm, 98% inhibition of biofilm	-	[27]
		Fisetin, phloretin, curcumin	*In vitro*, monomicrobial	-	[28]
		Curcumin	*In vitro*, polymicrobial (mixed biofilm of *A. baumannii* and *C. albicans*)	No toxicity in *Caenorhabditis elegans* model	[28]
		Citral	*In vitro*, monomicrobial biofilm, 200 µg/ml, Inhibited *A. baumannii* biofilms by 90%	-	[29]
		Imidazole from *Azadirachta indica* (Neem)	*In vitro*, Monomicrobial biofilm, 90% inhibition of ESBL *A. baumannii* biofilms	Binds to CsgA- a virulence factor of *A. baumannii*	[30]
		Cinnamaldehyde	*In vitro*, Monomicrobial biofilm, inhibition of carbapenem-resistant *A. baumannii* biofilm by 49.5%-71.2%	Confirmation of anti-biofilm activity by Scanning Electron Microscopy	[25]
		Thymol (THY), eugenol (EUG), and carvacrol (CAR)	*In vitro*, Monomicrobial biofilm	-	[21]
		Methyl 16-methyl heptadecanoate, 2-methox--4-vinyl phenol, 2-[5-ethenyl-5-methylox-lan-2-yl]propan-2-ol, 2,3,4-triacetyloxybutyl acetate, and methyl hexadecanoate from *Tinospora cordifolia* stem	*In vitro*, monomicrobial biofilm	Bioguided fractionation, GC-MS and Molecular docking study revealed the presence of major bioactives in the extract	[22]
		Zerumbone	*In vitro*, monomicrobial biofilm	Downregulation of biofilm-associated genes (*bap*) and virulence-associated (*adeA, adeB, adeC*)	[32]
		myristoleic (MoA) and palmitoleic (PoA)	In vitro, monomicrobial biofilm, 200 µg/ml, reduction in biofilm formation to 24% and 38% respectively	Decreased expression of the *abaR* (quorum sensing regulator)	[23]

	Animal	5-episinuleptolide from *Sinularialeptoclados*	*In vitro*, monomicrobial, 45-55% biofilm inhibition	Reduced expression of *pgaABCD* locus, which encodes the extracellular polysaccharide poly-β-[1, 6]---acetylglucosamine (PNAG), SEM study showed reduced extracellular polysaccharide matrix	[33]
		Magainin 2 isolated fromthe skin of *Xenopus laevis*	*In vitro,* monomicrobial biofilm, 2–8 μM, biofilm inhibition as well as biofilm development inhibition and removal activity in 5 MDR *A. baumannii* strains *viz.* KCTC 2508, *Acinetobacter baumannii* 719705, 244752, 907233, 409081, 892199	-	[34]
		aliphatics, alicyclic and aromatic from Sea anemone-*Stichodactylahaddoni*	*In vitro*, monomicrobal, 625 μg/ml, ~60% inhibition	-	[35]
	Bacteria	Staphylosan [dimannooleate] from *Staphylococcus saprophyticus* SBPS-15	*In vitro*, monomicrobial	Non-toxic to brine shrimp	[36]
		Dispersin-B from *Aggregatibacter actinomycetemcomitans*	*In vitro*, monomicrobial	-	[37, 38]
		Cahuitamycins C from *Streptomyces gandocaensis*	*In vitro*, monomicrobial	-	[39]
Pseudomonas aeruginosa	Plant	Rutin, Myricetin-3-O-rutinoside, kaempferol-3-O- rutinoside and iso quercitrin from *Pistacia Atlantica*	*In vitro* Polymicrobial	Antioxidant activity	[40]
		Zingerone from *Zingiber officinale*	*In vitro* Monomicrobial	-	[41, 42]
		Heptacosanoic acid, s-Dioxide, 3-Methyl 2-[--Oxopropyl] and 3-N-Hexylthiane s from *Syzygium cumini* L. Skeels	*In vitro* Monomicrobial Concentration: 900 μg/ml	Antioxidant Anti-diabetic	[43]
	Marine macroalga	Furanones C-30 and C-56 from *Delisea pulchra*	*In vivo* (model: mouse pulmonary infection)	-	[44]
		Triterpenoid ursolic acid, asiatic acid and corosolic acid from edible medicinal plants	*In vitro* Polymicrobial, 10 μg/ml	-	[45]
		AL-1 (14-alpha-lipoyl andrographolide) from *Andrographis paniculate*	*In vitro* Monomicrobial	Inhibition of pyocyanin production	[46, 47]
		Casbane diterpene from *Croton Nepetaefolius*Baill	*In vitro* Polymicrobial Concentration: 250 μg/ml	-	[47]
	Marine sponge	TAGE: Trans- bromoageliferin analogue 1], CAGE: Cis bromoageliferin analogue 2 from *Agelas conifer and Agelaceae*	*In vitro* Monomicrobial	-	[48]
		Lectin –FCL from *Fasciospongia cavernosa*	*In vitro* Monomicrobial	-	[49]
Shigella flexneri	Bacteria	Exopolysaccharides (L-EPSs) from *Lactobacillus plantarum* 12	*In vitro* Monomicrobial	-	[50]
	Plant	Lectin (AGL) from *Amaranthus gangeticus* seeds	*In vitro* Polymicrobial*: Shigella, E.coli,* S.aureus *E.coli*: 250, 500 and 1000 μg/ml	-	[51]
		Phenolics: Ferrulic acid	*In vitro* Monomicrobial	-	[52]

(Table 1) cont.....

Escherichia coli O157:H7	Plant	Beta -sitosterol glucoside (SG) from *Citrus* plants	*In vitro* Polymicrobial	-	[53]
		Caffeic acid, gallic acid and isothiocyanates (ITC) from Brassicaceae plant extracts	*In vitro* Monomicrobial:2000 µg/ml	-	[54]
		Ellagic acid from *Punica granatum* L peels	*In vitro* Polymicrobial: *Staphylococcus aureus*, *Escherichia coli*, and *Candida albicans* Concentration: <40 µg/ ml	Antioxidant Antibacterial Anti -inflammatory	[55].
Klebsiella pneumonia 05-506	Bacteria	ASK2 bioactive from *Streptomyces sp.*	*In vitro* and In vivo Monomicrobial	Cytotoxicity analysis: MTT	[56, 57]
Salmonella enterica serovar *Typhimurium*	Bacteria	Lectins Llp1 and Llp2 from *Lactobacillus rhamnosus*	*In vitro* Polymicrobial: *SalmonellaTyphimurium* and *E.coli*	-	[58]
	Plant	*Holarrhena antidysentrica* (Ha) and *Andrographis paniculata* (Ap)	*In vitro* Monomicrobial	Antioxidant	[59]
	Plant	Essential oils monoterpene hydrocarbons and phenolic monoterpenes from *Thymus vulgaris*, *Satureja montana*, and *Rosmarinus officinalis*	*In vitro* Monomicrobial	Antibacterial	[60]
	Plant	Quercetin-3-O-rhamnoside from *C. elaeagnoides* leaf extracts	*In vitro* Polymicrobial: *Salmonella* spp. and *Staphylococcus aureus* Concentration:1000 µg/mL	Antioxidant Antibacterial	[61]
	Fungi	*Flavourzyme* from *Aspergillus oryzae*	*In vitro* Polymicrobial: *SalmonellaTyphimurium*, *Escherichia coli*, and *Pseudomonas aeruginosa*	-	[62]

In the last few years, a plethora of natural sources have been explored [20]. Plant bioactives such as thymol (THY), eugenol (EUG), and carvacrol (CAR) showed a prominent loss of live *A. baumannii* cells within the biofilm. The effect of the compound was examined with the biofilm formed on the stainless steel and polystyrene microtiter plates [21]. Another study showed that plant *Tinospora cordifolia* extract diminished the development of *A. baumannii* biofilm. Further, the bio-guided fractionation, GC-MS and molecular docking studies revealed the presence of methyl 16-methyl heptadecanoate, 2-methoxy-4-vinyl phenol, 2-[- -ethenyl-5-methyloxolan-2-yl] propan-2-ol, 2,3,4-triacetyloxybutyl acetate, and methyl hexadecanoate in the extract [22]. Similarly, an extract of kiwi (*Actinidia deliciosa*) showed anti-biofilm activity against Carbapenem-resistant *A. baumannii*. Further, a TLC (thin layer chromatography) profile of the extract indicated the presence of sanquinarine (an alkaloid) and hydroxyflavone [a flavonoid]. Thus, the anti-biofilm activity of the kiwi extract can be attributed to sanquinarine and hydroxyflavone [20]. The pathogenicity of *A. baumannii* is also regulated by the quorum-sensing mechanism. Mono-unsaturated fatty acids such as myristoleic (MoA) and palmitoleic (PoA) acids are identified to be excellent *A. baumannii* biofilm inhibitors. These fatty acids (MoA, PoA) at the concentration of 0.02 mg/ml reduced biofilm formation in *A. baumannii* by up to 24% and 38%, respectively and investigation into its molecular mechanism showed decreased expression of the abaR (quorum sensing regulator) [23]. It was observed that fatty acids affect adhesion by manipulating cell membrane fluidity, reducing extracellular polysaccharide matrix and modulating quorum sensing [24]. Similarly, cinnamaldehyde showed strong antibacterial activity against planktonic *A. baumannii* and its MIC (minimum inhibitory concentration) and MBC (Minimum bactericidal concentration) were found to be 875 and 175 µg/ml. Further, the anti-biofilm assay demonstrated that at ½ minimum inhibitory concentration (MIC) cinnamaldehyde inhibited carbapenem-resistant *A. baumannii* biofilm by 49.5%-71.2%. However, at ¼ MIC, biofilm inhibition percentage was in the range of 18.5% to 29.6%. Anti-biofilm activity of cinnamaldehyde was confirmed by Scanning Electron Microscopy (SEM) [25].

It has been also found that propolin D, a prenylated flavanoid extracted from fruits of *Macaranga tanarius* (L.) inhibits *A. baumannii* biofilm and it showed minimal toxicity in *Caenorhabditis elegans* model [26], methanolic extract of *Carum copticum* inhibited biofilm formation by *A. baumannii* and *K. pneumoniae* by 98% and 19% respectively. Moreover, the GC-MS analysis showed the presence of pcymene (21%), Υ-terpinene (36%), and Thymol (40%) in the extract [27]. Moreover, the bioactives from flavonoid class such as fisetin, phloretin and curcumin showed concentration-dependent biofilm inhibition in *A. baumannii*. The anti-biofilm activity of curcumin was higher than gallium nitrate a common biofilm inhibitor and it also exhibited activity against mixed biofilm of *A. baumannii* and *C. albicans*. Further molecular docking established a correlation between the binding of flavonoid to the biofilm response regulator (BfmR) and the biofilm. The toxicity assessment study showed the non-toxic nature of the curcumin in an *in vivo Caenorhabditis elegans* model [28]. Citral is a major component of several essential oils and belongs to the class of monoterpene aldehyde. It has been recently demonstrated that citral (200 µg/ml) inhibits *A. baumannii* biofilms by 90% [29]. Moreover, *Azadirachta indica* (Neem), a plant that is recognized for its medicinal properties inhibited biofilms of Extended-spectrum beta-lactamase (ESBL) producing *A. baumannii*. A CsgA is one of the potent virulence factors prevalent in *A. baumannii* strains and hence, is considered an excellent target for biofilm inhibition. Further in silico docking studies into the identification of specific anti-biofilm bioactive from neem revealed the involvement of imidazole interaction with CsgA. It was also noticed that binding of imidazole to CsgA involves minimal docking energy and a high number of hydrogen bonds. However, validation through *in-vivo* studies is further required [30]. Similarly, the leaf extract of *Schinus terebinthifolia* at 256 µg/ml concentration showed 80% inhibition in the growth of carbapenem-resistant *A. baumannii* (CRAB). Further fractionation and characterization studies identified a bioactive compound of the extract which is pentagalloyl glucose (PGG) and its probable mechanism of action was found to be iron chelation. Besides, the compound did not lead to the production of resistant mutant till 21 days. Even though PGG showed excellent antimicrobial activity against CRAB, it did not affect the *A. baumannii* biofilm. PGG has few delivery challenges hence, it refrained from applications in therapeutics and can be used only in tropical applications [31]. However, Zerumbone showed dose-dependent biofilm inhibition in multidrug-resistant *A. baumannii*. These phenotypic results were validated by transcriptional analysis. The expression of biofilm-associated genes (*bap*) and virulence-associated genes (*adeA, adeB, adeC*) were significantly downregulated due to zerumbone [32].

However, a compound 5-episinuleptolide, extracted from a marine organism *Sinularia leptoclados* belonging to phylum *Cnidaria* showed significant biofilm inhibition in three multi-drug resistant (MDR) strains of *A. baumannii viz.* A. baumannii 29115, 68704 (resistant to 6 antibiotics and susceptible to colistin) and *A. baumannii* D4 (resistant to 8 antibiotics and sensitive to colistin). Moreover, the percent biofilm inhibition was in the range of 45-55%. As the minimal difference in the percent inhibition was observed between 24 hours and 48-hours of infections, it was concluded that 5-episinuleptolide remains active till 48 hours. Moreover, the study also stated that the compound did not eradicate *A. baumannii* biofilm, but inhibited biofilm formation in MDR *A. baumannii* and can be used as a prophylactic agent. Furthermore, gene expression studies revealed that the pgaABCD locus, synthesizing extracellular polysaccharide poly— [1, 6]--acetylglucosamine (PNAG), was downregulated, and SEM research revealed that the biofilm's extracellular matrix was substantially reduced after treatment with 5-episinuleptolide [33]. Likewise, the frog skin is a rich source of antimicrobial peptides. Magainin 2, a peptide extracted from the skin of *Xenopus laevis* (African clawed frog) at 2–8 µM concentration exhibited biofilm development inhibition and removal activity in 5 MDR *A. baumannii* strains isolated from patients at Eulji University Hospital (Seoul, Korea) *viz.* KCTC 2508, *Acinetobacter baumannii* 719705, 244752, 907233, 409081, 892199 [34]. Another study found that *Stichodactyla haddoni* (a sea anemone) extract possesses both biofilm inhibition and destruction activity at concentration 6.25 mg/ml. Furthermore, GC-MS analysis was employed to determine the composition of the extract. The extract contained three types of compounds aliphatics, alicyclic and aromatics. However, aliphatic compounds were abundant [35].

Similarly, bacteria are often explored for their bioactives. A glycolipid surfactant, Staphylosan (dimannooleate) synthesized by *Staphylococcus saprophyticus* SBPS-15 inhibited biofilm formation by *Acinetobacter baumannii* BHKH-11, *Pseudomonas aeruginosa* BHKH-19, *Micrococcus luteus* BHKH-39, *Bacillus subtilis* BHKH-7, *Marinobacter lipolyticus* BHKH-31 and *Serratia liquefaciens* BHKH-23. Since the compound did not show toxicity to brine shrimp, it can be used as an anti-biofilm compound [36]. The Gram-negative periodontal pathogen *Aggregatibacter actinomycetemcomitans* synthesized dispersin B which can hydrolyse mature *A. baumannii* biofilms [37, 38]. An extract derived from terrabacteria *Streptomyces gandocaensis* significantly inhibited biofilm formation by *A. baumannii*. Further analysis of the extract showed the presence of three metabolites cahuitamycins A-C wherein cahuitamycins C was relatively more efficient in inhibiting biofilm than other identified bioactives [39].

Natural Bioactive Against *Pseudomonas aeruginosa* Biofilm

P. aeruginosa produces virulence factors and has the potential to cause major health damages. Biofilm is the most significant of these variables. *P. aeruginosa* cells present inside the biofilm are resistant to conventional antimicrobial drugs, therefore, several studies recommend using a new generation of antibiotics. Due to the advent of multidrug-resistant (MDR) strains, biofilm inhibitors obtained from natural products or modified from natural compounds are now being tested.

The anti-biofilm activity was reported in large number of medicinal and edible plants. Methanolic leaf extract of *Pistacia atlantica* (Anacardiaceae) has bioactive components which showed an inhibitory effect on the biofilm production in *P. aeruginosa* PAO1 with no effects seen on its growth. The identification and characterisation of four bioactives from the extracts with strong anti-biofilm activity were made by HPLC. The identified bioactives from extracts rutin, myricetin-3-O-rutinoside, kaempferol-3-O- rutinoside and isoquercitrin. All the four bioactives extracted from *P. atlantica* can be used against *P. aeruginosa* biofilm infection. The active compounds are bound to LasR [a receptor protein involved in the quorum sensing], as per a molecular docking simulation. Rutin and myricetin 3-O-rutinoside inhibited the development of biofilm by *P. aeruginosa* by >90% at 310 µg/ml. However, isoquercetin (190 µg/ml) and kaempferol-3-O-rutinoside (300 µg/ml) reduced biofilm development by >90% and 70% respectively [40]. These bioactives in the methanolic extract of *P. atlantica* have potent anti-biofilm properties and may be used to treat MDR *P. aeruginosa* infections. Similarly, an extract of Ginger (*Zingiber officinale* Rosc.), which has been traditionally used to treat numerous ailments, exhibited a significant decrease in the biofilms of *P. aeruginosa*. Furthermore, the decreased level of bis-[3'-5']-cyclic dimeric guanosine monophosphate (2° messenger) leads to inhibition of biofilm and decrease in total polysaccharide production [41]. Zingerone, a bioactive component in the dry ginger root, showed biofilm inhibition and also increased susceptibility to ciprofloxacin in *Pseudomonas aeruginosa* PAO1. Besides, zingerone suppresses the motility (swarming, swimming, twitching) and thereby inhibiting *P. aeruginosa* initial attachment to a solid substratum. Zingerone functions by altering cell morphology, thus preventing the formation of extracellular polymeric substances *i.e.* EPS [42]. Kumar *et al.*, (2013) explored the anti-biofilm property of zingerone and provided a new method for preventing the development of biofilms. However, its molecular mechanisms need to be analysed to widen the applications of the compound. *Syzygium cumini* L. Skeels is well known for its anti-diabetic properties. *S. cumini* leaf extract using Ethyl acetate (EA) as solvent was prepared for further investigating its anti-biofilm ability against *P. aeruginosa* MCC 2081 and *S. aureus*. The active ethyl acetate fraction (EA) had no effect on the growth of two pathogens. Biofilms of *P. aeruginosa* and *S. aureus* were inhibited around 86% by using 900 µg/ml of EA. The reduction in biofilm formation was also verified by SEM analysis. Further investigation of EA by GC-MS revealed the presence of Heptacosanoic acid, 3-Methyl 2-[2-Oxopropyl] and 3-N-Hexylthiane which probably showed a considerable biofilm inhibition of *P. aeruginosa* [43]. Moreover, *P. aeruginosa* biofilms are also reduced by halogenated furanones *viz.* C-56, C-30 formed by *Delisea pulchra* [marine microalgae]. These were also meant to prevent the colonisation of lungs in mouse caused by *P. aeruginosa,* clearing the bacterial load and minimising the tissue damage [44]. Moreover, a combination of furanone and sodium dodecyl sulphate effectively clears biofilms by modulating their antibiotic sensitivity especially tobramycin which is a commonly used antibiotic in the care of patients with CF. Tobramycin destroyed 85-90% of biofilm cells pre-treated with furanone. Furthermore, *in vivo* experiments using a mouse pulmonary infection model also confirmed the antimicrobial activity of furanone C-30 [44].

Another study showed that the triterpenoid ursolic acid when used at a concentration of 10 µg/ml, inhibits the development of biofilms by *Pseudomonas aeruginosa* and some other pathogenic organisms. However, other structural analogues triterpenoids asiatic acid and corosolic acid showed higher activity in increasing *P. aeruginosa*'s susceptibility to ciprofloxacin as compared to Ursolic acid. These terpenoids have been isolated from a variety of edible and medicinal plants [45]. An herb *Andrographis paniculate* has a diterpenoid lactone: andrographolide, used to cure inflammation, pyrexia, and pain caused by infections of bacteria and viruses. Derivative of andrographolide, 14-alpha-lipoyl andrographolide (AL-1) was synthesised with antibacterial activity. The report by Zeng *et al.* (2011) demonstrated that AL-1 blocked biofilm development and sensitised *P. aeruginosa* to a number of antibiotics, resulting in different synergistic outcomes. Furthermore, when these antibiotics were combined with AL-1, the amount of EPS and pyocyanin was drastically decreased [46]. Moreover, the casbane diterpene, from *Croton Nepetaefolius* baill, reduced biofilm formation in *Pseudomonas aeruginosa* and also in other clinically relevant species. It was observed that 250 μg /ml concentration of the compound was effective in inhibiting biofilm formation by *P. aeruginosa* without compromising the viability of bacterial cells. Thus, less susceptible to bacterial resistance. Furthermore, the studies carried out to identify the molecular mechanism of the compound showed its action on the preliminary binding of the bacteria to the surface [47]. Besides, there are some fungal agents which have shown promising anti-biofilm activity.

Marine sponges, which belong to the phylum Porifera are predominantly explored nowadays due to their broad-spectrum profile for secondary metabolites with a variety of applications. Lectins are often isolated from marine sponges. They are mostly glycoproteins and possess a wide range of structures. Some of the natural compounds from marine sponges are being used as scaffolds in designing synthetic anti-biofilm compounds against *P. aeruginosa*. The examples of such bioactive scaffolds are given below. Bromoageliferin is an alkaloid derived from marine sponge (*Agelas conifer*, Agelaceae). Bromoageliferin belonging to oroid in class of bioactives possesses biological activity. Its analogues *viz.* TAGE (trans-bromoageliferin analogue 1) and CAGE (cis-bromoageliferin analogue 2) are also capable to reduce biofilm synthesis. Moreover, these analogues disperse pre-existing *P. aeruginosa* PAO1 biofilm without any growth-inhibiting effect. CAGE 2 at the concentration of 400 and 500 μM, was noted for reducing the biofilm mass. The anti-biofilm activity of these compounds needs to be further strongly supported by a detailed study on the action mechanism of 2-AI [48]. Likewise, lectin derived from *Fasciospongia cavernosa* was analysed for its anti-biofilm activity against the biofilms formed by *P. aeruginosa*. The lectin FCL (*Fasciospongia cavernosa* lectin) has a molecular weight of 80kDa, and was able to reduce the biofilm synthesis in *P. aeruginosa* and also in other pathogens such as *S. aureus*, *B. subtilis* [49].

Natural Bioactive Against *Enterobacteriaceae* biofilm

The frequent occurrence of clinical therapy failures is due to the emergence of antibacterial resistance. In this book chapter, we focus on the pathogenic organisms that belong to Enterobacteriaceae family which includes *Shigella* spp., *K. pneumoniae, E. coli*, and *Salmonella* spp.

Natural Bioactives Against *Shigella spp.* Biofilm

An enteric pathogen, *Shigella flexneri* is a major etiological agent of bacillary dysentery. As biofilms of *S. flexneri* mediate antibiotic resistance, these pose significant risks to human health. Moreover, the gap between AMR and novel antimicrobial production is widening. Plant extracts are active sources of effective antimicrobial compounds that can combat planktonic mass or biofilms of the pathogen. Phytochemical ferulic acid (FA) is a phenolic compound. It has been used in the food industry as a natural preservative. FA is investigated to affect the planktonic and biofilm formation in *S. flexneri*. On exposure to FA, the planktonic growth of *S. flexneri* underwent irreversible destruction leading to reduced cell viability, leaking of cytoplasmic contents, depolarization of cell membrane *etc*. As a result, FA hindered *S. flexneri* adhesion and biofilm formation greatly. Transcriptomic profiling showed variation in gene expression of *S. flexneri* biofilm after exposure to a subinhibitory level of FA. The studies of transcriptomics revealed downregulation of 533 differentially expressed genes (DEGs) and upregulation of 169 genes, in comparison to unexposed biofilms. Genes that are known to involve in adhesion, control of transcription, and in the synthesis of biofilm matrix were shown to be downregulated. On FA application, *S. flexneri* and its biofilm forming capability may be significantly suppressed [52]. Bioactives from probiotic organisms have also gained attention and are used as antimicrobial agents. *Lactobacillus plantarum* 12 exopolysaccharides (L-EPSs) could prominently decrease the synthesis of biofilm matrix of *S. flexneri* CMCC51574 and thus can be used as a preventive measure. Furthermore, a cell line study revealed that the compound acts on the adhesion of *S. flexneri* and also hinder its entry into the HT-29 cells. Monosaccharides such as glucose, mannose, xylose, glucuronic acid, galactose, and galactosamine were the components of L-EPS. Further, the separation of L-EPS into acidic (L-EPS2-1) and neutral (L-EPS2-1) was carried out using chromatography techniques. However, according to their anti-biofilm efficacy, the acidic L-EPS was superior to neutral. Moreover, it was found that L-EPS acts on the bacterial surface and modulates its physical properties. Besides, it regulates the expression of biofilm associated genes [50]. Likewise, *Eleusine coracana*, commonly known as Finger millet has numerous health benefits due to its nutritional value. A carbohydrate moiety, β-glucan (Ec-βG) isolated from the seeds of *Eleusine coracana* is reported to exhibit anti-biofilm activity against *S. sonnei* at 100 μg/ml. The anti-biofilm activity was further confirmed by confocal laser scanning microscopy [63].

Natural Bioactives Against *Escherichia coli* Biofilm

Food borne diseases such as hemolytic uremic syndrome and bloody diarrhoea are commonly caused by Enterohaemorrhagic *Escherichia coli* (EHEC). As the virulence factors produced by EHEC such as shiga toxin and resistance to conventional antibiotics increase the mortality rate there is an urge for novel and safe antimicrobials for the treatment of EHEC. A great number of natural bioactives with diverse biological activities like antibacterial and anti-biofilm formation can be exploited as potential candidates in the treatment of these pathogens. A study showed that six bioactives derived from citrus plants could suppress biofilm formation by *Escherichia coli* O157:H7. Amongst the six bioactives tested, β-sitosterol glucoside significantly inhibited EHEC biofilm. Furthermore, qRT-PCR analysis concluded that the compound could inhibit motility and biofilm formation by suppressing the *rssAB* gene and has mediated repression of flagellar master operon *flhDC* [53].

Similarly, caffeic acid, gallic acid and isothiocyanates isolated from *Brassicaceae* plant extracts can reduce biofilm formation by *E. coli* [54]. *Punica granatum L.* or Pomegranate peels primarily consist of tannins, phenols and flavonoids. It was found that pomegranate extract is able to inhibit biofilms of *E. coli*, *S. aureus* and *Candida albicans*. HPLC analysis identified the presence of ellagic acid (2,3,7,8-tetrahydroxy-chromeno[5,4,3-cde] chromene-5,10-dione) in the Pomegranate peels. Ellagic acid has been widely used as anticancer, antioxidant agent, however, its anti-biofilm activity was reported for the first time [55]. Ellagic acid showed growth inhibition at a concentration higher than 75 µg/ml and biofilm inhibition at sub-lethal concentration *i.e.* lower than 40 µg /ml. Thus, the potential of ellagic acid can be further investigated by *in vivo* studies [55]. Likewise, a lectin called AGL was derived from seeds of *Amaranthus gangeticus* by employing chromatography techniques. Maximum anti-biofilm activity achieved by AGL treatment was 82.85% at 1000 µg/ml [51].

Natural Bioactives against *Klebsiella Pneumonia* Biofilm

Klebsiella pneumonia 05-506 strain is reported to produce carbapenemase, thus making them resistant to conventional antibiotics, posing a major challenge to public health. *K. pneumoniae* is known to cause urinary tract especially catheter-associated infections.

A potential bioactive derived from *Streptomyces sp.* ASK2 was purified using HPLC to identify the active component that has an antagonistic property against MDR *K. pneumonia*. An aromatic compound was further purified. FT-IR showed the presence of two functional groups mainly C=O and OH [56]. The drug induced toxicity was studied by carrying out MTT assay in cultured zebrafish liver cells and the effective concentration of AKS2 was estimated as 48 µg/ml. In studies conducted by Lalitha *et al.,* (2017) the anti-biofilm ability of ASK2 was analysed on the basis of MIC and minimum biofilm eradication concentration (MBEC). Results showed that MBEC was 15 times higher than MIC [57].

Natural Bioactives against *Salmonella spp.* Biofilm

Bioactives isolated from *Andrographis paniculata* (Ap) and *Holarrhena antidysentrica* (Ha) inhibited biofilm formation by *Salmonella enterica* serovar *Typhimurium*. Moreover, identification of the bioactives was done using bioactivity fingerprint analysis and Attenuated Total Reflection (ATR) infrared spectroscopy. Both the bioactives inhibited *SalmonellaTyphimurium*, biofilm whereas the uptake of Propidium Iodide (PI) indicated that the integrity of the cell membrane was impaired on exposure to the above extracts for a span of an hour. Thus, they can be used to treat infections caused by the biofilms of *S. Typhimurium* [59].

Bacteria have diverse bioactives with potential applications as valuable products like biopharmaceuticals, biocontrol agents, biocatalysts, health supplements *etc.* Some of the bacterial bioactives having anti-biofilm activity are mentioned below. Lectins present in probiotic *Lactobacillus rhamnosus* are used as bioactive to inhibit the biofilm synthesis by *Salmonella* spp. Genome sequencing was carried out to estimate the presence of genes that code for lectin-like proteins. Two polypeptides with their conserved domains at N and C-terminal were identified as Lectin like protein (Llp) 1 and 2. Moreover, *S.Typhimurium* ATCC14028 biofilm inhibition assay showed 60% inhibition by LIp (10 µg/ml). However, Llp1 needed a higher concentration 50 µg/ml to attain significant reduction. Moreover, Llp1 inhibited *E. coli* UTI89 biofilm at lower concentrations. The study also stated that the anti-biofilm efficacy of purified lectins was higher than their crude extracts [58].

Essential oils of *Rosmarinus officinalis* L., *Thymus vulgaris* L. and *Satureja montana* L. contain monoterpene hydrocarbons, phenolic monoterpenes as the bioactives. A study showed that these bioactives impart anti-biofilm and anti-adhesive properties to EOs against *SalmonellaTyphimurium*. The inhibition of biofilm was tested using the 2, 3-bis (2-methyloxy-4-nitro-5-sulfophenyl)-2 H-tetrazolium-5-carboxanilide reduction assay [60]. Moreover, another study conducted by Miladi H *et.al.*, (2016) showed that *S. montana* and *T. vulgaris* essential oils have anti-biofilm activity and it is found to be higher than *R. officinalis* EO. Thyme EO act as natural food preservative agent by preventing biofilm formation in processed food. In Africa, traditional medicine *Combretum elaeagnoides* Klotzsch (Combretaceae) is used against infections and diarrhoea. The leaf extracts of *C. elaeagnoides* contain quercetin-3-O-rhamnoside, that was evaluated for its anti-biofilm and antioxidant activity. The quercetin-3-O-rhamnoside was able to act against all tested organisms at concentrations 30 - 125 µg/ml. On purification, it inhibited biofilm formation of *S.Typhimurium* and *S. aureus* with a greater percentage *i.e.* 50% at 1000 µg/mL [61]. Fungi can produce bioactives such as polysaccharides, proteoglycans, phenolic compounds, lectins, peptides, proteins, *etc.* These bioactive confers to antioxidant, antimicrobial, anti–inflammatory, antidiabetic, anticancer as well as anti-biofilm properties. Flavourzyme is a commercially derived peptidase from *Aspergillus oryzae*. This peptidase enzyme was able to reduce biofilm formation by S. Typhimurium on rubber and polyethylene surfaces *e.g.* Ultra-High Molecular

Weight polyethylene (UHMWPE). A significant reduction in young (24-h-old) and mature (72-h-old) biofilms of *S.Typhimurium*, *E.coli*, and *P. aeruginosa* was observed on treatment with flavourzyme. Its efficacy was compared with DNase I and was found to be higher [62]. Moreover, it was found that the flavourzyme acts on the polysaccharide (C-O-C) and amide (N-H) bonds in the biofilm matrix and further eradicates biofilms [62]. Reducing the microbial EPS formation and its non-toxic nature can aid in controlling microbial food contamination caused by biofilm formation. Therefore, it can be used as a novel method for controlling foodborne illness.

LIMITATIONS AND RESEARCH GAPS IN THE DISCOVERY OF NATURAL BIOACTIVES AGAINST BIOFILMS

Different compounds used as drugs that are derived from natural sources have provided ample benefits to pharma industries in terms of therapeutics against infectious diseases and cancer. Unfortunately, over the last few years, pharmaceutical firms have greatly reduced their natural product discovery efforts. Though there is a slow-down in the discovery of natural products, many new and fascinating biologically active compounds have been released in recent years. We assume that if natural products are tested for desirable therapeutic activities, significant progress will be made in discovering novel anti-biofilm drugs and other valuable medicines [64].

A significant number of herb extracts have been reported to demonstrate biofilm effects, but in the majority of these extracts, the bioactive molecule is still unknown and requires further investigation. To identify such bioactive molecules from extracts, the techniques employed for separation and extraction play a pivotal role. Sophisticated instrumentation techniques like HPLC, structure-based virtual screening can be useful in the characterization of specific bioactive from the extracts. Although, there are many potential bioactives as anti-biofilm agents, their detailed mechanisms of action remain to be understood. This adds to the limitation in the use of such bioactives. The molecular pathways and animal model studies of these agents need to be carried out to meet the paucity of knowledge regarding the mechanism of action. The majority of the clinical trials that are conducted on bioactives focus on its implication as anti-bacterial and anti-biofilm agent in patients concerning oral health or treatment of urinary tract infections. However, other infections are so far rarely studied. There is a need to include clinical trials related to other infectious diseases, along with the trials that mainly focus on the use of bioactives in denture and somatology. So far, anti-biofilm compounds acting against bacterial infection have not been approved by U.S. Food and Drug Administration yet [65]. Several active phases from I - IV of clinical trials for bioactives as an anti-biofilm agent have been conducted, but the findings of several completed clinical trials have yet to be published. More clinical trials of natural bioactives in inhibiting biofilm synthesis, suggest a promising future in the clinical application of natural anti-biofilm compounds. Also, plant bioactives are widely explored as compared to the other natural sources of bioactives, however, other sources also possess the potential to be used as antimicrobial agents.

Extensive research is needed to prove the efficacy of these natural bioactives as anti-biofilm agents, involving more *in vivo* studies. This will assist in addressing challenges during drug approval and application. Tissue cultures have been used as a substitute for *in vivo* biofilm experiments, but building a three-dimensional tissue culture is time-consuming and costly [66]. The use of animal models to study medical biofilms is advantageous because it includes an environment similar to the host system, including the components of the host defences and complex body fluids, which are difficult to mimic *in vitro* [67]. The *in vivo* studies are very crucial for understanding the therapeutic effect of bioactives in a biofilm with respect to its toxicity, bioavailability, clearance, absorbance and also optimising the concentration range.

Moreover, it is worthy to calculate the efficacy of bioactives in synergy with the current antibiotics being used, to maximise the effect in the eradication of clinically challenging biofilms. Studies on improving specificity, stability and safety also demand attention.

CONCLUSION

The pathogenic biofilms have developed resistance to conventional antibiotics and antimicrobials, creating a complicated challenge for clinicians as well as researchers. Treatment of such persistent biofilms has become cumbersome. To overcome the concern of antibiotic resistance, novel antimicrobial techniques are urgently needed. Natural resources are an abundant source of bioactives, allowing researchers to scan a large library for effective agents. Even though we have witnessed advancement in the screening of anti-biofilm bioactives in the last few decades, more studies on identifying the bioactives and their mechanism of action are still required. In addition, phase I–IV clinical trials on natural anti-biofilm bioactives require attention for rapid discovery. Thus, the therapeutic use of natural anti-biofilm agents has huge potential in the management of drug-resistant bacterial infections and will support health care industries all over the world. The chapter provides information on a novel approach of using bioactives as a preventive and therapeutic measure in combination with antibiotics to eradicate pathogenic biofilm formation and related infections. Since these natural bioactives are the plentiful source and an inspiration for numerous medical agents with their divergent biological activities. It provides the basis for future aspects of using efficient approaches for producing bioactives in high yield.

CONSENT FOR PUBLICATION

Not applicable.

CONFLICT OF INTEREST

The authors declare no conflict of interest, financial or otherwise.

ACKNOWLEDGEMENTS

AB supported by the junior research fellowship program of Symbiosis International (Deemed University). AP is supported by the ERASMUS+ under grant 598515-EPP-1-2018-1-IN-EPPKA2-CBHE-JP. The work was also supported by the Ramalingaswami fellowship program of the Department of Biotechnology, India under grant BT/RLF/Re-entry/41/2015; Major research project grant of Symbiosis International (Deemed University) under grant SIU/SCRI/MJRP-Approval/2019/1556.

REFERENCES

[1]   Guaadaoui A, Benaicha S, Elmajdoub N, Bellaoui M, Hamal A. What is a bioactive compound? A combined definition for a preliminary consensus. Int J Food Sci Nutr 2014; 3(3): 17-179.

[2]   Carbonell-Capella JM, Barba FJ, Esteve MJ, Frígola A. Quality parameters, bioactive compounds and their correlation with antioxidant capacity of commercial fruit-based baby foods. Food Sci Technol Int = Cienc y Tecnol los Aliment Int 2014; 20(7): 479-87.

[3]   Ham SS, Kim SH, Moon SY, *et al.* Antimutagenic effects of subfractions of Chaga mushroom (Inonotus obliquus) extract. Mutat Res Genet Toxicol Environ Mutagen 2009; 672(1): 55-9. [http://dx.doi.org/10.1016/j.mrgentox.2008.10.002] [PMID: 18992843]

[4]   Khezerlou A, Jafari SM. Nanoencapsulated bioactive components for active food packaging. Jafari SMBT-H of FN 2020; 493-532. Available from: https://www.sciencedirect.com/science/article/ pii/B9780128158661000133

[5]   Siriwardhana N, Kalupahana NS, Cekanova M, LeMieux M, Greer B, Moustaid-Moussa N. Modulation of adipose tissue inflammation by bioactive food compounds. J Nutr Biochem 2013; 24(4): 613-23.https://www.sciencedirect.com/science/article/pii/S0955286313000090 [http://dx.doi.org/10.1016/j.jnutbio.2012.12.013] [PMID: 23498665]

[6]   Ibañez E, Kubátová A, Señoráns FJ, Cavero S, Reglero G, Hawthorne SB. Subcritical water extraction of antioxidant compounds from rosemary plants. J Agric Food Chem 2003; 51(2): 375-82. [http://dx.doi.org/10.1021/jf025878j] [PMID: 12517098]

[7]   Jafari SM, Mahdavee Khazaei K, Assadpour E. 2019.http://europepmc.org/abstract/MED/31024717

[8]   Rodriguez-Jasso RM, Mussatto SI, Pastrana L, Aguilar CN, Teixeira JA. Microwave-assisted extraction of sulfated polysaccharides (fucoidan) from brown seaweed. Carbohydr Polym (Internet) 2011; 86(3): 1137-44. [http://dx.doi.org/10.1016/j.carbpol.2011.06.006]

[9]   Kadam SU, Tiwari BK, O'Donnell CP. Application of novel extraction technologies for bioactives

from marine algae. J Agric Food Chem 2013; 61(20): 4667-75.
[http://dx.doi.org/10.1021/jf400819p] [PMID: 23634989]

[10] Høiby N. A short history of microbial biofilms and biofilm infections. Acta Pathol Microbiol Scand Suppl 2017; 125(4): 272-5.
[http://dx.doi.org/10.1111/apm.12686] [PMID: 28407426]

[11] Høiby N, Bjarnsholt T, Givskov M, Molin S, Ciofu O. Antibiotic resistance of bacterial biofilms. Int J Antimicrob Agents 2010; 35(4): 322-32. https://www.sciencedirect.com/science/article/pii/S09248-579010000099
[http://dx.doi.org/10.1016/j.ijantimicag.2009.12.011] [PMID: 20149602]

[12] Di Somma A. Inhibition of Bacterial Biofilm Formation. In: Moretta A, editor. Rijeka: IntechOpen; 2020. p. Ch. 4.
[http://dx.doi.org/10.5772/intechopen.90614]

[13] Cepas V, López Y, Muñoz E, *et al.* Relationship Between Biofilm Formation and Antimicrobial Resistance in Gram-Negative Bacteria. Microb Drug Resist 2019; 25(1): 72-9.
[http://dx.doi.org/10.1089/mdr.2018.0027] [PMID: 30142035]

[14] Gilbert P, Allison DG, McBain AJ. Biofilms *in vitro* and *in vivo* : do singular mechanisms imply cross-resistance? J Appl Microbiol 2002; 92 (Suppl.): 98S-110S.
[http://dx.doi.org/10.1046/j.1365-2672.92.5s1.5.x] [PMID: 12000619]

[15] Shankar PR. Book review: Tackling drug-resistant infections globally. Arch Pharm Pract (Mumbai) 2016; 7(3): 110.
[http://dx.doi.org/10.4103/2045-080X.186181]

[16] Tanguy M, Kouatchet A, Tanguy B. Pichard, Fanello S, Joly-Guillou ML. Prise en charge d'une épidémie à Acinetobacter baumannii. Med Mal Infect (Internet) 2017; 47(6): 409-14.
[http://dx.doi.org/10.1016/j.medmal.2017.06.003] [PMID: 28734630]

[17] Zhen X, Lundborg CS, Sun X, Hu X, Dong H. Economic burden of antibiotic resistance in ESKAPE organisms: a systematic review. Antimicrob Resist Infect Control 2019; 8(1): 137.
[http://dx.doi.org/10.1186/s13756-019-0590-7] [PMID: 31417673]

[18] Patil A, Banerji R, Kanojiya P, Saroj SD. Foodborne ESKAPE Biofilms and Antimicrobial Resistance: lessons Learned from Clinical Isolates. Pathog Glob Health 2021; 115(6): 339-56.
[http://dx.doi.org/10.1080/20477724.2021.1916158] [PMID: 33851566]

[19] Chung PY, Toh YS. Anti-biofilm agents: recent breakthrough against multi-drug resistant *Staphylococcus aureus*. Pathog Dis 2014; 70(3): 231-9.
[http://dx.doi.org/10.1111/2049-632X.12141] [PMID: 24453168]

[20] Tiwari V, Tiwari D, Patel V, Tiwari M. Effect of secondary metabolite of Actinidia deliciosa on the biofilm and extra-cellular matrix components of Acinetobacter baumannii. Microb Pathog 2017; 110: 345-51.
[http://dx.doi.org/10.1016/j.micpath.2017.07.013] [PMID: 28705748]

[21] Pelletier RP. Effect of Plant-Derived Molecules on Acinetobacter baumannii. University of Connecticut 2012.

[22] Desai KB, Gala VC, John NR, Bhagwat AM, Datar AG, Kharkar PS. Attenuation of quorum sensing-regulated behaviour by *Tinospora cordifolia* extract & identification of its active constituents. Indian J Med Res 2016; 144(1): 92-103.
[http://dx.doi.org/10.4103/0971-5916.193295] [PMID: 27834332]

[23] Nicol M, Alexandre S, Luizet JB, *et al.* Unsaturated Fatty Acids Affect Quorum Sensing Communication System and Inhibit Motility and Biofilm Formation of Acinetobacter baumannii. Int J Mol Sci 2018; 19(1): 214.
[http://dx.doi.org/10.3390/ijms19010214] [PMID: 29320462]

[24] Kumar P, Lee JH, Beyenal H, Lee J. Fatty Acids as Antibiofilm and Antivirulence Agents. Trends

Microbiol 2020; 28(9): 753-68.
[http://dx.doi.org/10.1016/j.tim.2020.03.014] [PMID: 32359781]

[25]   Mohamed SH, Salem D, Azmy M, Fam NS. Antibacterial and antibiofilm activity J Appl Pharm Sci 2018; 8(11): 151-6.

[26]   Lee JH, Kim YG, Khadke SK, Yamano A, Woo JT, Lee J. Antimicrobial and antibiofilm activities of prenylated flavanones from *Macaranga tanarius*. Phytomedicine 2019; 63(April): 153033.
[http://dx.doi.org/10.1016/j.phymed.2019.153033] [PMID: 31352284]

[27]   Mohammadi M, Masoumipour F, Hassanshahian M, Jafarinasab T. Study the antibacterial and antibiofilm activity of Carum copticum against antibiotic-resistant bacteria in planktonic and biofilm forms. Microb Pathog 2019; 129(January): 99-105.
[http://dx.doi.org/10.1016/j.micpath.2019.02.002] [PMID: 30731188]

[28]   Raorane CJ, Lee JH, Kim YG, Rajasekharan SK, García-Contreras R, Lee J. Antibiofilm and antivirulence efficacies of flavonoids. Front Microbiol 2019; 10(May): 990.
[http://dx.doi.org/10.3389/fmicb.2019.00990] [PMID: 31134028]

[29]   Selvaraj A, Valliammai A, Muthuramalingam P, *et al.* Proteomic and Systematic Functional Profiling Unveils Citral Targeting Antibiotic Resistance, Antioxidant Defense, and Biofilm-Associated Two-Component Systems of Acinetobacter baumannii To Encumber Biofilm and Virulence Traits. mSystems 2020; 5(6): e00986-20.
[http://dx.doi.org/10.1128/mSystems.00986-20] [PMID: 33203690]

[30]   Iswarya Jaisankar A, Smiline Girija AS, Gunasekaran S, Vijayashree Priyadharsini J. Molecular characterisation of csgA gene among ESBL strains of *A. baumannii* and targeting with essential oil compounds from Azadirachta indica. J King Saud Univ Sci 2020; 32(8): 3380-7.
[http://dx.doi.org/10.1016/j.jksus.2020.09.025]

[31]   Dettweiler M, Marquez L, Lin M, *et al.* Pentagalloyl glucose from Schinus terebinthifolia inhibits growth of carbapenem-resistant *Acinetobacter baumannii*. Sci Rep 2020; 10(1): 15340.
[http://dx.doi.org/10.1038/s41598-020-72331-w] [PMID: 32948818]

[32]   Kim HR, Shin DS, Jang HI, Eom YB. Anti-biofilm and anti-virulence effects of zerumbone against *Acinetobacter baumannii*. Microbiology (Reading) 2020; 166(8): 717-26.
[http://dx.doi.org/10.1099/mic.0.000930] [PMID: 32463353]

[33]   Tseng SP, Hung WC, Huang CY, *et al.* 5-Episinuleptolide decreases the expression Of the extracellular matrix in early biofilm formation of multi-drug resistant Acinetobacter baumannii. Mar Drugs 2016; 14(8): 143.
[http://dx.doi.org/10.3390/md14080143] [PMID: 27483290]

[34]   Kim M, Kang N, Ko S, *et al.* Antibacterial and antibiofilm activity. Int J Mol Sci 2018; 19(10): 3041.
[http://dx.doi.org/10.3390/ijms19103041] [PMID: 30301180]

[35]   Hamayeli H, Hassanshahian M, Askari Hesni M. The antibacterial and antibiofilm activity of sea anemone (Stichodactyla haddoni) against antibiotic-resistant bacteria and characterization of bioactive metabolites. Int Aquatic Research 2019; 11(1): 85-97.
[http://dx.doi.org/10.1007/s40071-019-0221-1]

[36]   Balan SS, Mani P, Kumar CG, Jayalakshmi S. Structural characterization and biological evaluation of Staphylosan (dimannooleate), a new glycolipid surfactant produced by a marine *Staphylococcus saprophyticus* SBPS-15. Enzyme Microb Technol 2019; 120(120): 1-7.
[http://dx.doi.org/10.1016/j.enzmictec.2018.09.008] [PMID: 30396390]

[37]   Yan Z, Huang M, Melander C, Kjellerup BV. Dispersal and inhibition of biofilms associated with infections. J Appl Microbiol 2020; 128(5): 1279-88.
[http://dx.doi.org/10.1111/jam.14491] [PMID: 31618796]

[38]   Ghosh A, Jayaraman N, Chatterji D. Small-Molecule Inhibition of Bacterial Biofilm. ACS Omega 2020; 5(7): 3108-15.

[http://dx.doi.org/10.1021/acsomega.9b03695] [PMID: 32118127]

[39]   Park SR, Tripathi A, Wu J, Schultz PJ, Yim I, McQuade TJ, *et al.* Discovery of cahuitamycins as biofilm inhibitors derived from a convergent biosynthetic pathway. Nat Commun 2016; 7(10710): 1-11.
[http://dx.doi.org/10.1038/ncomms10710]

[40]   Kordbacheh H, Eftekhar F, Ebrahimi SN. Anti-quorum sensing activity of Pistacia atlantica against *Pseudomonas aeruginosa* PAO1 and identification of its bioactive compounds. Microb Pathog 2017; 110: 390-8.
[http://dx.doi.org/10.1016/j.micpath.2017.07.018] [PMID: 28712963]

[41]   Kim HS, Park HD. Ginger extract inhibits biofilm formation by *Pseudomonas aeruginosa* PA14. PLoS One 2013; 8(9): e76106.
[http://dx.doi.org/10.1371/journal.pone.0076106] [PMID: 24086697]

[42]   Kumar L, Chhibber S, Harjai K. Zingerone inhibit biofilm formation and improve antibiofilm efficacy of ciprofloxacin against *Pseudomonas aeruginosa* PAO1. Fitoterapia 2013; 90: 73-8.
[http://dx.doi.org/10.1016/j.fitote.2013.06.017] [PMID: 23831483]

[43]   Gupta K, Singh SP, Manhar AK, Saikia D, Namsa ND, Konwar BK, *et al.* Inhibition of Staphylococcus aureus and *Pseudomonas aeruginosa* Biofilm and Virulence by Active Fraction of *Syzygium cumini (L.)* Skeels Leaf Extract: In-Vitro and In Silico Studies. Indian J Microbiol (Internet). 2019;59(1):13–21. http://europepmc.org/abstract/MED/30728626

[44]   Hentzer M, Riedel K, Rasmussen TB, *et al.* Inhibition of quorum sensing in *Pseudomonas aeruginosa* biofilm bacteria by a halogenated furanone compound. Microbiology (Reading) 2002; 148(1): 87-102.
[http://dx.doi.org/10.1099/00221287-148-1-87] [PMID: 11782502]

[45]   Chung P. Plant-derived Compounds as Potential Source of Novel Anti-Biofilm Agents Against *Pseudomonas aeruginosa*. Curr Drug Targets 2017; 18(4): 414-20. http://www.eurekaselect.com/node/146483/article
[http://dx.doi.org/10.2174/1389450117666161019102025] [PMID: 27758704]

[46]   Zeng X, Liu X, Bian J, Pei G, Dai H, Polyak SW, *et al.* Synergistic effect of 14-alpha-lipoyl andrographolide and various antibiotics on the formation of biofilms and production of exopolysaccharide and pyocyanin by *Pseudomonas aeruginosa*. Antimicrob Agents Chemother (Internet. 2011;55(6):3015–7. http://europepmc.org/abstract/MED/21422201

[47]   Carneiro VA, dos Santos HS, Arruda FVS, Bandeira PN, Albuquerque MRJR, Pereira MO, *et al.* Casbane Diterpene as a Promising Natural Antimicrobial Agent against Biofilm. Molecules 2011.
[PMID: 21193844]

[48]   Huigens RW III, Richards JJ, Parise G, *et al.* Inhibition of *Pseudomonas aeruginosa* biofilm formation with Bromoageliferin analogues. J Am Chem Soc 2007; 129(22): 6966-7.
[http://dx.doi.org/10.1021/ja069017t] [PMID: 17500516]

[49]   Sadanandan R, Rauf AA. Isolation, Purification and Characterisation of a D-galactose and N-acetyl-D-galactosamine Specific Lectin from Marine Sponge *Fasciospongia cavernosa*. Protein Pept Lett 2018; 25(9): 871-7.
[http://dx.doi.org/10.2174/0929866525666180905111452] [PMID: 30182831]

[50]   Yinglong S, Mengying S, Lu F, Xue L, Xing S, Guangqing M, *et al.* Antibiofilm Activity of Lactobacillus plantarum 12 Exopolysaccharides against *Shigella flexneri*. Appl Environ Microbiol (Internet) 2021; 86(15): e00694-20.
[http://dx.doi.org/10.1128/AEM.00694-20]

[51]   Hasan I, Rahman SN, Islam MM, *et al.* A N-acetyl-D-galactosamine-binding lectin from Amaranthus gangeticus seeds inhibits biofilm formation and Ehrlich ascites carcinoma cell growth *in vivo* in mice. Int J Biol Macromol 2021; 181: 928-36. https://www.sciencedirect.com/science/article/pii/S0141-813021008047
[http://dx.doi.org/10.1016/j.ijbiomac.2021.04.052] [PMID: 33878355]

[52]   Kang J, Liu L, Liu Y, Wang X. Ferulic Acid Inactivates *Shigella flexneri* through Cell Membrane Destruction, Biofilm Retardation, and Altered Gene Expression. J Agric Food Chem (Internet) 2020; 68(27): 7121-31.
[http://dx.doi.org/10.1021/acs.jafc.0c01901]

[53]   Vikram A, Jayaprakasha GK, Uckoo RM, Patil BS. Inhibition of *Escherichia coli* O157:H7 motility and biofilm by β-Sitosterol glucoside. Biochimica et Biophysica Acta - General Subjects 2013; Vol. 1830: pp. 5219-28.

[54]   Hu WS, Min Nam D, Kim JS, Koo OK. Synergistic anti-biofilm effects of Brassicaceae plant extracts in combination with proteinase K against *Escherichia coli* O157:H7. Sci Rep 2020; 10(1): 21090.
[http://dx.doi.org/10.1038/s41598-020-77868-4]

[55]   Bakkiyaraj D, Nandhini JR, Malathy B, Pandian SK. The anti-biofilm potential of pomegranate (*Punica granatum* L.) extract against human bacterial and fungal pathogens. Biofouling 2013; 29(8): 929-37.
[http://dx.doi.org/10.1080/08927014.2013.820825] [PMID: 23906229]

[56]   Cheepurupalli L, Raman T, Rathore SS, Ramakrishnan J. Bioactive molecule from streptomyces sp. mitigates MDR *Klebsiella pneumoniae* in zebrafish infection model. Vol. 8. Front Microbiol 2017; 8: 614.
[http://dx.doi.org/10.3389/fmicb.2017.00614] [PMID: 28446900]

[57]   Lalitha C, Raman T, Rathore SS, Ramar M, Munusamy A, Ramakrishnan J. ASK2 bioactive compound inhibits MDR *Klebsiella pneumoniae* by antibiofilm activity. Front Cell Infect Microbiol 2017; 7(AUG): 346.
[http://dx.doi.org/10.3389/fcimb.2017.00346] [PMID: 28824881]

[58]   Mariya I. Lectin-Like Molecules of Lactobacillus RHAMNOSUS GG inhibit pathogenic *E.coli* and Salmonella biofilm formation.pdf. 2016. p. 1–24.

[59]   Tanwar A, Chawla R, Chakotiya AS, Thakur P, Goel R, Basu M, *et al.* Effect of Holarrhena antidysentrica (Ha) and Andrographis paniculata.pdf. 2016. p. 76–82.

[60]   Miladi H, Mili D, Ben Slama R, Zouari S, Ammar E, Bakhrouf A. Antibiofilm formation and anti-adhesive property of three mediterranean essential oils.pdf. 2016. p. 22–31.

[61]   Erhabor RC, Aderogba MA, Erhabor JO, Nkadimeng SM, McGaw LJ. *In vitro* bioactivity of the fractions and isolated compound from Combretum elaeagnoides leaf extract against selected foodborne pathogens. J Ethnopharmacol 2021; 273: 113981. https://www.sciencedirect.com/science/article/pii/S0378874121002087
[http://dx.doi.org/10.1016/j.jep.2021.113981] [PMID: 33647425]

[62]   Nahar S, Ha AJ, Byun KH, Hossain MI, Mizan MFR, Ha SD. Efficacy of flavourzyme against *Salmonella Typhimurium*, *Escherichia coli*, and *Pseudomonas aeruginosa* biofilms on food-contact surfaces. Int J Food Microbiol 2021; 336: 108897. https://www.sciencedirect.com/science/article/pii/S0168160520303913
[http://dx.doi.org/10.1016/j.ijfoodmicro.2020.108897] [PMID: 33091755]

[63]   Divyaa M, Karthikeyanb S, Ravic C, Marimuthu Govindarajand E. Isolation of β-glucan from Eleusine coracana and its antibiofilm, antidiabetic. 2020.

[64]   Baker DD, Chu M, Oza U, Rajgarhia V. The value of natural products to future pharmaceutical discovery. Nat Prod Rep 2007; 24(6): 1225-44.
[http://dx.doi.org/10.1039/b602241n] [PMID: 18033577]

[65]   Lu L, Hu W, Tian Z, *et al.* Developing natural products as potential anti-biofilm agents. Chin Med 2019; 14(1): 11.
[http://dx.doi.org/10.1186/s13020-019-0232-2] [PMID: 30936939]

[66] Miquel S, Lagrafeuille R, Souweine B, Forestier C. Anti-biofilm activity as a health issue. Front Microbiol 2016; 7(APR): 592.
[PMID: 27199924]

[67] Rumbaugh K, Carty N. *In Vivo* Models of Biofilm Infection. In: Biofilm Infections. 2010. p. 267–90.

CHAPTER 4

Bioactive Compounds in Alternative Therapeutics against COVID-19

Prachi Jain[1], Mukesh Kumar Sharma[2], Sicheng Liu[3,4], Rajani Sharma[5] and Pallavi Kaushik[1,*]

[1] *Department of Zoology, University of Rajasthan, Jaipur, Rajasthan, India*

[2] *Department of Zoology, SPC Government College, Ajmer, Rajasthan, India*

[3] *Department of General Surgery, Innovation Center for Minimally Invasive Techniques and Devices, Sir Run Run Shaw Hospital, Zhejiang University School of Medicine, Zhejiang, 310019, Hangzhou, China*

[4] *Institute of Translational Medicine, Zhejiang University School of Medicine, Zhejiang, 310029, Hangzhou, China*

[5] *Department of Microbiology, SMS Medical College, Jaipur, India*

Abstract: The COVID-19 pandemic has created a very difficult time for the whole world with utmost challenge and responsibility on the public health sector to provide symptomatic relief and timely treatment. This condition has stimulated immediate research on the mode of transmission and pathogenesis of the viral variants. As the composition of SARS CoV-2 is similar to SARS-CoV by more than 50%, therefore the management of COVID-19 can possibly be done by repurposing the existing drugs used to treat SARS-CoV infection. The management of SARS CoV-2 infection can be performed at the level of control, prophylaxis and treatment. Many bioactive compounds isolated from medicinal plants have been studied for efficacy in controlling COVID-19 infection by either repression of viral host cell adjunction and subsequent penetration or by repression of viral genomic replication. The bioactive compounds target specific viral or host cell molecules in order to control the spread of virus. Another prominent approach is the development of plant-based vaccines to control the COVID-19 infection and associated complications. The literature also provides evidence of some phytonutrients present in the food supplements which are responsible for increasing the antioxidant, anti-inflammatory, immuno-stimulatory and anti-viral activities in the host cells.

For the purpose of COVID prophylaxis and treatment, these phytonutrients can be administered in appropriate functional doses. The chapter is a compilation of research on SARS CoV-2 with its life cycle, pathogenesis, currently used drugs for treatment, including the synthetic ones and the medical herbs and the specific bioactive compounds found efficacious against COVID-19.

* **Corresponding author Pallavi Kaushik:** Department of Zoology, University of Rajasthan, Jaipur-302004, India; Tel: +91-98286 96079; E-mail: pallavikaushik512@gmail.com

Mukesh Kumar Sharma and Pallavi Kaushik (Eds.)

Keywords: COVID-19, Phytomedicine, Therapeutics, Bioactive compounds, Vaccines, Food supplements.

INTRODUCTION

In December 2019, WHO (World health organization) announced a novel virus called coronavirus named as SARS-CoV-2, responsible for COVID-19 epidemics [1]. This disease has spread throughout the world with a total number of corona-impacted patients exceeding 208 million and about 4.3 million fatalities by the mid of August 2021 as per WHO.

The world has also witnessed the SARS outbreak in late 2002 and 2003 which was caused by SARS-CoV (Severe Acute Respiratory Syndrome-coronavirus) Virus. SARS CoV is not similar to the other coronavirus as it spreads through common cold. COVID-19 acute respiratory syndrome spreads *via the* respiratory route. There were about seven human coronaviruses discovered, named as CoV229E, HCoV-OC43, HCoV-NL63, HKU1, SARS-CoV, MERS-CoV and SARS-CoV-2 [2].

As per the reports of WHO [2020], the cases of COVID-19 have been observed in all the seven continents reported in 197 countries, including China, Italy, Spain, United States, Germany, France, Iran, United Kingdom, and other Asian countries, such as South Korea, Japan, India, Thailand, and Pakistan (WHO 2021). Majority of infected cases have been reported in America, followed by Europe, South East Asia, Eastern Mediterranean, Western Pacific and Africa. According to a report of World Health Organization 2019, the first case of novel coronavirus was reported at the end of year 2019.

The mortality rates of SARS CoV and MERS CoV in the last two decades were of approximately 9.5% and 34.4%, respectively and SARS-CoV-2 (COVID-19) was declared to be third severe pandemic with country wise variable mortality rates. The immediate emergency action to control the virus transmission was to break the chain of infection by isolation of patients and social distancing along with country specific initiative of lockdowns to provide reasonable time to the researchers for the development and testing of drugs and vaccines [3].

The COVID-19 virus is a single stranded RNA virus. "Corona" is a *latin* word which means "Crown", as the virus bear typical crown like surface spikes. The major cause of spreading of this virus could be due to contamination from some wild animals in seafood markets, and later spread from asymptomatic carrier population to healthy individuals through close contact [4].

COVID-19: Features and Characteristics

Causative Agent

The causative agent of COVID 19 is a virus known as coronavirus, which is a member of the family Coronaviridae. Alphacoronavirus (α CoV), Betacoronavirus (βCoV), Deltacoronavirus (δCoV), Gammacoronavirus (γCoV) are four genera included in the subfamily coronavirinae. From these, the α and β strains are capable of infecting only mammals, while the others infect birds but can also infect mammals [5].

The shape of coronavirus is round, but it possesses the capacity to transform itself according to environmental conditions. The outer envelope is known as a capsular membrane with glycoprotein projections (S proteins) which covers the core of virus, consisting of matrix protein enclosing the genomic RNA (+ss RNA). The positive strand RNA has 5'capped and 3' polyadenylated ends and looks identical to the 18S mRNA. The S proteins on the viral envelope help in the attachment of the virus to the host cell and it possesses the antigenic epitopes which are recognized by neutralizing antibodies. The shape of the S protein is subjected to modification to make the fusion of the virus with the host cell easier [6]. Recent studies show that membrane exopeptidase angiotensin-converting enzyme (ACE-2) works as a receptor for S protein for entering the human cell [7].

HCoV-OC43, and HCoV-HKU1 (betaCoVs) HCoV-229E, and HCoV-NL63 (alphaCoVs) are common human CoV and cause infection of upper respiratory tract in immunocompetent individuals [8]. Genomics study of coronavirus, which was isolated from some patients of Wuhan, showed 89 percent nucleotide identity with BAT SARS-like-CoVZXC21 and 82 percent with that of human SARS-CoV. Therefore, the experts from "International Committee on Taxonomy of Viruses" named this virus SARS-CoV-2, which contains 29891 nucleotides, encoding for 9860 amino acids, although its origin is completely unknown. It was only proposed that its origination is from animals and has undergone zoonotic transmission [9].

Similar to other Coronaviruses, it is sensitive to UV rays and heat, it was studied that virus has the ability to resist lower temperatures below 0°C, the virus can be inactivated by different solvents like lipid solvents and also from ether (75%), peroxyacetic acid, chlorine-containing disinfectant, ethanol and chloroform except for chlorhexidine [8].

Life Cycle and Pathogenicity of Coronavirus

SARS CoV-2 shows symptoms like flu, of common cold and gastrointestinal problems. High infection leads to severe respiratory infection, renal failure, pneumonia, and even death. It is structurally similar to SARS CoV and MERS CoV [10]. The glycoprotein present on the outer surface of the virion splits into amino (N)-terminal S1 subunit, which helps the virus to take entry into the host cell and a carboxyl (C)-terminal S2 subunit has a transmembrane domain, and cytoplasmic domain and a fusion peptide which is responsible for membrane fusion of virus cell [11]. The S1 subunit of virus was further divided into two domain that is receptor binding domain (RBD) and N terminal domain (NTD), these domain facilitates the entry of virus and also neutralizes the reaction of vaccine or antisera on virus. The receptor ACE-2 (angiotensin–converting enzyme 2) is present on receptor binding domain, considered a basic peptide domain in the pathogenesis of the virus infection [12] (Fig. **1**).

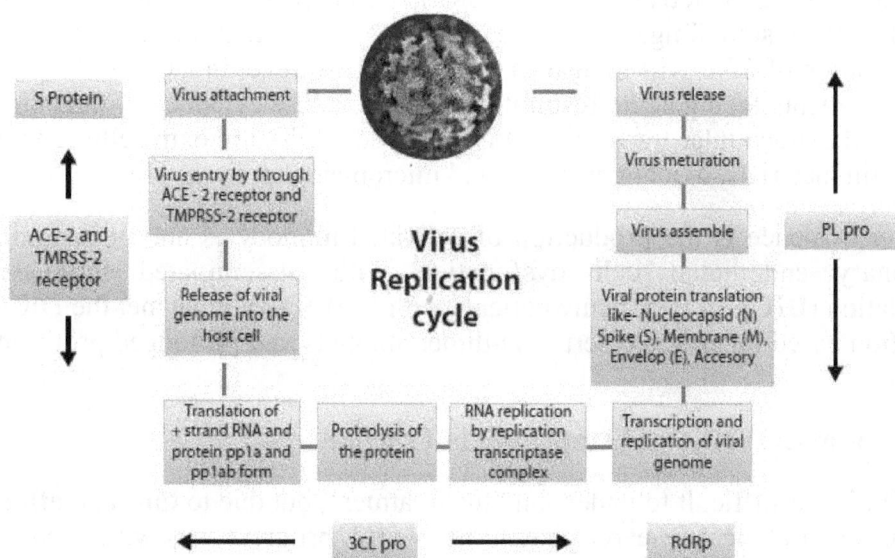

Fig. (1). Life cycle of corona virus and proteins involved in the process: S Protein (Spike protein), ACE-2 (Angiotensin converting enzyme-2), 3CL^{pro} (3-chymotrypsin-like protease), RdRp (RNA dependent RNA polymerase, PLpro (Papain like protease).

SARS CoV makes entry into the host cell by binding Spike protein to the ACE-2 receptor present on the alveolar epithelium of host. These ACE-2 receptors are also present on other cellular surfaces like upper esophagus, enterocytes from the ileum, myocardial cells, proximal tubular cells of the kidney, and urothelial cells of the bladder.

The pathogenicity of SARS CoV infection causes pneumonia in two stages. In the early stage, the morbidity conditions develop due to the replication and proliferation of virus in different body tissues, which results in tissue damage. In the later stage, the damage and morbidity are because of an activated immune system which recruits cells like T lymphocytes, neutrophils and monocytes, *etc.* in the affected region and subsequent release of different cytokines like tumor necrosis factor (TNFα) and various interleukins (IL-1,IL-6, IL-1β, IL-8, IL-12 and interferon -IFN-γ) [13].

The symptoms of the late stage of infection are manifested in corona-positive patients with an elevated proinflammatory response of neutrophils and macrophages in the bronchoalveolar lavage fluid (BALF) and along with high cytokines levels. These proinflammatory responses maintain the infection in lungs by increasing C reactive protein (CRP), through transcription activator 3 (STAT3)-IL-6 signalling. Therefore, it is observed that an increase in the concentration of CRP will increase the level of IL-6 level in COVID-19 patients [14]. In patients facing acute respiratory syndrome, the evidence of uncontrolled neutrophil extracellular traps (NETs) is observed. NETs are extracellular traps of chromatin materials, oxidant enzymes and microbicidal proteins [15].

Another evidence is the production of activated monocytes and neutrophils by pulmonary endothelial cell dysfunction with disseminated intravascular coagulation **(DIC)**. In fact, many patients with COVID-19 have met the DIC case definition based on elevated serum D-dimer amounts and prolonged prothrombin time [16].

Overview of COVID-19 Therapeutics in Practice

Initially, it was difficult to understand the treatment, but due to time and efforts of scientists and clinical research around the world, progress was witnessed in the management and development of therapies against COVID-19.

Currently, some therapeutic drugs are administered according to the physiology and symptoms. The main approach to find an effective drug for the treatment of COVID-19 is by testing the repurposed drug with anti-viral and anti-inflammatory properties to inhibit the overproduction of cytokines. One of the drugs used presently is Azithromycin, which is well known for its anti-inflammatory activity and it also increases the expression of interferon type I and type III in the patient who is infected with pulmonary disease. The azithromycin *in vitro* concentration EC_{50} (50% effective concentration) is 2.12μM following 72h incubation period post infection against SARS CoV-2 [17]. Other drugs include Chloroquine and hydroxychloroquine which are used worldwide as antimalarial drugs and also used for other immune disease like rheumatoid arthritis. These drugs show significant relief in pneumonia with shortening of disease course as per a China based study conducted on more than 100 patients [18]. Hydroxychloroquine is also a derivative chloroquine drug, but it is comparatively toxic with its half maximal inhibitory concentration of IC_{50} (0.72 µM) in inhibiting the SARS CoV-2 as per *in vitro* studies [19]. Both of these drugs block viral entry into the cell by inhibiting the glycosylation of the host receptor, inhibiting autophagy and lysosomal activity in the host cell [20]. Ivermectin is an antiparasitic drug which also shows anti-viral activity against Human immunodeficiency virus (HIV) and dengue virus. Ivermectin is also known to be an efficacious drug for controlling COVID-19 infections with the inhibitory concentration IC_{50} at 2µM in *in vitro* study [21]. In another *in vitro* study on Vero/hSLAM cells infected with SARS CoV-2, a single dose of drug showed about five thousand times reduction in viral load after 48h [22, 23].

Remdesivir is a broad spectrum drug and is a phosphoramidate nucleoside analogue. It is an effective drug as this decreases infection of SARS CoV-2 at low concentration (EC_{50} -0.77µM) [24]. First case of treatment of COVID-19 after use of intravenous (IV) remdesivir was reported in the United States. The effective result of the drug was also reported in hospitalized COVID-19 positive patients with oxygen saturation of 94% or less or who were in support of oxygen [25]. Remdesivir is the only medication that has been approved for COVID-19 infection by the U.S.FDA [23]. Favipiravir is another drug for the treatment of COVID-19 infection, approved in Japan (2014) for the treatment of the influenza virus [26]. This drug is a derivative of pyrazine carboxamide and of guanine analog, which show its activity against RdRp (RNA dependent RNA polymerase) of RNA virus and also inhibit the assembly of virion [27]. The EC_{50} of this drug is 61.88 µM and half cytotoxic concentration is over 400 µM [24]. Favipiravir is a more effective drug in comparison to umifenovir with 71.46% and 55.86% recovery rates respectively. In Wuhan, patients treated with this drug showed recovery an average of 2.5 days compared to the other patients on alternate medication (recovery in 4.2 days) [28]. Lopinavir-Ritonavir is the combination of two drugs that have been used as anti-viral agents with good efficacy against HIV (Human Immunodeficiency virus) type I Virus. Lopinavir is generally given in the combination with Ritonavir because of its lower bioavailability and also shows elevation in its half life with suppression of cytochrome P450 [29]. The treatment with a combination of two drugs gives favourable outcomes in patients having SARS infection and MERS-CoV infection in combination with IFN-β, [30]. Methyl prednisolone which is an alternative to natural corticosteroid is a classic immunosuppressive drug which help in decreasing pneumonia and is effective in acute respiratory distress syndrome [1]. Patient having a high infection and oxygen saturation level of less than 94% while breathing room air or patients in support of oxygen show high rate of recovery having received IV injection of methylprednisolone (0.5 mg/kg twice for 5 days) [17, 31].

Plasma therapy: Transfusion of plasma, collected from patients who recovered from COVID-19 and have developed antibodies to the infected patients, can either decrease infection or clinical severity. It is found to be safe efficacious method for therapy and post-exposure prophylaxis [32]. Research reports that concentration of antibodies increases from 40% in a week since beginning to 100% from day of onset which is a strong support for routine application and treatment [33].

Food Supplements Efficacious During COVID-19

For the effective treatment of COVID-19 some of the elements are very important taken as food supplements.

The metal Zinc (Zn) has been studied to be an important element against the virus because of its different biological involvements as it functions as a signalling molecule, structural element and also works as a cofactor [34]. After iron, zinc is the second most abundant trace metal in human body, and also it is the most essential component for the protein structure and its function [35]. Zinc supplements inhibit RdRp activity of SARS-coronavirus by inhibiting its replication. Zn helps in the reduction of acute respiratory infections by 35%. Therefore, zinc is considered a potential supplement in COVID-19 treatment because of its anti-viral, anti-inflammatory and antioxidant activities [34].

Vitamin D (Vit D) is also very essential for COVID-19 patients, as it helps in the stimulation of innate immunity and modulation of acquired immunity. A meta-analysis study shows that supplements of Vitamin D can help in the cure of acute respiratory syndrome [36]. Beneficial effects were shown in the individual who takes this vitamin in daily doses rather than those who consume bulk doses. Vitamin D increases the expression level of antioxidants, regulates balanced mitochondrial function and prevents oxidative stress and DNA damage [37]. Vitamin D shows affectivity against viral infection by suppression of virus induced inflammation and suppression of viral replication [34].

Similarly, Vitamin C which is a water-soluble vitamin also called ascorbic acid is an essential vitamin for the treatment of viral infection because of its antioxidant properties important for boosting immune system [38]. The IV dose of vitamin C is effective for COVID- 19 treatment by suppressing the cytokine release [39]. A study also shows that consumption of vitamin C in combination of quercetin gives synergistic antioxidant, anti-viral and immune-modulatory effects. Therefore, by boosting the immune system and antioxidant activity, intake of food supplements containing vitamin C seems very helpful in treating the infection [34].

Another compound is Curcumin which shows broad spectrum effect like antioxidant, antibacterial, antifungal and anti-viral activity. It shows the anti-viral effect by different mechanisms, like inhibiting the entry of virus into the host cell; inhibiting the replication of virus, disrupting the signalling pathway or by inhibiting the encapsulation of virus or viral assembly [40]. Recent study shows that curcumin inhibits the ACE-2, which is the potential receptor for viral entry. Curcumin stimulates interferon production and activates host immunity. As antioxidant it neutralizes the reactive radicals and boosts the synthesis of antioxidant enzymes [41]. So, curcumin act as a potential supplement in food which can boost immunity to fight against infection.

Cinnamaldehyde is a natural organic compound present in essential oils which is known for its anti-inflammatory properties. It is also responsible to decrease the production prostaglandins (PGEs) by downregulating the production of IL-1b instigated COX-2 pursuit, thus helping in decreasing the hyper-inflammation in lungs [42].

Probiotics are also helpful in protection of COVID-19. Probiotics are good microorganisms which can improve the functioning of gastrointestinal system. It was observed that probiotics show an impact on systemic and local immune responses in the lungs and other mucosal sites at distal mucosal sites. A study on probiotics has reported that consumption of *Bifidobacterium* and *Lactobacillus* helps in clearing the infection of influenza virus from the respiratory tract [43]. Thus, the use of probiotics can be considered useful in the treatment of SARS CoV-2 infection, as these act as adjuvants to fight the COVID-19 induced disease [34].

Some Natural Products and Phytomedicines used for Treatment of COVID-19

Herbs have been used all over the world for years to cure many diseases for ages as their use is considered safe due to no or low side effects. Phyto-constituents of herbal products are used as an important tool for the development of novel anti-viral agents which can also be effective against COVID-19 (Figs. **3** and **4**) [44]. The alcoholic extract of *Sambucus formosana* shows potent anti-viral properties with IC_{50} value of 1.17 µg/ml, against the coronavirus [45]. The natural products have more beneficial effects compared to synthetic products that are made from chemicals, because these products contain different bioactive molecules, formed by interrelated activity between enzymes, vitamins, and minerals. On the other hand, the use of man-made artificially fabricated medicines have certain unwanted impacts, making their use disadvantageous [46].

The compounds from medicinal plants such as, apigenin-7-glucoside, catechin, naringenin, kaempferol, oleuropein, luteolin, demethoxycurcumin, diosmin and epigallocatechin have been studied for their efficacies against COVID-19 [47, 48]. Many bioactive molecules have been studied and explored for their uses in treatment of COVID-19 patients, some of which are represented in Fig. (**2**) with their isolation source and specific targets.

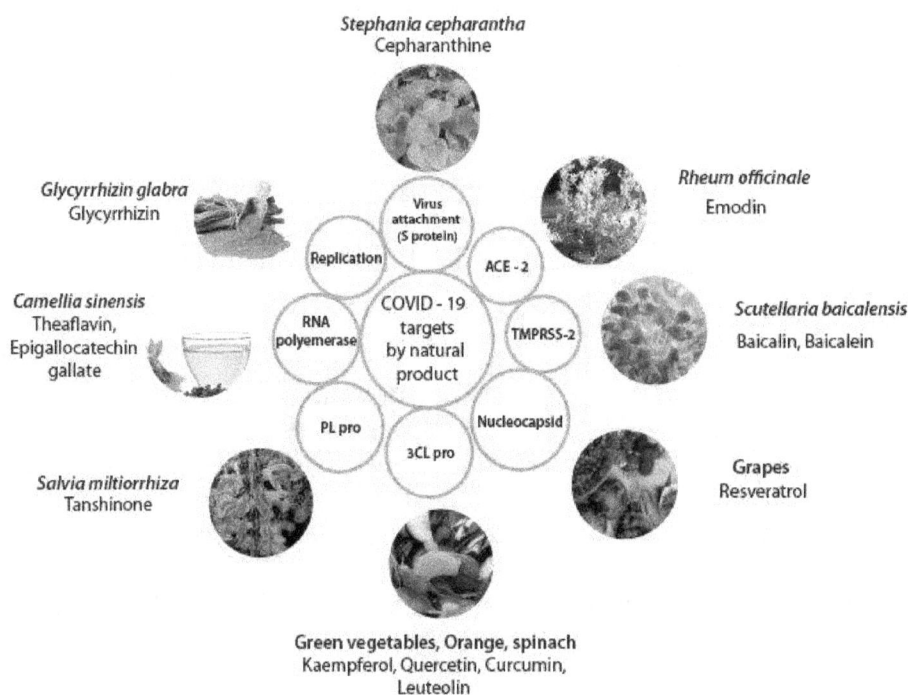

Fig. (2). Some bioactive compounds used for treatment of COVID- 19 along with their isolation source and specific viral targets.

A descriptive note on the most important bioactive compounds which have been proved efficacious against COVID- 19 is mentioned in the following text.

Quercetin

Quercetin is a natural compound present in fruits and vegetables. It shows different activities like anti-inflammatory, anti-oxidant, anti-viral, anti-allergic, anti-cancer, mood-enhancing as well as vasoprotective. Quercetin acts as viral inhibitor by causing breakdown of SARS CoV 3CLpro protein. So, it is expected that quercetin would show anti-viral activity to SARS CoV-2 because sequence of 3CLpro in SARS CoV2 is similar to SARS CoV [49]. 3CLpro is a virus protease which help in assembly and replication in host cell by cleaving viral peptides [50]. It is also reported that quercetin shows good affinity to viral spike protein, RdRp, ACE-2, and PL pro which are the main targets for anti-viral action against SARS CoV-2. It is available at low cost as well as wide range of sources, so it is very beneficial to test its efficiency against SARS CoV-2 infection [20].

Glycyrrhizic Acid

Glycyrrhizic acid is a natural product found in licorice plant root. It is very effective against different viruses like herpes simplex virus, human immunodeficiency virus and other coronaviruses. Therefore, it was assumed that the extract of licorice root would also be effective against SARS CoV-2 [51]. Further, research has shown that the replication of SARS CoV-2 is completely blocked by glycyrrhizin at a concentration of 0.5 mg/mL (combined pre- and post-entry conditions) or 1 mg/mL (post-entry conditions). The half maximal concentration EC_{50} was estimated 0.44 mg/mL, which suggests that glycyrrhizin is an important effectual agent to control SARS-CoV-2 [52]. Glycyrrhizic acids had shown good effect on SARS CoV. Both SARS CoV-2 and SARS CoV have similar structure of different subclasses. SARS CoV-2 and SARS CoV have the same receptor for ACE-2, this suggests that glycyrrhizic acid will show an efficacious effect on SARS CoV-2 treatment [53]. Molecular docking of glycyrrhizic acid suggests that it possesses the potential to treat COVID-19 due to its binding to ACE-2 with binding energy of -7.0 kcal/mol. Glycyrrhizic acid show binding potential with other targets also like Spike protein, RdRp, 3CLpro and PLpro with the energy of 6.5 kcal/mol, -7.2 kcal/mol, -6.9 kcal/mol and -7.3 kcal/mol. Study also reported that Glycyrrhizic acid is very useful in treating bacterial infection, autoimmune diseases by immune-modulatory activity, oxidative stress, inflammation and acute lung injury [54].

Baicalin and Baicalein

These are the bioactive compounds obtained from the plant *Scutellaria baicalensis Georgi* [50]. Both of these bioactive compounds possess potent anti-viral properties. In *in vitro* susceptibility tests it was reported that Baicalin reduced the plaque forming unit by 50% at EC_{50} of 12.5 µg/mL at 48 hrs in prototype SARS CoV virus infected fRhK-4 cell lines [55]. Its activity against SARS CoV-2 is assumed because of structural similarity of SARS CoV-2 with SARS COV. Baicalin shows binding affinity with ACE-2 and also with PLpro, these are the key targets for the treatment of SARS CoV-2. In SARS CoV-2 a highly conserved region Mpro is responsible for production of viral protein and baicalein has the property to bind this region with high affinity [50]. Baicalein is also used in traditional Chinese medicine as a broad anti-viral agent which shows inhibitory activity against the purified 3CLpro of SARS CoV-2 and anti-viral activity in Vero cell culture. Both of these compounds are also reported as novel inhibitors of SARS CoV-2 3CLpro with anti-viral activity in the SARS CoV-2 infected cells [50]. So, baicalin is an effective compound to protect cell from corona induced tissue damage as well control of inflammation by suppression of cell infiltration, with reduction in levels of cytokines such as IL-1β and TNF-α and altogether improves the respiratory efficiency of lungs [56].

Luteolin

This is a flavonoid found in herbs (China) used in treatment of cancer in traditional Chinese medicines and contains properties like anti-inflammatory, antioxidant and anti-viral. Study show that luteolin hampers the life cycle of virus by blocking the absorption and internalization of influenzae virus and ultimately the viral replication is disrupted [57]. Because of its action against virus it was assumed that it would show affectivity against SARS CoV-2 which was confirmed by docking studies. The binding energy of luteolin to ACE-2 was -7.1kcal/mol [20]. By this study we can conclude that luteolin contains effective anti-viral properties which can be also utilized to control COVID-19. The luteolin extracted from *Torreya nucifera* acts as an inhibitor 3CLpro [58], which is another way of treatment for SARS CoV-2. Although, further studies need to be performed for developing effective therapeutics against SARS CoV-2 infection.

Andrographolide

It is a compound isolated from the herb, *Andrographis paniculata*, which shows different properties like anti-viral, anti-bacterial, anti-tumor, anti-parasitic, and anti-hyperglycemic. It shows activity against different virus by inhibiting various intracellular pathways like unfolding of protein response, oxidative stress, autophagy, *etc* [59]. By studying anti-viral activity against SARS CoV-2 it reveals that key targets of andrographolide are Spike protein, ACE-2, 3CLpro, RdRp and PLpro, which help to inactivate SARS CoV-2. Andrographolide was also studied by *in silico* computational docking tools wherein it effectively docked against the inhibitor region of the prominent protease of SARS-CoV-2 virus with the score of -3.094357 Kcal/mol [60].

Propolis

It is a resinous natural product formed by honey bees using exudates of plants. There are different types of propolis which are considered valuable due to their therapeutic potential. Propolis shows high affinity with the ACE-2 receptor present on host cell surface and blocks the entry of virus into the host cell [61]. Limonin, quercetin and kaempferol are propolis compounds which show high docking scores. Kaempferol is an effective component of propolis, as it is involved in the inhibition of host cell surface protease TMPRSS2 (transmembrane serine protease 2) [62].

Cepharanthine (CEP)

It is an alkaloid derivative from plant *Stephania cepharantha* Hayata. It is known to exhibit anti-inflammatory, anti-oxidative, immune-modulating, anti-parasitic, and anti-viral activities. It acts by suppressing nuclear factor-kappa B (NF-κB) activation as well as lipid peroxidation, production of nitric oxide, cytokine, and expression of cyclo-oxygenase. All these play crucial role in viral response and its replication [63]. The *in vitro* study on cell line VeroE6/TMPRSS2 infected with SARS CoV-2 show that cepharanthine inhibits viral entry and replication by binding to the spike protein and interferes with ACE-2 receptor. The studies using cepharanthine were also conducted on cell lines like Vero cells and Calu-3 human lung cells, these cell lines also showed decrease in virus infection but the mechanism was unknown [64, 65].

Theaflavin (TF) and Epigallocatechin Gallate (EGCG)

Theaflavin (TF) and epigallocatechin gallate (EGCG), compounds are found in Tea (green or oolong). Tea catechins are polyphenolics present in green tea and are mainly responsible for its biological impacts. EGCG is regarded as typical tea catechin with the maximum activity [66]. All TFs and EGCG can inhibit 3CLpro and also exhibit higher binding potential to the target. TFs also exhibit higher binding potential with Ribose binding domain in SARS CoV-2, by forming hydrophobic and hydrogen bonding with the sites of viral S protein. It also exhibits RdRp suppression and ACE-2 binding potential. Therefore, EGCG and TFs can act as potential anti-viral agent which can be used for cure and prophylaxis of COVID-19 [67].

Emodin

Emodin is an important bioactive compound extracted from medicinal plants of genus *Rheum* and *Polygonum* which potentially blocks S protein and ACE-2 interaction. It also possesses anti-diuretic, anti-bacterial and vaso-relaxant effect with anti-inflammatory, anti-carcinogenic and anti-proliferative properties. It exhibits anti-viral effect by suppressing casein kinase 2 activity that is generally utilized by many viruses for the phosphorylation of proteins that are crucial for their growth and life. The estimated IC_{50} dose of emodin is 200 μM [68].

Resveratrol

It is a potential anti-inflammatory and antioxidant agent abundantly present in red wine, red grapes, dark chocolate and peanut butter [69]. It is also found in cranberries, blueberries, and grapes. Resveratrol can modulate the coagulating cascade and interferes with platelet activation and aggregation. It acts a potent agent against SARS-CoV-2 and HCoV-229 (Human corona virus-229) with very low toxicity [70].

Tanshinones

Various derivatives of tanshinones are found to possess pharmacologically important properties. These are derived from the roots of *Salvia miltiorrhiza* Bunge. Cryptotanshinone, tanshinone I and GRL0617 have been found to suppress SARS-CoV-2 PLpro with IC_{50} dose in the range of 1.39 to 5.63 μmol/L. These compounds also exhibit strong anti-viral activities in cell-based assays. The anti-cancer drug YM155, which is undergoing clinical trials, shows strong anti-viral potential with EC_{50} dose of 170 nmol/L. As per reports, all of the isolated tanshinones are good inhibitors of both cysteine proteases [71]. Tanshinone I and dihydrotanshinone I are strong 3CLpro and PLpro inhibitors and thus are suggested to help in control of viral infection [72].

Targets of Bioactive Compounds against COVID-19

SARS CoV genome shows 70% similarity to the genome of SARS CoV-2 and because of this similarity the drugs which are applicable to cure SARS CoV are tried against SARS CoV-2 [73]. Thus, repurposing of natural product or molecule which was used SARS CoV may be used for the treatment and control of COVID 19 [74]. The bioactive compounds pose inhibitory or suppressive action against the COVID-19 infection by either blocking the viral attachment and entry into the host cell or by inhibiting the replication and assembly of virus particle after entry into the host. These mechanisms of virus inhibition are explained in the following text.

(i) Inhibition of Host Cell Attachment and Penetration of COVID-19

Entry of coronavirus in the host cell is known to be an important determinant of pathogenesis and viral infectivity and also a major target for human intervention strategies and host immune surveillance. The entry of virus in cell requires the prior binding to a cell surface receptor, for viral attachment which is mediated by virus surface anchored spike protein (S-protein) [75]. The S protein modifies the primary viral entry and anchorage on host cells utilizing the receptor-binding domain in the S1 subunit and then fusion into host cells *via* the S2 subunit through the host ACE-2 receptor [76]. Although, the subtypes of corona virus identify different receptors [77]. The entry-activating proteases of SARS CoV comprise of cell surface proteases like TMPRSS2 and lysosomal protease like cathepsins [78].

The beginning of the COVID- 19 infection commences with the attachment of virus and further fusion with membrane of the host cell which involves the S (Spike) protein of CoV. Thus, the control on virus infection and spread using anti-viral drugs and vaccines need to be chiefly focused on these two processes [79]. The bioactive compounds emodin and hesperidin show their efficacy as anti-viral agent by blocking the binding of S protein to ACE-2 but this blockage is dose dependent [80, 81]. Similarly, caffeic acid is also found to be as important compound with anti-viral activity as this can inhibit the entry of virus by impeding interaction of coronavirus NL63 (HCoV-NL63) with ACE-2 receptor and heparan sulphate proteoglycans (co-receptor) on the host cell surface [77].

(ii) Viral Genome Replication and Protein Synthesis Machinery

RNA dependent RNA polymerase also called RNA replicases are known to be important proteases because they can assist the replication of RNA from RNA template. RdRps are present in all RNA virus which assist in replication, synthesis (mRNA) and RNA recombination. RdRp is an important target for anti-viral activity against coronavirus [82]. Other proteases like **3CLpro** and **PLpro** are important enzymes that help in the synthesis of structural as well as non-structural proteins, which are essential for the viral replication and packaging and subsequent formation of new viruses. Thus, targeting these two proteases can control the viral replication and formation of new viruses, subsequently reducing or controlling viral load and spread in the infected individual [83]. Another important structural protein is the **N protein** which plays a key role in structural organization of virus particles. It binds to the viral genomic RNA and helps in its incorporation of genetic materials in the CoV protein capsid. N protein primarily incorporates the viral genome, thus it is also considered as an important target for anti-viral agents and its breakdown can possibly hamper the viral assembly with a subsequent reduction in viral proliferation [84].

Papain-like protease (PLpro) present in SARS CoV is responsible for its assembly and replication and ultimately for the survival of the virus, thus it is used as an important target for the drug. High affinity with PLpro has been found in compounds extracted from galangal (*Alpinia officinarum* Hance), ginger (*Zingiber officinale* Roscoe) and curcuma (*Curcuma longa* L.) in *in silico* study indicating their anti-viral potential [85]. 3CLpro is also a conserved protease in SARS CoV-2 which controls its replication. Molecular docking of African plants showed that plant contains alkaloids and terpenoids which are a potential inhibitor of 3CLpro. The inhibitors of SARS CoV 3CLpro are Cryptoquindoline, 6-Oxoisoiguesterin, 10-Hydroxyusambarensine and 22-Hydroxyhopan-3-one [86].

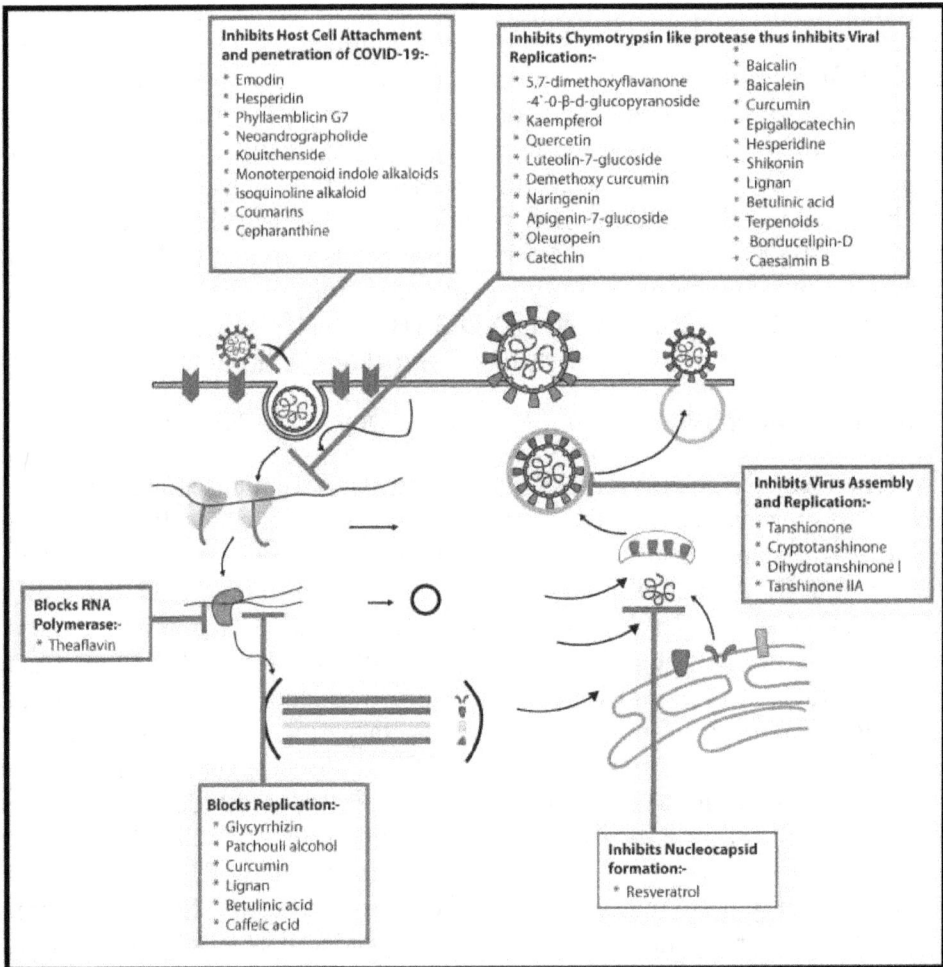

Fig. (3). Molecular targets of various bioactive compounds against COVID-19.

By molecule docking assay eight natural polyphenols were identified, these are quercetin, naringenin, caffeine, oleuropein, ellagic acid, benzoic acid, resveratrol, and gallic acid polyphenols used as inhibitors of SARS CoV-2 RdRp. Natural compound cepharanthine extracted from Stephania (*Stephania tetrandra* S.Moore) is an alkaloid tetrandrine that contains antioxidant and anti-inflammatory activities. Cepharanthine has the property of binding the active pockets of NSP12-NSP8 in SARS CoV-2, NSP 12 is an important RdRp for the replication of virus and needs to bind its cofactors NSP7 and NSP8 to activate replication machinery [87, 88].

Suppression of virus entry into host cells can also be controlled by use of flavonols myricetin and linebacker due to their S protein binding potential, helicases and other proteases along with interactive potential with ACE-2 receptor resulting in conformational change and thus impairing the virus entry [89]. The reports of docking study show comparable docking scores of bioactives galangin, morin and myricetin as compared to the currently used drugs abacavir and hydroxychloroquine as standard drugs [90].

Another approach of anti-viral therapy is the target molecule helicase which is involved in viral replication and proliferation. Myricetin and scutellarein are natural compounds with potential to suppress the SARS CoV helicase by targeting ATPase activity [91, 92].

The two major bioactive compounds Tryptanthrin and indigodole B [5aR-ethyltryptanthrin], present in the extract of *Strobilanthes cusia* (Nees) Kuntze can potentially inhibit the viral replication and protein synthesis along with minimum cytotoxicity with IC_{50} values of 1.52 and 2.60 µM, respectively [93].

As discussed earlier 3CLpro and PLpro viral protease also play an important role in the replication of virus and act as a potential drug target for the development of anti-coronavirus agents [94]. Some of the most effective herbal bioactives which inhibit these two proteases include N-cis-feruloyltyramine, quercetin, cryptotanshinone, kaempferol, tanshinone-IIa, isobavachalcone, pectolinarin, helichrysetin, herbacetin, and quercetin 3-β-D-glucoside [93, 95]. Table 1 is an exhaustive compilation of efficacious bioactive compounds against COVID-19 with their source of isolation, function and target molecules.

Vaccines Development by Natural Product

The evolution of COVID-19 vaccines is essential to control and curb the menace caused by the pandemic. The vaccines using spike glycoprotein or RBD (Ribose binding domain) of virion have the ability to interrupt the interaction between the host and virus particle. This as an antigenic molecule which can stimulate the production of antibodies and neutralize the pathogen in the initial stages of infection. Many of the COVID-19 ongoing projects of vaccine development globally are taking S protein as target antigen [107]. Another approach is to use plant-made vaccines which seem as the best solution to eradicate any disease as such vaccines will be more approachable for population with easy administration through oral route [108].

Table 1. Targets of various natural compounds against SARS CoV-2.

Targets Classification	Targets for SARS CoV-2	Function	Bioactive Molecules	Natural Material	Refs.
Host Cell Attachment and Penetration of COVID-19	**ACE-2 inhibitors**	ACE-2 acts as receptor for SARS-CoV-2 and aids in its entry into the host cell	Emodin Hesperidin	*Rheum officinale C. aurantium*	[96] [20]
	TMPRSS2 INHIBITOR	It is a serine protease TMPRSS-2 for S protein priming used for entry in host cell	Phyllaemblicin G7, Neoandrographolide Kouitchenside Monoterpenoid indole alkaloids Isoquinoline alkaloid Coumarins	*Phyllanthus emblica Andrographis paniculata Swertia kouitchensis Strychnos nux-vomica Corydalis govaniana, Nerium oleander Fumaria indica Edgeworthia gardneri*	[97] [98] [99]
	Viral attachment S protein	Spike or S proteins projecting out from viral surface aids the virus in attachment and fusion with host membrane.	Cepharanthine	*Stephania cepharantha*	[100]

(Table 1) cont.....

Targets Classification	Targets for SARS CoV-2	Function	Bioactive Molecules	Natural Material	Refs.
Viral Genome Replication and Protein Synthesis Machinery	**CLpro**	3-chymotrypsin-like protease (3CLpro) is a conserved protease in SARS CoV-2. This can cleave the polyprotein residue at 11 sites and produce non-structural proteins involved in viral replication.	**Flavonoid** Baicalein, Baicalin, 5,7-dimethoxy flavanone -4′-O-β-d-glucopyranoside, kaempferol, quercetin, luteolin-7-glucoside, demethoxycurcumin, naringenin, apigenin-7-glucoside, oleuropein, catechin, curcumin, epigallocatechin Hesperidine Shikonin Lignan Betulinic acid	*Scutellaria spp* Lauraceae, Lamiaceae, Apiaceae, Leguminosae	[101] [50]
			Terpenoids bonducellpin D caesalmin B	*Caesalpinia spp*	
	RNA polymerase inhibitor	RNA-dependent RNA polymerase (RdRp) is encoded by virus and catalyzes RNA synthesis from RNA templates.	Theaflavin	*Camellia sinensis*	[102] [103]
	Replication	RdRp, Nsp12 the zinc-binding helicase (HEL, Nsp13) other enzymes involved in modification of viral RNA	Glycyrrhizin Patchouli alcohol Curcumin Lignan Betulinic acid Caffeic Acid	*Glycyrrhizin glabra* Patchouli oil Turmeric Flaxseeds, Sesame seeds *Betula pubescens Eucalyptus globulus.*	[104]

(Table 1) cont.....

Targets Classification	Targets for SARS CoV-2	Function	Bioactive Molecules	Natural Material	Refs.
Viral Genome Replication and Protein Synthesis Machinery	Nucleocapsid	The structural protein of virus which complexes with viral genomic RNA is nucleocapsid. It is involved in viral assembly and transcription rate enhancement.	Resveratrol	Grapes	[105] [106]
	PLpro	Papain like protease are responsible for virus assembly and replication	Tanshinone Cryptotanshinone Dihydrotanshinone I Tanshinone IIA	*Salvia spp*	[106]

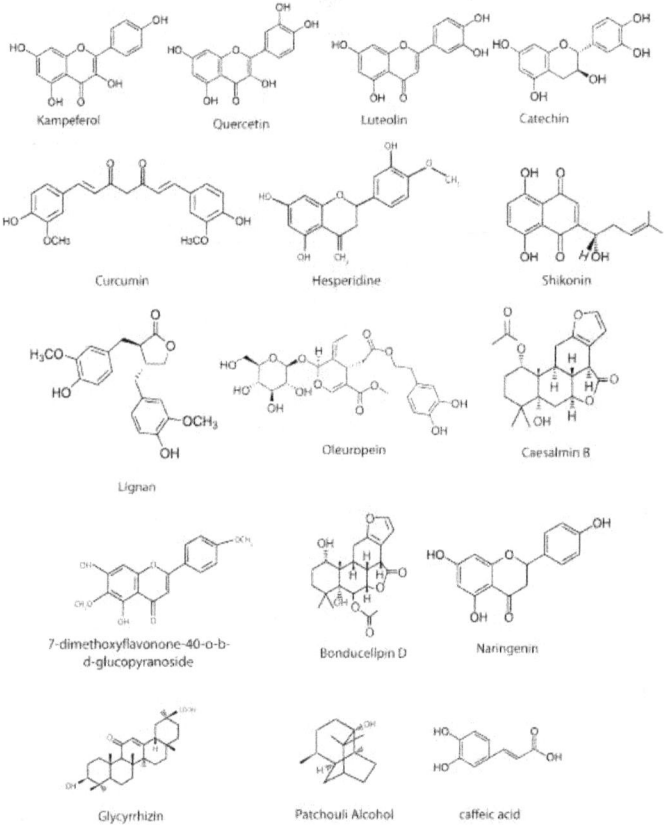

Kampeferol   Quercetin   Luteolin   Catechin

Curcumin   Hesperidine   Shikonin

Lignan   Oleuropein   Caesalmin B

7-dimethoxyflavonone-40-o-b-d-glucopyranoside   Bonducellpin D   Naringenin

Glycyrrhizin   Patchouli Alcohol   caffeic acid

(Fig. 4) contd.....

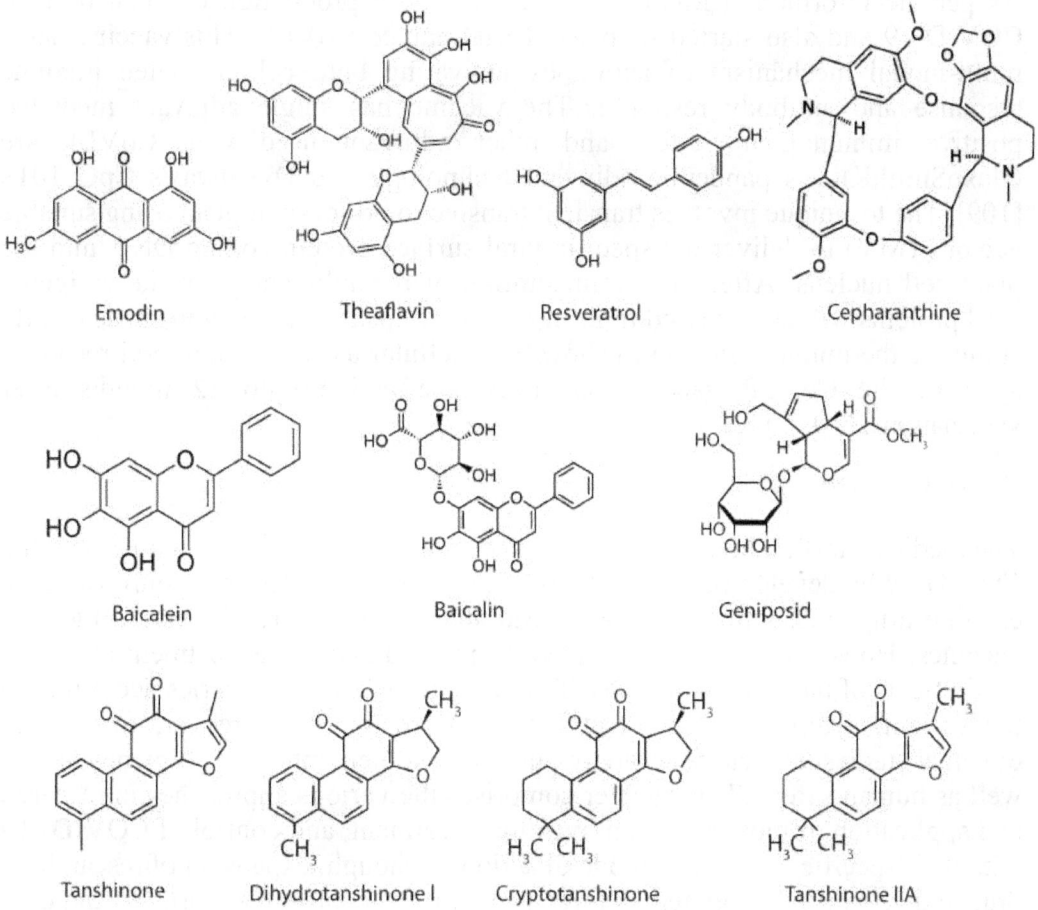

Fig. (4). Molecular structure of bioactive compounds effective against COVID-19.

As per the information Medicago Inc. started the production of plant derived COVID-19 and also started its phase I trial named CoVLP. This vaccine has a multi-modal mechanism of action by activating both cell mediated immune response and antibody response. The vaccine has single adjuvant mediated positive immunogenic effect and other adjuvant used with CoVLP are GlaxoSmithKline's pandemic adjuvant technology and Dynanvax's CpG 1018 [109]. The technique involves transient transfection of desired plant using suitable vector (TMV) to deliver the specific viral surface protein coding DNA into the plant cell nucleus. After the administration of recombinant plant the antigenic viral proteins will are released in form of bio-encapsulation and will subsequently stimulate the immune system to show both cellular as well as humoral response against. The CoVLP vaccine has proved effective upto 12 months after vaccination [110, 111].

CONCLUSION

The medical staff and researchers are making tremendous efforts to alleviate the COVID-19 by developing the methods of tests and diagnosis and repurposing the existing drugs to control the viral spread and also to create effective drugs and vaccines. However, many studies have concluded about the treatment and anti-viral effects of natural compounds. The method for treatment varies according to the variant, symptoms and effectiveness of treatment. Moreover, for further effectual studies, clinical trials are required to test their anti CoV efficiency and as well as human safety. This chapter comprises the various approaches in research and application of bioactives in prevention, treatment, and control of COVID- 19 with their specific targets and mode of action. Although, expansion of research on drug and vaccine development is further required to control the mortality and cure morbidity for the benefit of mankind.

CONSENT FOR PUBLICATION

Not applicable.

CONFLICT OF INTEREST

The authors declare no conflict of interest, financial or otherwise.

ACKNOWLEDGEMENTS

Declared none.

REFERENCES

[1]   Huang C, Wang Y, Li X, *et al.* Clinical features of patients infected with 2019 novel coronavirus in Wuhan, China. Lancet 2020; 395(10223): 497-506.

[http://dx.doi.org/10.1016/S0140-6736(20)30183-5] [PMID: 31986264]

[2]   Mohamadian M, Chiti H, Shoghli A, Biglari S, Parsamanesh N, Esmaeilzadeh A. COVID-19: Virology, biology and novel laboratory diagnosis. J Gene Med 2021; 23(2): e3303.
[http://dx.doi.org/10.1002/jgm.3303] [PMID: 33305456]

[3]   Ashour HM, Elkhatib WF, Rahman MM, Elshabrawy HA. Insights into the Recent 2019 Novel Coronavirus (SARS-CoV-2) in Light of Past Human Coronavirus Outbreaks. Pathogens 2020; 9(3): 186.
[http://dx.doi.org/10.3390/pathogens9030186] [PMID: 32143502]

[4]   Baloch S, Baloch MA, Zheng T, Pei X. The Coronavirus Disease 2019 (COVID-19) Pandemic. Tohoku J Exp Med 2020; 250(4): 271-8.
[http://dx.doi.org/10.1620/tjem.250.271] [PMID: 32321874]

[5]   Almaghaslah D, Kandasamy G, Almanasef M, Vasudevan R, Chandramohan S. Review on the coronavirus disease (COVID-19) pandemic: Its outbreak and current status. Int J Clin Pract 2020; 74(11): e13637.
[http://dx.doi.org/10.1111/ijcp.13637] [PMID: 32750190]

[6]   Luk HKH, Li X, Fung J, Lau SKP, Woo PCY. Molecular epidemiology, evolution and phylogeny of SARS coronavirus. Infect Genet Evol 2019; 71: 21-30.
[http://dx.doi.org/10.1016/j.meegid.2019.03.001] [PMID: 30844511]

[7]   Zhou P, Yang XL, Wang XG, *et al.* A pneumonia outbreak associated with a new coronavirus of probable bat origin. Nature 2020; 579(7798): 270-3.
[http://dx.doi.org/10.1038/s41586-020-2012-7] [PMID: 32015507]

[8]   Cascella M, Rajnik M, Aleem A, Dulebohn SC, Di Napoli R. Features, Evaluation, and Treatment of Coronavirus (COVID-19StatPearls. Treasure Island, FL: StatPearls Publishing 2021.http://www.ncbi.nlm.nih.gov/books/NBK554776/ Internet

[9]   Andersen KG, Rambaut A, Lipkin WI, Holmes EC, Garry RF. The proximal origin of SARS-CoV-2. Nat Med 2020; 26(4): 450-2.
[http://dx.doi.org/10.1038/s41591-020-0820-9] [PMID: 32284615]

[10]   Sharma A, Tiwari S, Deb MK, Marty JL. Severe acute respiratory syndrome coronavirus-2 (SARS-CoV-2): a global pandemic and treatment strategies. Int J Antimicrob Agents 2020; 56(2): 106054.
[http://dx.doi.org/10.1016/j.ijantimicag.2020.106054] [PMID: 32534188]

[11]   Du L, He Y, Zhou Y, Liu S, Zheng BJ, Jiang S. The spike protein of SARS-CoV — a target for vaccine and therapeutic development. Nat Rev Microbiol 2009; 7(3): 226-36.
[http://dx.doi.org/10.1038/nrmicro2090] [PMID: 19198616]

[12]   Song W, Gui M, Wang X, Xiang Y. Cryo-EM structure of the SARS coronavirus spike glycoprotein in complex with its host cell receptor ACE2. PLoS Pathog 2018; 14(8): e1007236.
[http://dx.doi.org/10.1371/journal.ppat.1007236] [PMID: 30102747]

[13]   Azkur AK, Akdis M, Azkur D, *et al.* Immune response to SARS-CoV-2 and mechanisms of immunopathological changes in COVID-19. Allergy 2020; 75(7): 1564-81.
[http://dx.doi.org/10.1111/all.14364] [PMID: 32396996]

[14]   Qin C, Zhou L, Hu Z, *et al.* Dysregulation of Immune Response in Patients With Coronavirus 2019 (COVID-19) in Wuhan, China. Clin Infect Dis 2020; 71(15): 762-8.
[http://dx.doi.org/10.1093/cid/ciaa248] [PMID: 32161940]

[15]   Zuo Y, Yalavarthi S, Shi H, *et al.* Neutrophil extracellular traps in COVID-19. JCI Insight 2020; 5(11): 138999.
[PMID: 32329756]

[16]   Harrison AG, Lin T, Wang P. Mechanisms of SARS-CoV-2 Transmission and Pathogenesis. Trends Immunol 2020; 41(12): 1100-15.
[http://dx.doi.org/10.1016/j.it.2020.10.004] [PMID: 33132005]

[17]   dos Santos WG. Natural history of COVID-19 and current knowledge on treatment therapeutic options. Biomed Pharmacother 2020; 129: 110493.
[http://dx.doi.org/10.1016/j.biopha.2020.110493] [PMID: 32768971]

[18]   Gao J, Tian Z, Yang X. Breakthrough: Chloroquine phosphate has shown apparent efficacy in treatment of COVID-19 associated pneumonia in clinical studies. Biosci Trends 2020; 14(1): 72-3.
[http://dx.doi.org/10.5582/bst.2020.01047] [PMID: 32074550]

[19]   Yao X, Ye F, Zhang M, *et al.* In Vitro Antiviral Activity and Projection of Optimized Dosing Design of Hydroxychloroquine for the Treatment of Severe Acute Respiratory Syndrome Coronavirus 2 (SARS-CoV-2). Clin Infect Dis 2020; 71(15): 732-9.
[http://dx.doi.org/10.1093/cid/ciaa237] [PMID: 32150618]

[20]   Huang F, Li Y, Leung ELH, *et al.* A review of therapeutic agents and Chinese herbal medicines against SARS-COV-2 (COVID-19). Pharmacol Res 2020; 158: 104929.
[http://dx.doi.org/10.1016/j.phrs.2020.104929] [PMID: 32442720]

[21]   Yang SNY, Atkinson SC, Wang C, *et al.* The broad spectrum antiviral ivermectin targets the host nuclear transport importin $\alpha/\beta 1$ heterodimer. Antiviral Res 2020; 177: 104760.
[http://dx.doi.org/10.1016/j.antiviral.2020.104760] [PMID: 32135219]

[22]   Caly L, Druce JD, Catton MG, Jans DA, Wagstaff KM. The FDA-approved drug ivermectin inhibits the replication of SARS-CoV-2 *in vitro.* Antiviral Res 2020; 178: 104787.
[http://dx.doi.org/10.1016/j.antiviral.2020.104787] [PMID: 32251768]

[23]   Tarighi P, Eftekhari S, Chizari M, Sabernavaei M, Jafari D, Mirzabeigi P. A review of potential suggested drugs for coronavirus disease (COVID-19) treatment. Eur J Pharmacol 2021; 895: 173890.
[http://dx.doi.org/10.1016/j.ejphar.2021.173890] [PMID: 33482181]

[24]   Wang M, Cao R, Zhang L, *et al.* Remdesivir and chloroquine effectively inhibit the recently emerged novel coronavirus (2019-nCoV) *in vitro.* Cell Res 2020; 30(3): 269-71.
[http://dx.doi.org/10.1038/s41422-020-0282-0] [PMID: 32020029]

[25]   Grein J, Ohmagari N, Shin D, *et al.* Compassionate Use of Remdesivir for Patients with Severe Covid-19. N Engl J Med 2020; 382(24): 2327-36.
[http://dx.doi.org/10.1056/NEJMoa2007016] [PMID: 32275812]

[26]   Scavone C, Brusco S, Bertini M, *et al.* Current pharmacological treatments for COVID-19: What's next? Br J Pharmacol 2020; 177(21): 4813-24.
[http://dx.doi.org/10.1111/bph.15072] [PMID: 32329520]

[27]   Furuta Y, Komeno T, Nakamura T. Favipiravir (T-705), a broad spectrum inhibitor of viral RNA polymerase. Proc Jpn Acad, Ser B, Phys Biol Sci 2017; 93(7): 449-63.
[http://dx.doi.org/10.2183/pjab.93.027] [PMID: 28769016]

[28]   2020.https://europepmc.org/article/ppr/ppr118169

[29]   Chu CM, Cheng VCC, Hung IFN, *et al.* Role of lopinavir/ritonavir in the treatment of SARS: initial virological and clinical findings. Thorax 2004; 59(3): 252-6.
[http://dx.doi.org/10.1136/thorax.2003.012658] [PMID: 14985565]

[30]   Arabi YM, Asiri AY, Assiri AM, *et al.* Treatment of Middle East respiratory syndrome with a combination of lopinavir/ritonavir and interferon-$\beta 1$b (MIRACLE trial): statistical analysis plan for a recursive two-stage group sequential randomized controlled trial. Trials 2020; 21(1): 8.
[http://dx.doi.org/10.1186/s13063-019-3846-x] [PMID: 31900204]

[31]   Khani E, Khiali S, Entezari-Maleki T. Potential COVID-19 Therapeutic. J Clin Pharmacol 2021; 61(4): 429-60.
[http://dx.doi.org/10.1002/jcph.1822] [PMID: 33511638]

[32]   Bloch EM, Shoham S, Casadevall A, *et al.* Deployment of convalescent plasma for the prevention and treatment of COVID-19. J Clin Invest 2020; 130(6): 2757-65.

[http://dx.doi.org/10.1172/JCI138745] [PMID: 32254064]

[33]   Zhao J, Yuan Q, Wang H, *et al.* Antibody Responses to SARS-CoV-2 in Patients With Novel Coronavirus Disease 2019. Clin Infect Dis 2020; 71(16): 2027-34.
[http://dx.doi.org/10.1093/cid/ciaa344] [PMID: 32221519]

[34]   Mrityunjaya M, Pavithra V, Neelam R, Janhavi P, Halami PM, Ravindra PV. Immune-Boosting, Antioxidant and Anti-inflammatory Food Supplements Targeting Pathogenesis of COVID-19. Front Immunol 2020; 11: 570122.https://www.ncbi.nlm.nih.gov/pmc/articles/PMC7575721/
[http://dx.doi.org/10.3389/fimmu.2020.570122] [PMID: 33117359]

[35]   Lambert SA, Jolma A, Campitelli LF, *et al.* The Human Transcription Factors. Cell 2018; 172(4): 650-65.
[http://dx.doi.org/10.1016/j.cell.2018.01.029] [PMID: 29425488]

[36]   Martineau AR, Jolliffe DA, Hooper RL, *et al.* Vitamin D supplementation to prevent acute respiratory tract infections: systematic review and meta-analysis of individual participant data. BMJ 2017; 356: i6583.
[http://dx.doi.org/10.1136/bmj.i6583] [PMID: 28202713]

[37]   Lemire JM, Archer DC, Beck L, Spiegelberg HL. Immunosuppressive actions of 1,25-dihydroxyvitamin D3: preferential inhibition of Th1 functions. J Nutr 1995; 125(6) (Suppl.): 1704S-8S.
[PMID: 7782931]

[38]   Carr A, Maggini S. Vitamin C and Immune Function. Nutrients 2017; 9(11): 1211.
[http://dx.doi.org/10.3390/nu9111211] [PMID: 29099763]

[39]   Carr AC. A new clinical trial to test high-dose vitamin C in patients with COVID-19. Crit Care 2020; 24(1): 133.
[http://dx.doi.org/10.1186/s13054-020-02851-4] [PMID: 32264963]

[40]   Catanzaro M, Corsini E, Rosini M, Racchi M, Lanni C. Immunomodulators Inspired by Nature: A Review on Curcumin and Echinacea. Molecules 2018; 23(11): 2778.https://www.ncbi.nlm.nih.gov/pmc/articles/PMC6278270/
[http://dx.doi.org/10.3390/molecules23112778] [PMID: 30373170]

[41]   Zahedipour F, Hosseini SA, Sathyapalan T, *et al.* Potential effects of curcumin in the treatment of COVID -19 infection. Phytother Res 2020; 34(11): 2911-20.
[http://dx.doi.org/10.1002/ptr.6738] [PMID: 32430996]

[42]   Guo JY, Huo HR, Zhao BS, *et al.* Cinnamaldehyde reduces IL-1β-induced cyclooxygenase-2 activity in rat cerebral microvascular endothelial cells. Eur J Pharmacol 2006; 537(1-3): 174-80.
[http://dx.doi.org/10.1016/j.ejphar.2006.03.002] [PMID: 16624280]

[43]   Baud D, Dimopoulou Agri V, Gibson GR, Reid G, Giannoni E. Using Probiotics. Front Public Health 2020; 8: 186.
[http://dx.doi.org/10.3389/fpubh.2020.00186] [PMID: 32574290]

[44]   Ahmad A, Rehman MU, Alkharfy KM. An alternative approach to minimize the risk of coronavirus (Covid-19) and similar infections. Eur Rev Med Pharmacol Sci 2020; 24(7): 4030-4.
[PMID: 32329879]

[45]   Weng JR, Lin CS, Lai HC, *et al.* Antiviral activity of *Sambucus FormosanaNakai* ethanol extract and related phenolic acid constituents against human coronavirus NL63. Virus Res 2019; 273: 197767.
[http://dx.doi.org/10.1016/j.virusres.2019.197767] [PMID: 31560964]

[46]   Singh YD, Jena B, Ningthoujam R, Panda S, Priyadarsini P, Pattanayak S, *et al.* Potential bioactive molecules from natural products to combat against coronavirus 2020.

[47]   Khaerunnisa S, Kurniawan H, Awaluddin R, Suhartati S, Soetjipto S. Potential Inhibitor of COVID-19 Main Protease (Mpro) From Several Medicinal Plant Compounds by Molecular Docking Study. 2020. Available from: https://www.preprints.org/manuscript/202003.0226/v1

[48]   Adem S, Eyupoglu V, Sarfraz I, Rasul A, Ali M. Identification of Potent COVID-19 Main Protease (Mpro) Inhibitors from Natural Polyphenols: An *in Silico* Strategy Unveils a Hope against CORONA. 2020. Available from: https://www.preprints.org/manuscript/202003.0333/v1

[49]   Wu W, Li R, Li X, *et al.* Quercetin. Viruses 2015; 8(1): 6.
[http://dx.doi.org/10.3390/v8010006] [PMID: 26712783]

[50]   Su H, Yao S, Zhao W, Li M, Liu J, Shang W, *et al.* Discovery of baicalin and baicalein bioRxiv 2020; 2020.04.13.038687.

[51]   Huang W, Chen X, Li Q, *et al.* Inhibition of intercellular adhesion in herpex simplex virus infection by glycyrrhizin. Cell Biochem Biophys 2012; 62(1): 137-40.
[http://dx.doi.org/10.1007/s12013-011-9271-8] [PMID: 21874590]

[52]   van de Sand L, Bormann M, Alt M, *et al.* Glycyrrhizin Effectively Inhibits SARS-CoV-2 Replication by Inhibiting the Viral Main Protease. Viruses 2021; 13(4): 609.https://www.ncbi.nlm.nih.gov/pmc/articles/PMC8066091/
[http://dx.doi.org/10.3390/v13040609] [PMID: 33918301]

[53]   Chen H, Du Q. Potential Natural Compounds for Preventing SARS-CoV-2 2019.https://www.preprints.org/manuscript/202001.0358/v3

[54]   Gomaa AA, Abdel-Wadood YA. The potential of glycyrrhizin and licorice extract in combating COVID-19 and associated conditions. Phytomedicine Plus 2021; 1(3): 100043.
[http://dx.doi.org/10.1016/j.phyplu.2021.100043] [PMID: 35399823]

[55]   Chen F, Chan KH, Jiang Y, *et al. In vitro* susceptibility of 10 clinical isolates of SARS coronavirus to selected antiviral compounds. J Clin Virol 2004; 31(1): 69-75.
[http://dx.doi.org/10.1016/j.jcv.2004.03.003] [PMID: 15288617]

[56]   Song J, Zhang L, Xu Y, *et al.* The comprehensive study on the therapeutic effects of baicalein for the treatment of COVID-19 in vivo and in vitro. Biochem Pharmacol 2021; 183: 114302.
[http://dx.doi.org/10.1016/j.bcp.2020.114302] [PMID: 33121927]

[57]   Yan H, Ma L, Wang H, *et al.* Luteolin decreases the yield of influenza A virus *in vitro* by interfering with the coat protein I complex expression. J Nat Med 2019; 73(3): 487-96.
[http://dx.doi.org/10.1007/s11418-019-01287-7] [PMID: 30758716]

[58]   Ryu YB, Jeong HJ, Kim JH, *et al.* Biflavonoids from Torreya nucifera displaying SARS-CoV 3CLpro inhibition. Bioorg Med Chem 2010; 18(22): 7940-7.
[http://dx.doi.org/10.1016/j.bmc.2010.09.035] [PMID: 20934345]

[59]   Paemanee A, Hitakarun A, Wintachai P, Roytrakul S, Smith DR. A proteomic analysis of the anti-dengue virus activity of andrographolide. Biomed Pharmacother 2019; 109: 322-32.
[http://dx.doi.org/10.1016/j.biopha.2018.10.054] [PMID: 30396090]

[60]   Enmozhi SK, Raja K, Sebastine I, Joseph J. Andrographolide as a potential inhibitor of SARS-CoV-2 main protease: an *in silico* approach. J Biomol Struct Dyn 2020; 1-7.
[http://dx.doi.org/10.1080/07391102.2020.1760136] [PMID: 32329419]

[61]   Berretta AA, Silveira MAD, Cóndor Capcha JM, De Jong D. Propolis and its potential against SARS-CoV-2 infection mechanisms and COVID-19 disease. Biomed Pharmacother 2020; 131: 110622.
[http://dx.doi.org/10.1016/j.biopha.2020.110622] [PMID: 32890967]

[62]   Vardhan S, Sahoo SK. Searching inhibitors for three important proteins of COVID-19 2020.http://arxiv.org/abs/2004.08095 [q-bio]Internet

[63]   Rogosnitzky M, Okediji P, Koman I. Cepharanthine: a review of the antiviral potential of a Japanese-approved alopecia drug in COVID-19. Pharmacol Rep 2020; 72(6): 1509-16.
[http://dx.doi.org/10.1007/s43440-020-00132-z] [PMID: 32700247]

[64]   Jeon S, Ko M, Lee J, *et al.* Identification of Antiviral Drug Candidates against SARS-CoV-2 from FDA-Approved Drugs. Antimicrob Agents Chemother 2020; 64(7): e00819-20.

[http://dx.doi.org/10.1128/AAC.00819-20] [PMID: 32366720]

[65] Ko M, Jeon S, Ryu W-S, Kim S. Comparative analysis of antiviral efficacy of FDA-approved drugs against SARS-CoV-2 in human lung cells: Nafamostat is the most potent antiviral drug candidate. bioRxiv 2020; 2020.05.12.090035.
[http://dx.doi.org/10.1101/2020.05.12.090035]

[66] Jang M, Park YI, Cha YE, *et al.* Tea Polyphenols EGCG and Theaflavin Inhibit the Activity of SARS-CoV-2 3CL-Protease *In Vitro*. Evid Based Complement Alternat Med 2020; 2020: 1-7.
[http://dx.doi.org/10.1155/2020/5630838] [PMID: 32963564]

[67] Mhatre S, Srivastava T, Naik S, Patravale V. Antiviral activity of green tea and black tea polyphenols in prophylaxis and treatment of COVID-19: A review. Phytomedicine 2021; 85: 153286.
[http://dx.doi.org/10.1016/j.phymed.2020.153286] [PMID: 32741697]

[68] Ho T, Wu S, Chen J, Li C, Hsiang C. Emodin blocks the SARS coronavirus spike protein and angiotensin-converting enzyme 2 interaction. Antiviral Res 2007; 74(2): 92-101.
[http://dx.doi.org/10.1016/j.antiviral.2006.04.014] [PMID: 16730806]

[69] Kelleni MT. Resveratrol-zinc nanoparticles or pterostilbene-zinc: Potential COVID-19 mono and adjuvant therapy. Biomed Pharmacother 2021; 139: 111626.
[http://dx.doi.org/10.1016/j.biopha.2021.111626] [PMID: 33894625]

[70] Pasquereau S, Nehme Z, Haidar Ahmad S, *et al.* Resveratrol. Viruses 2021; 13(2): 354.
[http://dx.doi.org/10.3390/v13020354] [PMID: 33672333]

[71] Zhao Y, Du X, Duan Y, *et al.* High-throughput screening identifies established drugs as SARS-CoV-2 PLpro inhibitors. Protein Cell 2021; 12(11): 877-88.
[http://dx.doi.org/10.1007/s13238-021-00836-9] [PMID: 33864621]

[72] Kim CH. Anti–SARS-CoV-2 Natural Products as Potentially Therapeutic Agents. Front Pharmacol 2021; 12: 590509.https://www.frontiersin.org/articles/10.3389/fphar.2021.590509/full
[http://dx.doi.org/10.3389/fphar.2021.590509] [PMID: 34122058]

[73] Gallelli L. 2020.https://clinicaltrials.gov/ct2/show/NCT04322344

[74] Wang D, Huang J, Yeung AWK, *et al.* The Significance of Natural Product Derivatives and Traditional Medicine for COVID-19. Processes (Basel) 2020; 8(8): 937.
[http://dx.doi.org/10.3390/pr8080937]

[75] Shang J, Wan Y, Luo C, *et al.* Cell entry mechanisms of SARS-CoV-2. Proc Natl Acad Sci USA 2020; 117(21): 11727-34.
[http://dx.doi.org/10.1073/pnas.2003138117] [PMID: 32376634]

[76] Liu S, Xiao G, Chen Y, *et al.* Interaction between heptad repeat 1 and 2 regions in spike protein of SARS-associated coronavirus: implications for virus fusogenic mechanism and identification of fusion inhibitors. Lancet 2004; 363(9413): 938-47.
[http://dx.doi.org/10.1016/S0140-6736(04)15788-7] [PMID: 15043961]

[77] Remali J, Aizat WM. A Review on Plant Bioactive Compounds and Their Modes of Action Against Coronavirus Infection. Front Pharmacol 2021; 11: 589044. https://www.ncbi.nlm.nih.gov/pmc/articles/PMC7845143/
[http://dx.doi.org/10.3389/fphar.2020.589044] [PMID: 33519449]

[78] Li F. Receptor recognition and cross-species infections of SARS coronavirus. Antiviral Res 2013; 100(1): 246-54.
[http://dx.doi.org/10.1016/j.antiviral.2013.08.014] [PMID: 23994189]

[79] Walls AC, Park YJ, Tortorici MA, Wall A, McGuire AT, Veesler D. Structure, Function, and Antigenicity of the SARS-CoV-2 Spike Glycoprotein. Cell 2020; 181(2): 281-292.e6.
[http://dx.doi.org/10.1016/j.cell.2020.02.058] [PMID: 32155444]

[80] Schwarz S, Wang K, Yu W, Sun B, Schwarz W. Emodin inhibits current through SARS-associated

coronavirus 3a protein. Antiviral Res 2011; 90(1): 64-9.
[http://dx.doi.org/10.1016/j.antiviral.2011.02.008] [PMID: 21356245]

[81]   Fuzimoto AD, Isidoro C. The antiviral and coronavirus-host protein pathways inhibiting properties of herbs and natural compounds - Additional weapons in the fight against the COVID-19 pandemic? J Tradit Complement Med 2020; 10(4): 405-19.
[http://dx.doi.org/10.1016/j.jtcme.2020.05.003] [PMID: 32691005]

[82]   Durai P, Batool M, Shah M, Choi S. Middle East respiratory syndrome coronavirus: transmission, virology and therapeutic targeting to aid in outbreak control. Exp Mol Med 2015; 47(8): e181-1.
[http://dx.doi.org/10.1038/emm.2015.76] [PMID: 26315600]

[83]   Báez-Santos YM, St John SE, Mesecar AD. The SARS-coronavirus papain-like protease: structure, function and inhibition by designed antiviral compounds. Antiviral Res 2015; 115: 21-38.
[http://dx.doi.org/10.1016/j.antiviral.2014.12.015] [PMID: 25554382]

[84]   Cong Y, Kriegenburg F, de Haan CAM, Reggiori F. Coronavirus nucleocapsid proteins assemble constitutively in high molecular oligomers. Sci Rep 2017; 7(1): 5740.
[http://dx.doi.org/10.1038/s41598-017-06062-w] [PMID: 28720894]

[85]   Goswami D, Kumar M, Ghosh SK, Das A. Natural Product Compounds in *Alpinia officinarum* and Ginger are Potent SARS-CoV-2 Papain-like Protease Inhibitors. 2020.

[86]   Gyebi GA, Ogunro OB, Adegunloye AP, Ogunyemi OM, Afolabi SO. Potential inhibitors of coronavirus 3-chymotrypsin-like protease (3CLpro): an *in silico* screening of alkaloids. J Biomol Struct Dyn 2020; 1-13.
[http://dx.doi.org/10.1080/07391102.2020.1764868] [PMID: 32367767]

[87]   Weber C, Opatz T. Bisbenzylisoquinoline Alkaloids. Alkaloids Chem Biol 2019; 81: 1-114.
[http://dx.doi.org/10.1016/bs.alkal.2018.07.001] [PMID: 30685048]

[88]   Huang J, Tao G, Liu J, Cai J, Huang Z, Chen J. Current Prevention of COVID-19. Front Pharmacol 2020; 11: 588508.https://www.ncbi.nlm.nih.gov/pmc/articles/PMC7597394/
[http://dx.doi.org/10.3389/fphar.2020.588508] [PMID: 33178026]

[89]   Mouffouk C, Mouffouk S, Mouffouk S, Hambaba L, Haba H. Flavonols as potential antiviral drugs targeting SARS-CoV-2 proteases (3CLpro and PLpro), spike protein, RNA-dependent RNA polymerase (RdRp) and angiotensin-converting enzyme II receptor (ACE2). Eur J Pharmacol 2021; 891: 173759.
[http://dx.doi.org/10.1016/j.ejphar.2020.173759] [PMID: 33249077]

[90]   Pandey P, Khan F, Rana AK, Srivastava Y, Jha SK, Jha NK. A drug repurposing approach towards elucidating the potential of flavonoids Biointerface Res Appl Chem 2021; 11(1) https://covid19.elsevierpure.com/en/publications/a-drug-repurposing-approach-tow-rds-elucidating-the-potential-of- [Internet].

[91]   Jang KJ, Jeong S, Kang DY, Sp N, Yang YM, Kim DE. A high ATP concentration enhances the cooperative translocation of the SARS coronavirus helicase nsP13 in the unwinding of duplex RNA. Sci Rep 2020; 10(1): 4481.
[http://dx.doi.org/10.1038/s41598-020-61432-1] [PMID: 32161317]

[92]   Yu MS, Lee J, Lee JM, *et al.* Identification of myricetin and scutellarein as novel chemical inhibitors of the SARS coronavirus helicase, nsP13. Bioorg Med Chem Lett 2012; 22(12): 4049-54.
[http://dx.doi.org/10.1016/j.bmcl.2012.04.081] [PMID: 22578462]

[93]   Tsai YC, Lee CL, Yen HR, *et al.* Antiviral Action of Tryptanthrin Isolated from *Strobilanthes cusia* Leaf against Human Coronavirus NL63. Biomolecules 2020; 10(3): 366.https://www.ncbi.nlm.nih.gov/pmc/articles/PMC7175275/
[http://dx.doi.org/10.3390/biom10030366] [PMID: 32120929]

[94]   Zhang D, Wu K, Zhang X, Deng S, Peng B. *In silico* screening of Chinese herbal medicines with the potential to directly inhibit 2019 novel coronavirus. J Integr Med 2020; 18(2): 152-8.

[http://dx.doi.org/10.1016/j.joim.2020.02.005] [PMID: 32113846]

[95]   Jo S, Kim S, Shin DH, Kim MS. Inhibition of SARS-CoV 3CL protease by flavonoids. J Enzyme Inhib Med Chem 2020; 35(1): 145-51.
[http://dx.doi.org/10.1080/14756366.2019.1690480] [PMID: 31724441]

[96]   Kai H, Kai M. Interactions of coronaviruses with ACE2, angiotensin II, and RAS inhibitors—lessons from available evidence and insights into COVID-19. Hypertens Res 2020; 43(7): 648-54.
[http://dx.doi.org/10.1038/s41440-020-0455-8] [PMID: 32341442]

[97]   Hoffmann M, Kleine-Weber H, Schroeder S, *et al.* SARS-CoV-2 Cell Entry Depends on ACE2 and TMPRSS2 and Is Blocked by a Clinically Proven Protease Inhibitor. Cell 2020; 181(2): 271-280.e8.
[http://dx.doi.org/10.1016/j.cell.2020.02.052] [PMID: 32142651]

[98]   Wu C, Liu Y, Yang Y, *et al.* Analysis of therapeutic targets for SARS-CoV-2 and discovery of potential drugs by computational methods. Acta Pharm Sin B 2020; 10(5): 766-88.
[http://dx.doi.org/10.1016/j.apsb.2020.02.008] [PMID: 32292689]

[99]   Vivek-Ananth RP, Rana A, Rajan N, Biswal HS, Samal A. *In Silico* Identification of Potential Natural Product Inhibitors of Human Proteases Key to SARS-CoV-2 Infection. Molecules 2020; 25(17): 3822.
[http://dx.doi.org/10.3390/molecules25173822] [PMID: 32842606]

[100] Duan L, Zheng Q, Zhang H, Niu Y, Lou Y, Wang H. The SARS-CoV-2 Spike Glycoprotein Biosynthesis, Structure, Function, and Antigenicity: Implications for the Design of Spike-Based Vaccine Immunogens. Front Immunol 2020; 11: 576622. https://www.frontiersin.org/articles/10.3389/fimmu.2020.576622/full
[http://dx.doi.org/10.3389/fimmu.2020.576622] [PMID: 33117378]

[101] Tahir ul Qamar M, Alqahtani SM, Alamri MA, Chen L-L. Structural basis of SARS-CoV-2 3CLpro and anti-COVID-19. J Pharm Anal 2020; 10(4): 313-9.
[http://dx.doi.org/10.1016/j.jpha.2020.03.009] [PMID: 32296570]

[102] Buonaguro L, Tagliamonte M, Tornesello ML, Buonaguro FM. SARS-CoV-2 RNA polymerase as target for antiviral therapy. J Transl Med 2020; 18(1): 185.
[http://dx.doi.org/10.1186/s12967-020-02355-3] [PMID: 32370758]

[103] Boozari M, Hosseinzadeh H. Natural products for COVID -19 prevention and treatment regarding to previous coronavirus infections and novel studies. Phytother Res 2021; 35(2): 864-76.
[http://dx.doi.org/10.1002/ptr.6873] [PMID: 32985017]

[104] Romano M, Ruggiero A, Squeglia F, Maga G, Berisio R. A Structural View of SARS-CoV-2 RNA Replication Machinery: RNA Synthesis, Proofreading and Final Capping. Cells 2020; 9(5): 1267.https://www.ncbi.nlm.nih.gov/pmc/articles/PMC7291026/
[http://dx.doi.org/10.3390/cells9051267] [PMID: 32443810]

[105] McBride R, van Zyl M, Fielding B. The coronavirus nucleocapsid is a multifunctional protein. Viruses 2014; 6(8): 2991-3018.
[http://dx.doi.org/10.3390/v6082991] [PMID: 25105276]

[106] Xian Y, Zhang J, Bian Z, *et al.* Bioactive natural compounds against human coronaviruses: a review and perspective. Acta Pharm Sin B 2020; 10(7): 1163-74.
[http://dx.doi.org/10.1016/j.apsb.2020.06.002] [PMID: 32834947]

[107] Prompetchara E, Ketloy C, Palaga T. Immune responses in COVID-19 and potential vaccines: Lessons learned from SARS and MERS epidemic. Asian Pac J Allergy Immunol 2020; 38(1): 1-9.
[PMID: 32105090]

[108] Sohrab SS, Suhail M, Kamal MA, Husen A, Azhar EI. Recent Development and Future Prospects of Plant-Based Vaccines. Curr Drug Metab 2017; 18(9): 831-41.
[http://dx.doi.org/10.2174/1389200218666170711121810] [PMID: 28699508]

[109] Balfour H. 2020.https://www.europeanpharmaceuticalreview.com/news/124092/plant-based-covid-19-vaccine-enters-phase-i-trials/

[110] Ward BJ, Gobeil P, Séguin A, *et al.* Phase 1 randomized trial of a plant-derived virus-like particle vaccine for COVID-19. Nat Med 2021; 27(6): 1071-8.
[http://dx.doi.org/10.1038/s41591-021-01370-1] [PMID: 34007070]

[111] Rawat K, Kumari P, Saha L. COVID-19 vaccine: A recent update in pipeline vaccines, their design and development strategies. Eur J Pharmacol 2021; 892: 173751.
[http://dx.doi.org/10.1016/j.ejphar.2020.173751] [PMID: 33245898]

CHAPTER 5

Plant Based Bioactive Molecules in Diabetes with Their Therapeutic Mechanism

Amit Kumar Dixit[1,*], Qadir Alam[1], Deepti Dixit[2], Parvathy G. Nair[3] and P.V.V. Prasad[1]

[1] *Central Ayurveda Research Institute-CCRAS, Ministry of Ayush, Kolkata, India*

[2] *School of Biochemistry, Devi Ahilya University, Khandwa Road, Indore, Madhya Pradesh, India*

[3] *National Ayurveda Research Institute for Panchakarma, Cheruthuruthy, Thrisuur, Kerala, India*

Abstract: Plant based bioactive compounds are the secondary metabolites that are produced by them to perform their non-essential functions. They provide an ample source of nutraceuticals and therapeutics for humans. The research on these compounds is on trend these days and most of the research suggests their importance as therapeutic agents and as prophylactic agents against many diseases. Easy accessibility, and better efficacy with lesser adverse effects of bioactive compounds have made their research trending. Diabetes is the oldest known metabolic disease which requires a multimodal treatment approach for its management. The available drugs and treatment options are still unable to control the complications and economic burden faced by the patients. Many plants have been used traditionally for the management of diabetes worldwide. Now it has been well established that the plants provide a rich reservoir of bioactive compounds which have the potential to modulate various pathways involved in the regulation of blood glucose. This chapter discusses the common groups of plant derived bioactive compounds, their sources, and their mechanistic antidiabetic role.

Keywords: Bioactive compounds, Diabetes, Medicinal plants, Phytocompounds, Therapeutic potential.

INTRODUCTION

A bioactive compound is a substance which produces some biological activities when taken by an organism. They have the potential to modulate metabolic processes, which can aid in achieving better health conditions [1]. Thus, we can say that bioactive compounds of plant origin are the secondary metabolites which poses some pharmacological or toxicological effects in man and animals [2].

---

* **Corresponding author Amit Kumar Dixit:** Central Ayurveda Research Institute, Central Council for Research in Ayurvedic Sciences, Ministry of Ayush, Government of India, Kolkata, India; Tel: +91-89205 74307; E-mail: deepdixit20@gmail.com

Mukesh Kumar Sharma and Pallavi Kaushik (Eds.)

Different plant based food that we consume like grains, fruits, vegetables, legumes, and seeds, all may contain numerous bioactive compounds. The bioactive compounds have been under consumption since the beginning of man's existence.

As there are many archaeological findings of remains of seeds and legumes in dental pieces of Neanderthal fossils, which proves the food intake of vegetable origin, including plants, fruits, and vegetables by them [3]. There is evidence in the historical books like in Chinese traditional medicines books and Ayurveda mentioning about the herbs and roots, and their application for medicinal use. There are still many preparations which include plants and roots which are still in use in the modern times as well [4].

With the development of analytical techniques like nuclear magnetic resonance spectrometry (NMR), chromatographic techniques like gas chromatography (GC), mass spectrometry (MS), high-performance liquid chromatography (HPLC), liquid chromatography-mass spectrometry (LCMS) which aids in the isolation of single bioactive compound its purification, as well as its structure elucidation from plant extracts have become available [2]. Thus, we came to know about the phytochemical profiling of any plant based extract [5]. Based on their chemistry, the bioactive compounds can be classified as glycosides, carotenoids, flavonoids, saponins, alkaloids, saponins, phytosterols, polyphenols. Since vitamins and minerals elicit pharmacological effects, these can also be categorized as bioactive compounds [6].

Bioactive compounds have been implicated in numerous diseases, as disease modulator as, therapeutic agents, prophylactic medications and as nutraceutical supplement. These are known to affect various metabolic pathways and thus affecting functions of various organs and organ systems of body [7]. There is a plethora of examples which prove the therapeutic potential of bioactive compounds. Falcarinol and falcarindiol, which are bioactive compounds obtained from carrot, possess anti-inflammatory effects [8]. Some of the bioactive compounds namely, resveratrol, curcumin, catechins, *etc.* are known to have an anti-ageing effect by their ability to directly inhibit oxidizing agents like reactive oxygen species and inflammatory pathways [9]. Polyphenolic bioactive compounds can modulate the transcription factors like mitogen activated kinase, which is crucial for cell division process [9, 10]. 6-Shogaol, ginkgolide, quercetin, *etc.* have the ability to interact with various neuronal receptors, thus inducing the synthesis of neurotropic factors that promote regeneration, growth, and neuronal survival, reducing the rate of progression of neurodegenerative diseases [11]. Bioactive compounds are well known immunomodulators, as they can affect the B cells and T cells proliferation, thus they play an important role in immune related diseases and different types of cancers [12].

Diabetes mellitus (DM) can be considered as one of the oldest and most commonly known endocrine disorder, which is characterized by an elevation of the blood glucose levels that requires its frequent monitoring and proper control [5]. DM can be classified into many types, however, the most common types are type 1 and type 2 Diabetes mellitus. Type 1 DM is mainly associated with the failure of insulin production due to destruction of insulin-secreting pancreatic β-cells by cytotoxic T Cell (CD8+) mediated autoimmunity whereas, the type 2 DM is the result of insulin resistance and reduction of insulin production [5, 13]. DM in the later stages leads to complications like nephropathy, neuropathies, cardiovascular disorders and the patient becomes prone to a number of infections as well [14]. As per WHO data, a third leading cause of morbidity and mortality after heart attack and cancer is due to DM. In the year 2014, there were 8.5% of adults aged 18 and more had DM. In the year 2012, 2.2 million deaths were due to high blood glucose and in the year 2016, DM caused 6 million deaths. There was 5% increase in premature mortality from DM between the years 2000 and 2016. As per World Health organization people with DM were more prone to COVID-19 as there was 33.8% comorbidity.

The plant based bioactive compounds are known to have better efficacy, a wide availability, and fewer adverse effects which make them more in demand as compared to the synthetic medicines for the management of DM [15]. There are more than 1200 plants with known antidiabetic properties. Out of them, 400 plants have proven the antidiabetic properties after appropriate research and investigation [16]. Bioactive compounds are excellent antioxidants, for example, α and β carotene, ascorbic acid (vitamin c), lutein, lycopene, *etc.* help in managing the complications like endothelial dysfunction and atherosclerosis in the patients with DM [17]. Polyphenolic compounds and vitamin E are other essential bioactive compounds with the ameliorative potential against oxidative stress related to diabetic risk [18]. Several phytochemicals have been associated with benefits to people with DM, including cinnamaldehyde, epigallocatechin, and chlorogenic acid, showing hypoglycemic effects, α-amylase inhibitor and insulin sensitizer, respectively [19]. The available evidence from *in-vitro* and animal studies suggested the protective effects of cinnamon as an antitumor, anti-inflammatory, antioxidant, antimicrobial, and cholesterol lowering agent, as a treatment of infectious diseases, and for the prevention of cardiovascular diseases [20]. There is well-documented profile of pharmacological effects of cinnamon for the treatment of type 2 DM [21]. Moreover, the bioactive compounds can be an adjuvant and therapeutic option for multimodal treatment for managing DM due to their better safety and efficacy profiles.

This chapter highlights the groups of bioactive compounds which are obtained from plants, their sources, and pharmacological actions involved in the regulation of blood glucose.

Bioactives Compounds with their Pharmacological Actions Involved in the Regulation of Blood Glucose

Alkaloids

Alkaloids are a group of diverse low-molecular-weight bioactive compounds derived mostly from amino acids, chemically composed of one or more carbon rings containing a nitrogen atom inside the ring owing to its bitter taste and potent bioactivity [22]. They are diverse categories of alkaloids out of which some of the common ones are tropane alkaloids, indole alkaloids, quinolone alkaloids, pyrrolidine alkaloids, isoquinoline alkaloids, and izidine alkaloids [23]. Berberine (Fig. **1**), an alkaloid which is extracted from *Tinospora cordifolia*, increases hexokinase and phosphofructokinase activity which facilitates glucose transport and boosts carbohydrate digestion and absorption [24]. Methanolic extract of *Adhatodavasica* containing alkaloids vasicine (Fig. **2**) and vasicinol (Fig. **3**) has shown to reduce glucose absorption by inhibiting intestinal α-glucosidase in the animal [25]. *Aegle marmelos* contains the alkaloids, namely marmesin (Fig. **4**), aegelin (Fig. **5**) and marmelosin (Fig. **6**) which can regenerate the pancreatic β cells and enhance insulin secretion [26]. Similar activities have been shown by harmine (Fig. **7**), nor-harmine (Fig. **8**) which are alkaloids obtained from *Tribulus terrestris [27]*. Betaine (Fig. **9**), achyranthine (Fig. **10**) and β ecdysone (Fig. **11**), which are isolated from *Achyranthes aspera* have modulatory effects on sugar digestion and absorption process [28].

Glycosides

Glycosides are the bioactive compounds which are composed of two moieties a glycone or a sugar moiety and anaglycone or a non-sugar moiety connected by a glycosidic bond [29]. Both the glycone as well as aglycone possess different functions in the plants and have biological activities. Some of the known glycosides like stevioside (Fig. **12**), rutin (Fig. **13**), gymnemic acid I (Fig. **14**), puerarin (Fig. **15**), *etc.* which are contained in *Gymnema sylvestre*, are well known antihyperglycemic bioactive compounds [30]. Glycosides like ginsenoside (Fig. **16**), gymnemosides (Fig. **17**), momordin (Fig. **18**), momordicine I (Fig. **19**), momorcharaside A (Fig. **20**), have known antidiabetic effect, they act by enhancing insulin secretion and glycogen synthesis [27]. *Tinospora cordifolia* contains one of the important glycosides like cordifolide A (Fig. **21**), cordifole, tinosporide (Fig. **22**), and columbin (Fig. **23**), which regulates glucose biosynthesis and metabolism pathway [31]. Anthraquinone glycoside from rhubarb preparation helped ameliorate insulin resistance by regulating of the gut microbiota, and activation of the glucagon like peptide-/cyclic adenosine monophosphate or GLP-1/cAMP pathway [32].

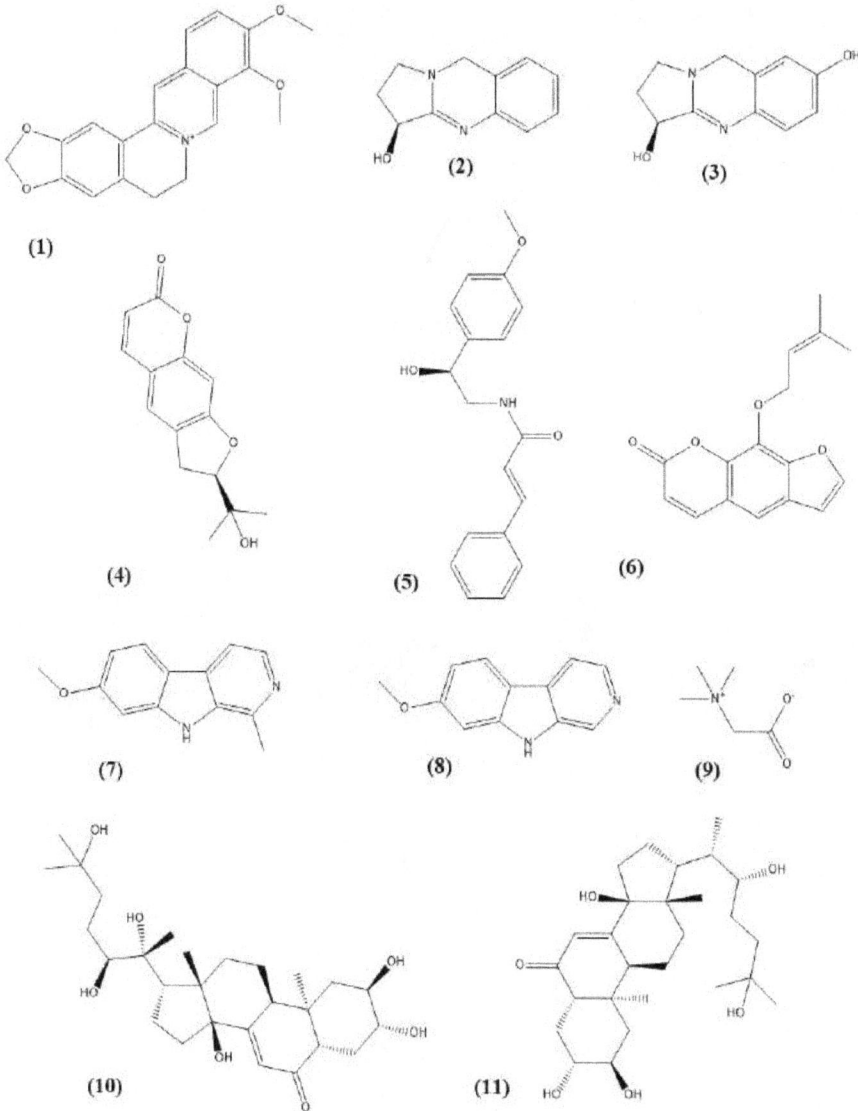

Fig. (1). Chemical structures of bioactive compounds of alkaloids phytochemical class.

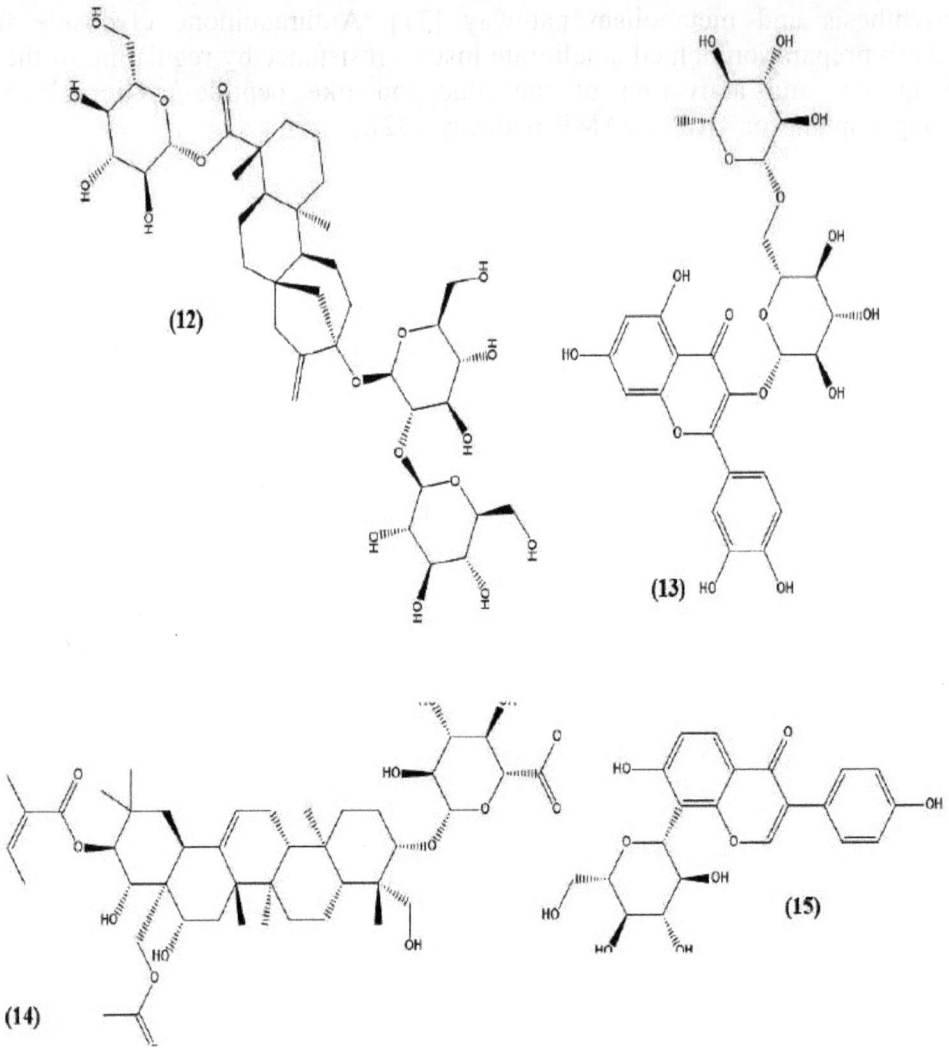

(12)

(13)

(14)

(15)

(Fig. 2) contd.....

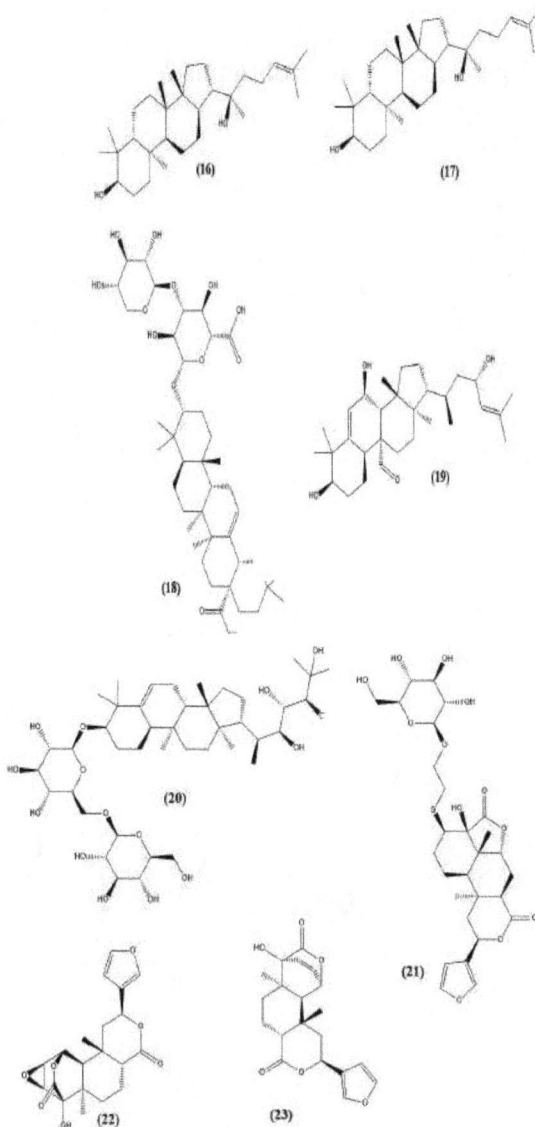

Fig. (2). Chemical structures of bioactive compounds of glycosides phytochemical class.

Phenolic

Phenolic bioactive compounds are a type of secondary metabolites which chemically contain groups hydroxyl (-OH) functional group attached to an aromatic ring directly. Some of the common polyphenolic compounds are classified as flavonoids, coumarins, lignans, chalcones, xanthones, tannins *etc*. The well-known phenolics include: ellagic acid, quercetin, resorcinol (Fig. **24**), catechins (Fig. **25**), ferulic acid, caffeic acid *etc*. They are very common in plants but some of them are also produced by microorganisms [33].

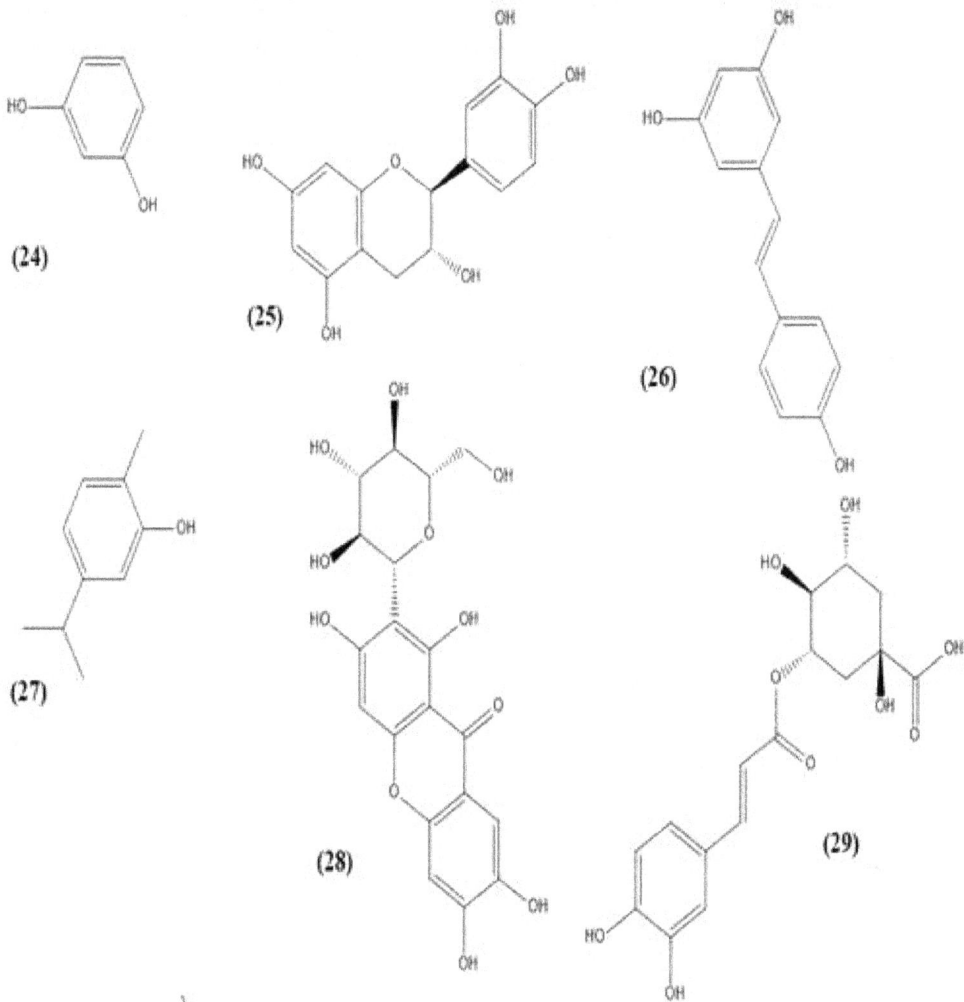

(24)

(25)

(26)

(27)

(28)

(29)

(Fig. 3) contd.....

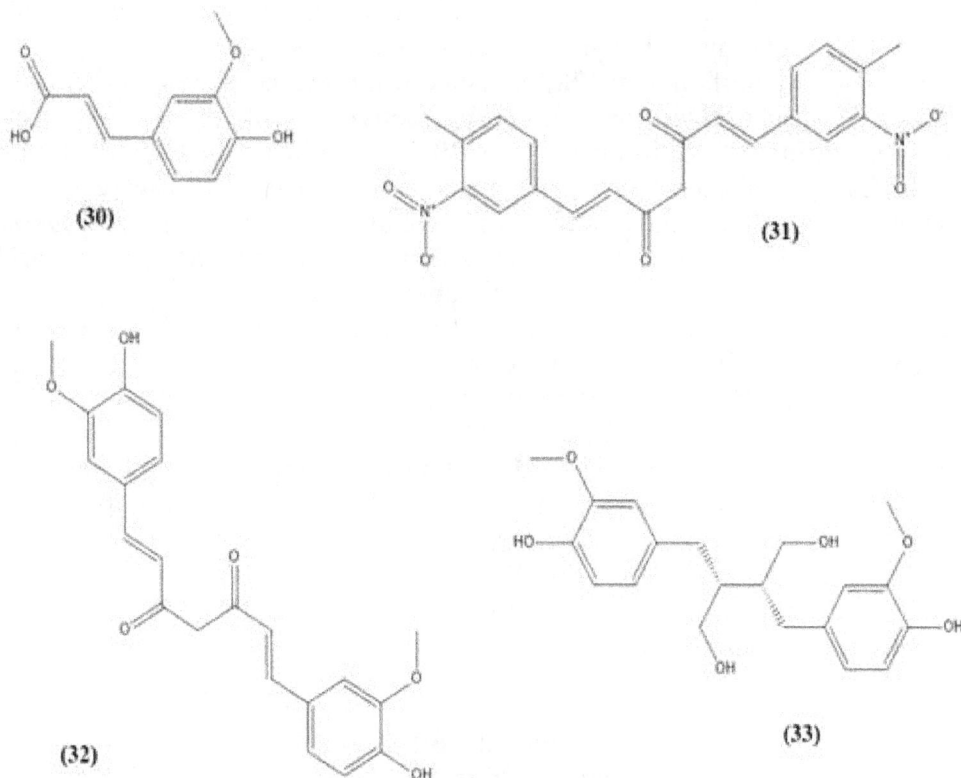

Fig. (3). Chemical structures of bioactive compounds of polyphenols phytochemical class.

Resveratrol (Fig. **26**) is a phenolic bioactive compound which is a phytoalexin, and it is synthesized by plants in stressful conditions. It is abundantly present in red grapes, cranberry juices, red wine, peanuts, pistachios, and blueberries. Resveratrol has anti-hyperglycemic effects which are mainly exerted by increasing the action of the glucose transporter specifically GLUT4, in the cytoplasmic membrane [34]. It has been shown to suppress the postprandial glucagon responses when administered for a duration of one month [35] and it has improved HbA1c after the completion of three months treatment, suggesting an improvement of glycemic control [36]. It has shown to have protective actions in diabetic neuropathy, which were earlier attributed to the intrinsic radical scavenger properties only. However, recently various novel mechanisms like upregulation of Sirtuin 1 (SIRT1), Nuclear factor erythroid 2-related factor 2 (Nrf2), and inhibition of Nuclear factor-kappa B(NF-κB) *etc.* have been found which are implicated in this [37].

Carvacrol (Fig. **27**) and linalool are present in *Ocimum sanctum* regulating glucose by modulating carbohydrate digestion and absorption as well as insulin secretion [38]. Mangiferin (Fig. **28**) extracted from salacia species and *Mangifera indica* tree has α-glucosidase-inhibiting activity, making it an effective antidiabetic agent [38]. Chlorogenic (Fig. **29**) and ferulic acids (Fig. **30**) stimulate glucose transporters and thus these manage the plasma glucose levels [39]. Curcumin is one of the most active components present in turmeric (*Curcuma longa*), is in the limelight because of its potential as a therapeutic agent in various diseases, including DM. It shows antidiabetic activity primarily by reducing glycemia and hyperlipidemia as observed in rodent models and it is relatively inexpensive and safe as well [40]. Curcuminoids (Fig. **31**) are derived from turmeric extract and have significantly suppressed the increased blood glucose levels by PPAR-γ activation and stimulated human adipocyte differentiation in type 2 DM [41]. Curcumin (Fig. **32**) is known to improve peripheral insulin resistance in an insulin-resistant animal model by reducing proinflammatory nuclear factors like NF-κB *etc* [42]. Diabetic neuropathy and nephropathy are the disorders that are associated with DM. These conditions occur as a result of diabetic microvascular injury, elevated AGEs, and activated protein kinase C, and curcumin has shown to suppress the development of diabetic-related complications in rat models [43].

Clinical trial studies further confirmed the effect of curcumin on end-stage renal disease and showed that curcumin could reduce the growth factors, inflammatory markers, and nephrotic complications [44].

Lignans are a bioactive compounds subgroup of nonflavonoid polyphenols which are formed of two β-β-linked phenylpropane units [45]. Also, plant lignans like secoisolariciresinol (Fig. **32**), and matairesinol have powerful antioxidant activity which is higher than vitamin E when compared, and thus they can be effective in the treatment of several reactive oxygen species manifested diseases like cardiovascular disease, coronary heart disease, and diabetes [46].

Flavonoids

Flavonoids are chemically poly-hydroxy and poly-phenolic bioactive compounds which have a wide-range presence in the plant kingdom. Flavonoids are classified into categories like flavanols, flavones and flavanones, and they have shown numerous medicinal effects, including antidiabetic properties *via* enhanced insulin secretion. Some of the common flavonoids are epigallocatechin gallate (EGCG) (Fig. **34**), epigallocatechin (Fig. **35**), epicatechin (Fig. **36**), quercetin (Fig. **37**), apigenin (Fig. **38**), rutin (Fig. **39**), and naringenin (Fig. **40**) [38]. Some of the soy isoflavones, such as genistein (Fig. **41**), daidzein (Fig. **42**) are peroxisome proliferator-activated receptors (PPARs) activators which are known to modulate the glucose and fat homeostasis in the body [47]. Flavonoids from citrus fruits like hesperidin (Fig. **43**) and naringin (Fig. **44**) are known to possess anti-glycemic effects by targeting glycogen synthesis, glycolysis and gluconeogenesis [48].

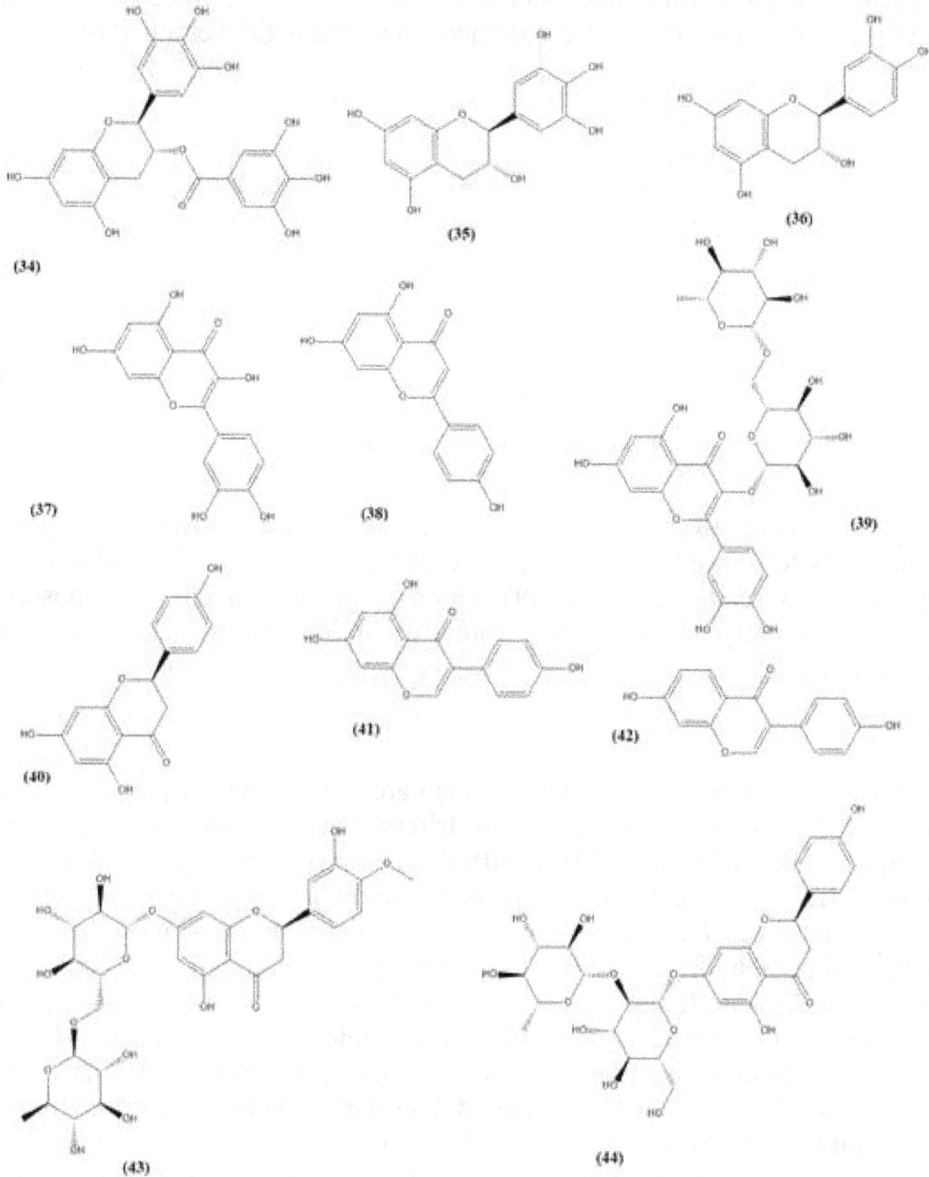

Fig. (4). Chemical structures of bioactive compounds of flavonoids phytochemical class.

Coumarins

Coumarins are a large class of C6-C3 derivatives belonging to the benzo-α-pyrone group, which are present in the free form or in the combined form found in higher plants such as Rutaceae and Umbelliferae family [49]. Osthole (Fig. **45**), esculin (Fig. **46**), and fraxetin (Fig. **47**) which are a type of coumarins, have been shown to improve the glomerular and islet structure of diabetic mice with reduced mesangial matrix and glomerular basement membrane thickening [50].

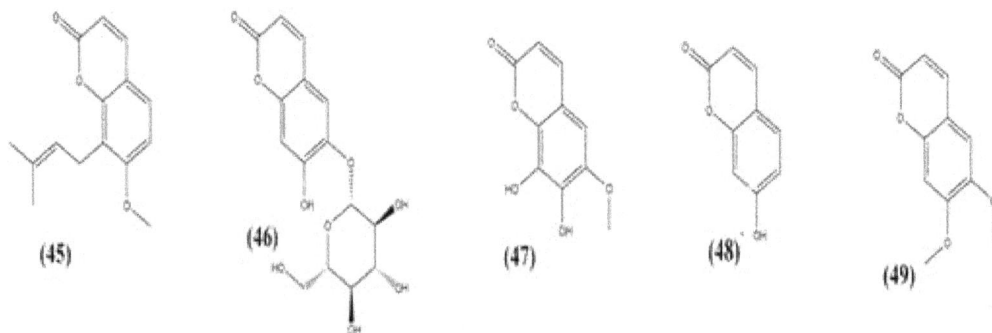

Fig. (5). Chemical structures of bioactive compounds of coumarins phytochemical class.

Umbelliferone (Fig. **48**), another variant of coumarin also known to bring blood glucose levels to normal level in the mice diabetes model [51]. A derivative of coumarin called scoparone (Fig. **49**) which is present in chestnut, possesses antidiabetic property mediated by protective action on the pancreas against inflammation [52].

Saponins

Saponins are the bioactive compounds which are predominantly present in plants and chemically they occur as polycyclic triterpenes or steroids with glycosides [53]. Saponins like stigmasterol (Fig. **50**), diosgenin (Fig. **51**), quercitol (Fig. **52**), gymnemic acid, *etc.* are known to possess potent antihyperglycaemic activity [54]. Diosgenin from *Trigonella foenumgraecum* works by regulating the glucose transport and carbohydrate metabolism process [55]. Gymnemic acid which is an important constituent found in *G. sylvestre* leaves, causes hypoglycemia and thereby helps in the management of DM. Gymnemic acid stimulates the pancreas and increases insulin secretion [56]. Gymnema leaf extract contains another hypoglycemic bioactive compound called 'Gurmarin', which alters the ability of the taste buds to taste sweet, thereby inhibiting the sweet taste sensation, it ultimately limits their sweet intake [57]. Gymnema leaf extract at the molecular level has proven to alleviate the endoplasmic reticulum or ER stress and facilitates insulin signal transduction mechanism [58]. Panaxan A, B, C, D, E are the steroidal saponin moieties obtained from the extract of *Panax quinquefolium* and have shown protective effects on pancreas by restoring the β-cell of pancreas and facilitates insulin secretion [59].

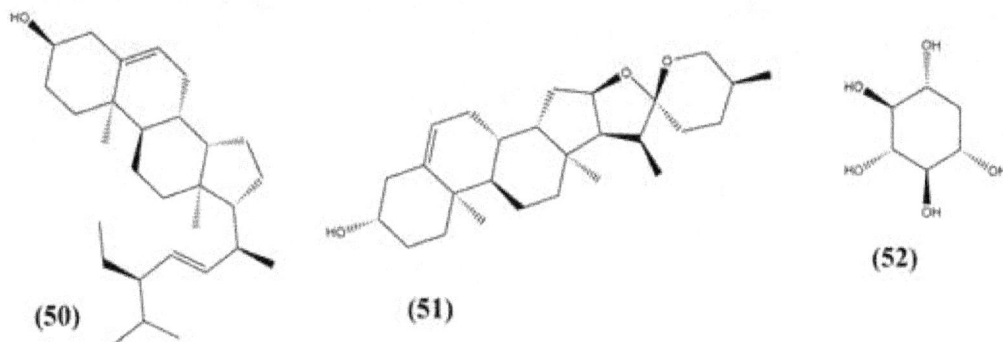

(50)   (51)   (52)

Fig. (6). Chemical structures of bioactive compounds of saponins phytochemical class.

Vitamins

Vitamins are essential bioactive compounds that need to be ingested in small amounts in order to complete the human diet [6, 60]. The vitamins including A, B, C, D, and E have been shown to strengthen human body by acting as an immunomodulator and thus strengthening the body by preventing from various diseases [61]. Tocopherol (Fig. **53**) (precursor of Vitamin E) and carotenoids (Fig. **54**) (precursors of Vitamin A), the two common natural vitamins which can be obtained from the seeds of *Cucurbita pepo* (pumpkin) and carrot. Tocopherol and carotenoids have been shown to have antidiabetic effects on experimental diabetic models [62]. Besides fish, mushrooms are often considered as another valuable source of vitamin D (Fig. **55**), in particular of vitamin D_2 (Fig. **56**). However, the major natural vitamin D metabolite in fungi and yeast [63]. Vitamin D has a strong implication in the pathogenesis of DM specifically in type 2 DM [64]. Vitamin D level and β-cell functioning are positively correlated. Vitamin D deficiency leads to type 2 DM and people with type 2 DM are also prone to vitamin D deficiency and related pathologies. Vitamin D supplementation improves fasting plasma glucose and insulin level [65]. Vitamin C, commonly called as ascorbic acid, which is abundantly present in citrus fruits is known to decrease blood glucose [66]. Biotin (Fig. **57**) (Vitamin H), when administered as an adjuvant with other mainline antidiabetic medication has shown better glucose level regulation in obese patients with type 2 DM [67].

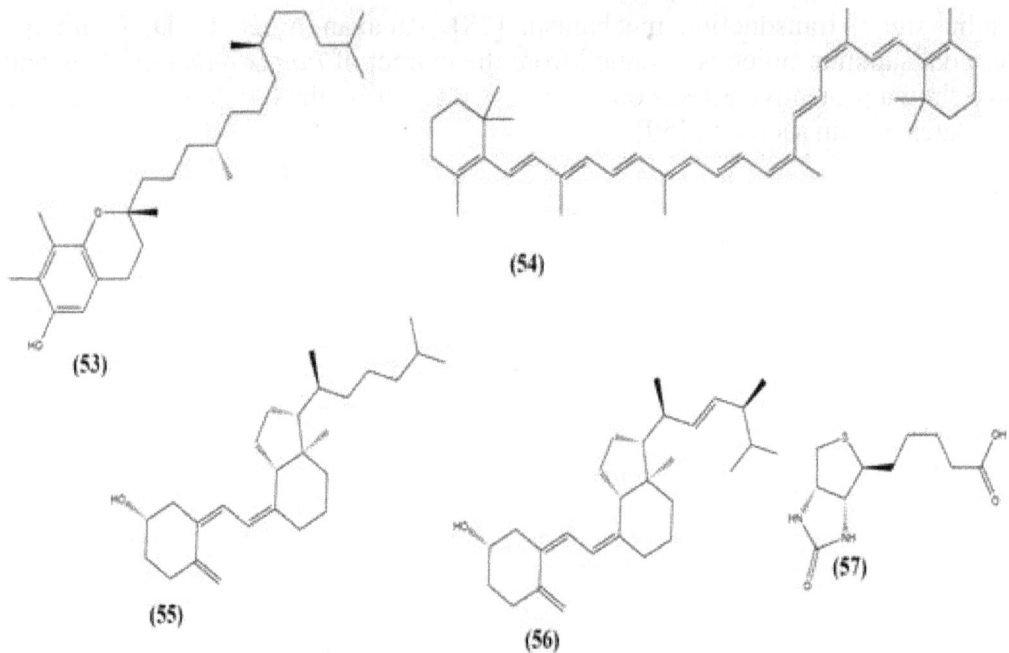

Fig. (7). Chemical structures of bioactive compounds - vitamins.

Other Compounds /Metabolites

Berry fruits are a rich source of anthocyanins which have potency to alleviate hyperglycemia, mostly *via* glucosidase inhibitory activity [68]. Allicin (Fig. **58**), and alliin (Fig. **59**) are sulfur containing bioactive compounds which are obtained from *Allium sativum* and possess antidiabetic activity. These ameliorate high blood glucose level by promoting glycogen synthesis and thus making less glucose available in the blood [69]. *Momordica charantia* contains an amino acid-based bioactive compound called polypeptide-P is which reduces hyperglycemia by both the mechanisms, which are by promoting insulin secretion as well as glycogen synthesis [70]. Another bioactive compound which is a dimeric guianolides called as lactucain C (Fig. **60**) have pancreatic cyto-regenerative effects on β cells and thus enhances insulin biosynthesis and secretion. It is obtained from *Lactuca indica*, and contains another important furofuran lignan called lactucaside (Fig. **61**), which also possesses antidiabetic effects [71].

Seaweeds

Seaweeds are not a phytochemical class, but as these are a rich source of bioactive compounds obtained from the sea, the chapter would not have been completed without its discussion. Seaweeds contain carotenoids, polysaccharides, vitamins, polyphenols, phycobilins, phycocyanins, and many other phytoconstituents which are all known to possess beneficial applications for good health [72]. It has been found that intake of *Fucus vesiculosus* and *Ascophyllum nodosum* was linked with improved insulin regulation and sensitivity in clinical trials. These seaweeds contain dietary fibers, monounsaturated fatty acids and polyunsaturated fatty acids, commonly known as MUFA (Fig. **62**) and PUFA (Fig. **63**), respectively [73], all of them are known to regulate blood glucose levels [74].

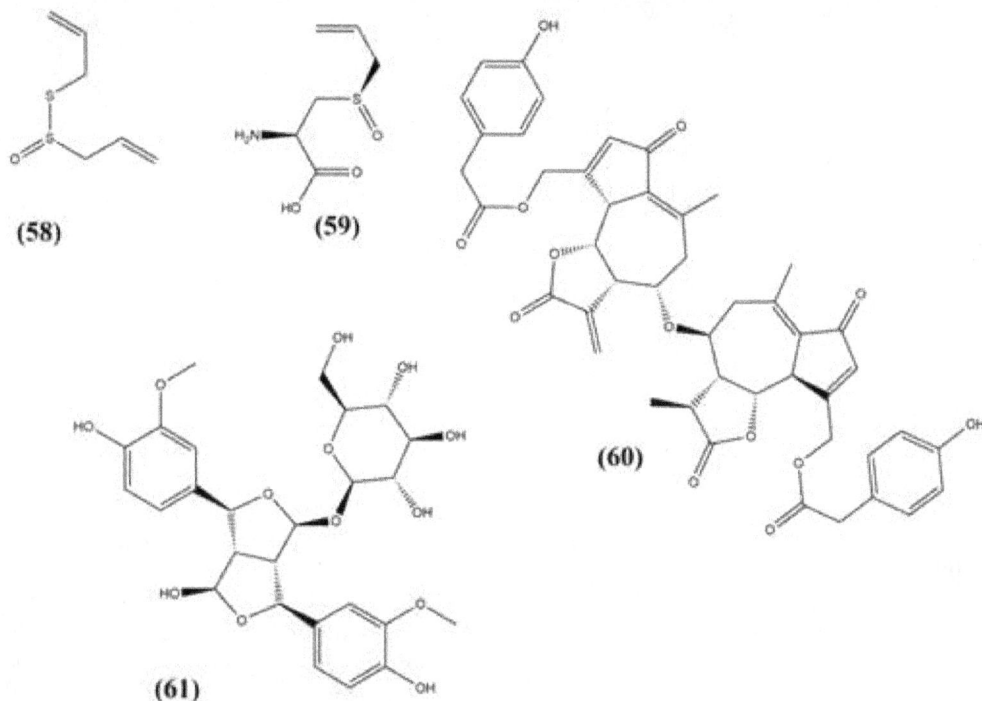

Fig. (8). Chemical structures of other metabolites bioactive compounds of plant origin.

Some bioactive compounds from seaweeds, namely eckol (Fig. **64**), dieckol (Fig. **65**), phloroglucinol (Fig. **66**), phloroeckol (Fig. **67**), phlorotannin (Fig. **68**) *etc.*, work by inhibiting important enzymes involved in glucose absorption (α-glucosidase) and excretion (DPP-4) [75]. Along with this, these stimulate incretin hormones and ameliorate insulin sensitivity and which are crucial processes in diabetes [73]. Moreover, the extracts from the seaweed are also known to exert anti-diabetic effects by enhancing the glucose uptake by the cell, and by providing cytoprotection to the pancreatic β-cells [76, 77].

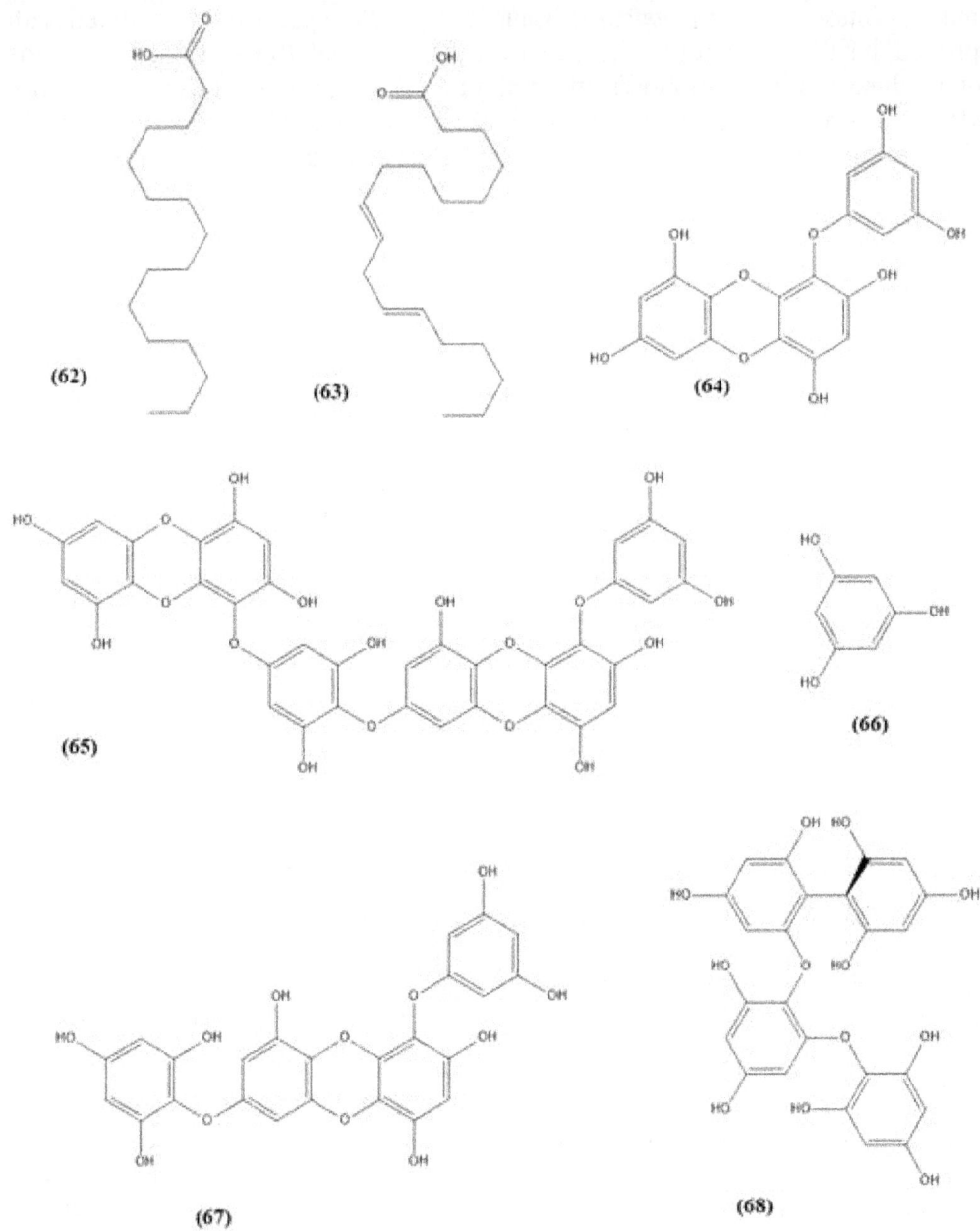

Fig. (9). Chemical structures of bioactive compounds obtained from seaweeds.

Some antidiabetic plants with their mechanism of action have been tabulated (Table **1**). An overall pictorial representation of the mechanism of action of various plant based bioactive compounds has been presented (Fig. **69**). Similarly, Fig. (**70**) shows inhibitory action of plant based antidiabetic compounds in various pathways related to DM.

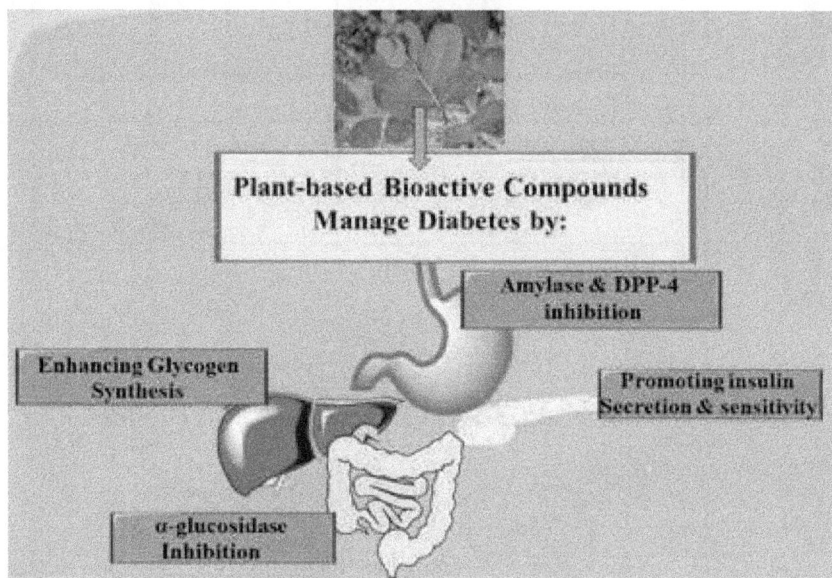

Fig. (10). Mechanism of action of plant based bioactive compounds.

Table 1. Antidiabetic Plant based bioactive compounds with their mechanism of action.

Mechanism of Action	Bioactive Compound	Plant Source	References
α-glucosidase inhibition	Vasicine and vasicinol Mangiferin Anthocyanins	*Adhatodavasica* *Salaciachinensis, Mangifera* *indica* Black berries	[25] [38] [68]
Enhancing Glycogen synthesis	Momordinmomordicine I, momorcharaside A, polypeptide-P hesperidin and naringin Allicin, and alliin	*Momordica charantia* Citrus fruits *Allium Sativum*	[27] [71] [48] [69]
Promoting insulin secretion	Lactucain C Polypeptide-P Vitamin D quercetin, apigenin, rutin	*Latuca indica* *Momordica charantia* Mushroom Flavanoid containing plants like buckwheat, citrus fruits.	[73] [72] [62] [38]

(Table 1) cont.....

Cytoprotecting and regenerating β cells	Panaxan A, B, C	*Panax quinquefolium*	[53]
	Marmesin, aegelin, marmelosin	*Aegle marmelos*	[26]
	Scoparone	Chestnut	[59]
	Dieckol, Phloroglucinol	Seaweeds	[69]
	Lactucain C	*Latuca indica*	[73]
Ameliorating insulin sensitivity	Phloroeckol, Phlorotannin	Seaweeds	[68]
	phycobilins, phycocyanins	Seaweeds	[65]
	curcumin	*Curcuma longa*	[42]
	Anthraquinone glycoside	Aloe vera (*Aloe barbadensis*)	[32]
	chlorogenic acid	*Cinnamomum verum*	[19]
Modulating Glucose transport	Berberine	*Tinosporacordifolia*	[24]
	Resveratrol	*Berries*	[34]
	Chlorogenic and ferulic acids	*Cinnamom*	[39]
	Diosgenin	*Trigonellafoenum*	[49]

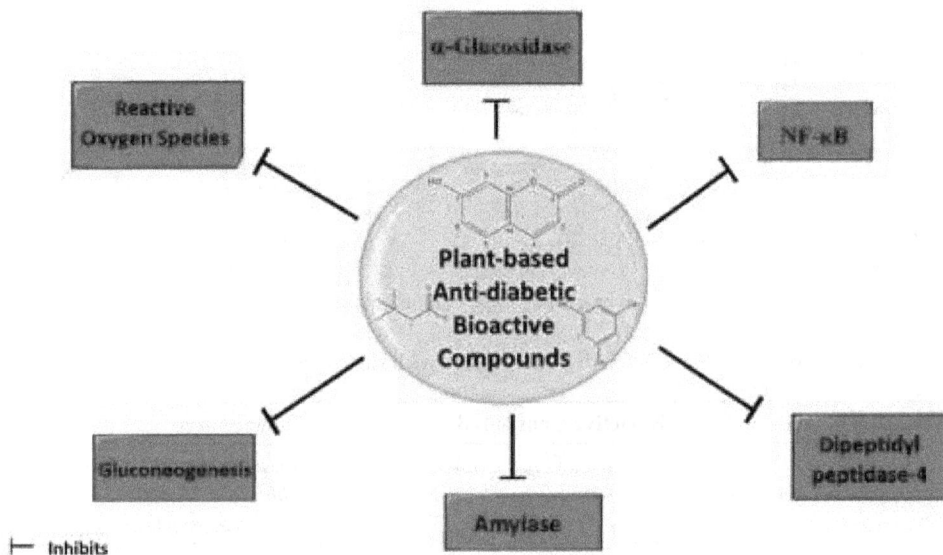

Fig. (11). Inhibitory action of plant based antidiabetic compounds in various pathways related to diabetes.

CONCLUDING REMARKS

Diabetes mellitus is a metabolic disorder manifested by a reduction in the production of insulin or reinforcement in the resistance to its action. DM is still a major cause of morbidity, mortality, and an economic burden to the world. Although, the medical field has developed much, but still there is no exact cure for the same. Nature has given us the diversity of plants and infinite bioactive compounds. Interestingly, the most common modern-era medicines constitute drugs like aspirin, quinine, digitalis, vincristine, taxol, *etc*. are plant based only. In this chapter, we have compiled up information on a list of bioactive compounds which are known to have antidiabetic effects with investigated molecular mechanisms, but still, further detailed studies would help to establish their mechanisms of actions and would ensure their safety as well. These bioactive compounds will ensure a much better multimodal treatment approach which is requisite for the management of DM. Also, the accessibility and comparative better efficacy and safety profile of the bioactive compounds make them better substitutes and adjuvants for the management of DM. Consumption of food and medicinal plants containing bioactive compounds could help not only diabetes but also help improve health, delaying aging, and better memory as well.

CONSENT FOR PUBLICATION

Not applicable.

CONFLICT OF INTEREST

The authors declare no conflict of interest, financial or otherwise.

ACKNOWLEDGEMENTS

The authors are thankful to Dr. N. Srikanth, Director General, Central Council for Research in Ayurvedic Sciences, Ministry of AYUSH, Government of India for his continuous encouragement, guidance and support.

REFERENCES

[1]   Guaadaoui A, Benaicha S, Elmajdoub N, Bellaoui M, Hamal A. What is a bioactive compound? A combined definition for a preliminary consensus. Int J Food Sci Nutr 2014; 3(3): 174-9.
        [http://dx.doi.org/10.11648/j.ijnfs.20140303.16]

[2]   Zhao Y, Wu Y, Wang M. Bioactive Substances of Plant Origin 30. Handbook of food chemistry, 2015, 967.

[3]   Henry AG, Brooks AS, Piperno DR. Microfossils in calculus demonstrate consumption of plants and cooked foods in Neanderthal diets (Shanidar III, Iraq; Spy I and II, Belgium). Proc Natl Acad Sci USA 2011; 108(2): 486-91.
        [http://dx.doi.org/10.1073/pnas.1016868108] [PMID: 21187393]

[4]   Petrovska BB. Historical review of Medicinal Plants usage. Pharmacognosy Reviews 2012; 6(11): 1-5.

[5]   Bernhoft A. A brief review on bioactive compounds in plants. Bioactive compounds in plants-benefits and risks for man and animals, 2010, 50, 11-17.

[6]   Hamzalıoğlu A, Gökmen V. Interaction between Bioactive Carbonyl Compounds and Asparagine and Impact on Acrylamide.Acrylamide in Food: Analysis, Content and Potential Health Effects. 2016; pp. 355-76.
        [http://dx.doi.org/10.1016/B978-0-12-802832-2.00018-8]

[7]   Dabeek WM, Marra MV. Dietary quercetin. Nutrients 2019; 11(10): 2288.
        [http://dx.doi.org/10.3390/nu11102288] [PMID: 31557798]

[8]   Teodoro AJ. Bioactive compounds of Food: Their role in the prevention and treatment of Disease.

Oxidative Medicine and Cellular Longevity 2019; 1-4.

[9]   Hernandez DF, Cervantes EL, Luna-Vital DA, Mojica L. Food-derived bioactive compounds with anti-aging potential for nutricosmetic and cosmeceutical products. Crit Rev Food Sci Nutr 2020; 1-16.
[PMID: 32772550]

[10]   Si H, Liu D. Dietary antiaging phytochemicals and mechanisms associated with prolonged survival. J Nutr Biochem 2014; 25(6): 581-91.
[http://dx.doi.org/10.1016/j.jnutbio.2014.02.001] [PMID: 24742470]

[11]   Venkatesan R, Ji E, Kim SY. Phytochemicals that regulate neurodegenerative disease by targeting neurotrophins: a comprehensive review. Biomed Res In 2015; 2015: 814068.

[12]   Ortega AMM, Campos MRS. Bioactive compounds as therapeutic alternatives.M.R.S. Campos (Ed.), Bioactive Compounds, Woodhead Publishing (2019), pp. 247-264.
[http://dx.doi.org/10.1016/B978-0-12-814774-0.00013-X]

[13]   Wise J. Metrformin is backed as first line therapy for type 2 diabetes. The BMJ 2016; (353): i2236.

[14]   Kumar A, Bharti SK, Kumar A. Type 2 diabetes mellitus: the concerned complications and target organs. Apollo Medicine 2014; 11(3): 161-6.
[http://dx.doi.org/10.1016/j.apme.2014.01.009]

[15]   Chang CL, Lin Y, Bartolome AP, Chen Y-C, Chiu S-C, Yang W-C. Herbal therapies for type 2 diabetes mellitus: chemistry, biology, and potential application of selected plants and compounds. Evidence-Based Complementary and Alternative Medicine 2013; 2013: 378657.
[http://dx.doi.org/10.1155/2013/378657]

[16]   Alarcon-Aguilara FJ, Roman-Ramos R, Perez-Gutierrez S, Aguilar-Contreras A, Contreras-Weber CC, Flores-Saenz JL. Study of the anti-hyperglycemic effect of plants used as antidiabetics. J Ethnopharmacol 1998; 61(2): 101-10.
[http://dx.doi.org/10.1016/S0378-8741(98)00020-8] [PMID: 9683340]

[17]   Tan BL, Norhaizan ME, Liew WPP, Sulaiman Rahman H. Antioxidant and oxidative stress. Front Pharmacol 2018; 9: 1162.
[http://dx.doi.org/10.3389/fphar.2018.01162] [PMID: 30405405]

[18]   Dembinska-Kiec A, Mykkänen O, Kiec-Wilk B, Mykkänen H. Antioxidant phytochemicals against type 2 diabetes. British Journal of Nutrition, 2008, 99, (E-S1), ES109-ES117.

[19]   Zhu R, Liu H, Liu C, *et al.* Cinnamaldehyde in diabetes: A review of pharmacology, pharmacokinetics and safety. Pharmacol Res 2017; 122: 78-89.
[http://dx.doi.org/10.1016/j.phrs.2017.05.019] [PMID: 28559210]

[20]   Rao PV, Gan SH. Cinnamon: a multifaceted medicinal plant. Evidence-Based Complementary and Alternative Medicine 2014; 2014: 642942.
[http://dx.doi.org/10.1155/2014/642942]

[21]   Gruenwald J, Freder J, Armbruester N. Cinnamon and Health. Crit Rev Food Sci Nutr 2010; 50(9): 822-34.
[http://dx.doi.org/10.1080/10408390902773052] [PMID: 20924865]

[22]   Fattorusso E, Taglialatela-Scafati O. Modern alkaloids: structure, isolation, synthesis, and biology. John Wiley & Sons, 2007.

[23]   Dey P. Kundu, A.; Kumar, A.; Gupta, M.; Lee, B.M.; Bhakta, T.; Dash, S.; Kim, H.S.Recent Advances in Natural Products Analysis. Elsevier 2020; pp. 505-67.
[http://dx.doi.org/10.1016/B978-0-12-816455-6.00015-9]

[24]   Singh S, Pandey S, Srivastava S, Gupta V, Patro B, Ghosh A. Chemistry and medicinal properties of Tinospora cordifolia. Guduchi 2003.

[25]   Gao H, Huang YN, Gao B, Li P, Inagaki C, Kawabata J. Inhibitory effect on α-glucosidase by Adhatoda vasica Nees. Food Chem 2008; 108(3): 965-72.

[http://dx.doi.org/10.1016/j.foodchem.2007.12.002] [PMID: 26065759]

[26]   Kamalakkannan N, Prince PSM. The effect of Aegle marmelos fruit extract in streptozotocin diabetes: a histopathological study. J Herb Pharmacother 2005; 5(3): 87-96.
[http://dx.doi.org/10.1080/J157v05n03_08] [PMID: 16520300]

[27]   Cooper EJ, Hudson AL, Parker CA, Morgan NG. Effects of the β-carbolines, harmane and pinoline, on insulin secretion from isolated human islets of Langerhans. Eur J Pharmacol 2003; 482(1-3): 189-96.
[http://dx.doi.org/10.1016/j.ejphar.2003.09.039] [PMID: 14660022]

[28]   Akhtar MS, Iqbal J. Evaluation of the hypoglycaemic effect of Achyranthes aspera in normal and alloxan-diabetic rabbits. J Ethnopharmacol 1991; 31(1): 49-57.
[http://dx.doi.org/10.1016/0378-8741(91)90143-2] [PMID: 2030593]

[29]   Shah A, Varma C, Patankar S, Kadam V. Plant Glycosides and Aglycones Displaying Antiproliferative and Antitumour Activities – A Review. Curr Bioact Compd 2013; 9(4): 288-305.
[http://dx.doi.org/10.2174/1573407209999131231095332]

[30]   Adki KM. Kulkarni, Y.A. Structure and Health Effects of Natural Products on Diabetes. Springer 2021; pp. 81-102.
[http://dx.doi.org/10.1007/978-981-15-8791-7_5]

[31]   Noor H, Ashcroft SJH. Insulinotropic activity ofTinospora crispa extract: effect on ß-cell Ca2+ handling. Phytother Res 1998; 12(2): 98-102.
[http://dx.doi.org/10.1002/(SICI)1099-1573(199803)12:2<98::AID-PTR195>3.0.CO;2-F]

[32]   Cheng FR, Cui HX, Fang JL, Yuan K, Guo Y. Ameliorative effect and mechanism of the purified anthraquinone-glycoside preparation from Rheum Palmatum L. on type 2 diabetes mellitus. Molecules 2019; 24(8): 1454.
[http://dx.doi.org/10.3390/molecules24081454] [PMID: 31013790]

[33]   Pandey KB, Rizvi SI. Plant polyphenols as dietary antioxidants in human health and disease. Oxid Med Cell Longev 2009; 2(5): 270-8.
[http://dx.doi.org/10.4161/oxim.2.5.9498] [PMID: 20716914]

[34]   Michael LF, Wu Z, Cheatham RB, *et al.* Restoration of insulin-sensitive glucose transporter (GLUT4) gene expression in muscle cells by the transcriptional coactivator PGC-1. Proc Natl Acad Sci USA 2001; 98(7): 3820-5.
[http://dx.doi.org/10.1073/pnas.061035098] [PMID: 11274399]

[35]   Bhatt JK, Thomas S, Nanjan MJ. Resveratrol supplementation improves glycemic control in type 2 diabetes mellitus. Nutr Res 2012; 32(7): 537-41.
[http://dx.doi.org/10.1016/j.nutres.2012.06.003] [PMID: 22901562]

[36]   Poulsen MM, Vestergaard PF, Clasen BF, *et al.* High-dose resveratrol supplementation in obese men: an investigator-initiated, randomized, placebo-controlled clinical trial of substrate metabolism, insulin sensitivity, and body composition. Diabetes 2013; 62(4): 1186-95.
[http://dx.doi.org/10.2337/db12-0975] [PMID: 23193181]

[37]   Kumar A, Negi G, Sharma SS. Neuroprotection by resveratrol in diabetic neuropathy: concepts & mechanisms. Curr Med Chem 2013; 20(36): 4640-5.
[http://dx.doi.org/10.2174/09298673113209990151] [PMID: 24206125]

[38]   Hannan JMA, Marenah L, Ali L, Rokeya B, Flatt PR, Abdel-Wahab YHA. Ocimum sanctum leaf extracts stimulate insulin secretion from perfused pancreas, isolated islets and clonal pancreatic β-cells. J Endocrinol 2006; 189(1): 127-36.
[http://dx.doi.org/10.1677/joe.1.06615] [PMID: 16614387]

[39]   Ong KW, Hsu A, Tan BKH. Chlorogenic acid stimulates glucose transport in skeletal muscle *via* AMPK activation: a contributor to the beneficial effects of coffee on diabetes. PLoS One 2012; 7(3): e32718.
[http://dx.doi.org/10.1371/journal.pone.0032718] [PMID: 22412912]

[40]　Pérez-Torres I, Ruiz-Ramírez A, Baños G, El-Hafidi M. Hibiscus sabdariffa Linnaeus (Malvaceae), curcumin and resveratrol as alternative medicinal agents against metabolic syndrome. Cardiovascular & Hematological Agents in Medicinal Chemistry (Formerly Current Medicinal Chemistry-Cardiovascular & Hematological Agents), 2013, 11, (1), 25-37.

[41]　Kuroda M, Mimaki Y, Nishiyama T, *et al.* Hypoglycemic effects of turmeric (*Curcuma longa L.* rhizomes) on genetically diabetic KK-Ay mice. Biol Pharm Bull 2005; 28(5): 937-9.
[http://dx.doi.org/10.1248/bpb.28.937] [PMID: 15863912]

[42]　Yekollu SK, Thomas R, O'Sullivan B. Targeting curcusomes to inflammatory dendritic cells inhibits NF-κB and improves insulin resistance in obese mice. Diabetes 2011; 60(11): 2928-38.
[http://dx.doi.org/10.2337/db11-0275] [PMID: 21885868]

[43]　Joshi RP, Negi G, Kumar A, *et al.* SNEDDS curcumin formulation leads to enhanced protection from pain and functional deficits associated with diabetic neuropathy: An insight into its mechanism for neuroprotection. Nanomedicine 2013; 9(6): 776-85.
[http://dx.doi.org/10.1016/j.nano.2013.01.001] [PMID: 23347896]

[44]　Khajehdehi P, Pakfetrat M, Javidnia K, *et al.* Oral supplementation of turmeric attenuates proteinuria, transforming growth factor-β and interleukin-8 levels in patients with overt type 2 diabetic nephropathy: A randomized, double-blind and placebo-controlled study. Scand J Urol Nephrol 2011; 45(5): 365-70.
[http://dx.doi.org/10.3109/00365599.2011.585622] [PMID: 21627399]

[45]　Ayres DC, Loike JD. Lignans: chemical, biological and clinical properties. Cambridge university press 1990.
[http://dx.doi.org/10.1017/CBO9780511983665]

[46]　Mishra S, Verma P. Flaxseed- Bioactive compounds and health significance. IOSR J Humanit Soc Sci 2013; 17(3): 46-50.
[http://dx.doi.org/10.9790/0837-1734650]

[47]　Li Y, Qi Y, Huang TH, Yamahara J, Roufogalis BD. Pomegranate flower: a unique traditional antidiabetic medicine with dual PPAR-α/-γ activator properties. Diabetes Obes Metab 2008; 10(1): 10-7.
[PMID: 18095947]

[48]　Jung UJ, Lee MK, Jeong KS, Choi MS. The hypoglycemic effects of hesperidin and naringin are partly mediated by hepatic glucose-regulating enzymes in C57BL/KsJ-db/db mice. J Nutr 2004; 134(10): 2499-503.
[http://dx.doi.org/10.1093/jn/134.10.2499] [PMID: 15465737]

[49]　Jain P, Joshi H. Coumarin: chemical and pharmacological profile. J Appl Pharm Sci 2012; 2(6): 236-40.

[50]　Li H, Yao Y, Li L. Coumarins as potential antidiabetic agents. J Pharm Pharmacol 2017; 69(10): 1253-64.
[http://dx.doi.org/10.1111/jphp.12774] [PMID: 28675434]

[51]　Ramesh B, Pugalendi KV. Antihyperglycemic effect of umbelliferone in streptozotocin-diabetic rats. J Med Food 2006; 9(4): 562-6.
[http://dx.doi.org/10.1089/jmf.2006.9.562] [PMID: 17201645]

[52]　Kim EK, Kwon KB, Lee JH, *et al.* Inhibition of cytokine-mediated nitric oxide synthase expression in rat insulinoma cells by scoparone. Biol Pharm Bull 2007; 30(2): 242-6.
[http://dx.doi.org/10.1248/bpb.30.242] [PMID: 17268059]

[53]　Howes MJR, Perry NSL, Houghton PJ. Plants with traditional uses and activities, relevant to the management of Alzheimer's disease and other cognitive disorders. Phytother Res 2003; 17(1): 1-18.
[http://dx.doi.org/10.1002/ptr.1280] [PMID: 12557240]

[54]　Ponnachan P, Paulose C, Panikkar K. Effect of leaf extract of Aegle marmelose in diabetic rats 1993.

[55] Khosla P, Gupta D, Nagpal R. Effect of Trigonella foenum graecum (Fenugreek) on serum lipids in normal and diabetic rats. Indian J Pharmacol 1995; 27(2): 89.

[56] Persaud SJ, Al-Majed H, Raman A, Jones PM. Gymnema sylvestre stimulates insulin release *in vitro* by increased membrane permeability. J Endocrinol 1999; 163(2): 207-12.
[http://dx.doi.org/10.1677/joe.0.1630207] [PMID: 10556769]

[57] Vaidya S. Review on gymnema: an herbal medicine for diabetes management. Pharmacia 2011; 1(2): 37-42.

[58] Li Y, Sun M, Liu Y, Liang J, Wang T, Zhang Z. Gymnemic acid alleviates type 2 diabetes mellitus and suppresses endoplasmic reticulum stress *in vivo* and *in vitro*. J Agric Food Chem 2019; 67(13): 3662-9.
[http://dx.doi.org/10.1021/acs.jafc.9b00431] [PMID: 30864442]

[59] Ma SW, Benzie IF, Chu TT, Fok BS, Tomlinson B, Critchley LA. Effect of *Panax ginseng* supplementation on biomarkers of glucose tolerance, antioxidant status and oxidative stress in type 2 diabetic subjects: results of a placebo-controlled human intervention trial. Diabetes Obes Metab 2008; 10(11): 1125-7.
[http://dx.doi.org/10.1111/j.1463-1326.2008.00858.x] [PMID: 18355331]

[60] Webb ME, Marquet A, Mendel RR, Rébeillé F, Smith AG. Elucidating biosynthetic pathways for vitamins and cofactors. Nat Prod Rep 2007; 24(5): 988-1008.
[http://dx.doi.org/10.1039/b703105j] [PMID: 17898894]

[61] Aslam MF, Majeed S, Aslam S, Irfan J. Vitamins: Key role players in boosting up immune response—A mini review. Vitam Miner 2017; 6(1): 2376-1318.

[62] Bharti SK, Kumar A, Sharma NK, *et al.* Tocopherol from seeds of Cucurbita pepo against diabetes: Validation by *in vivo* experiments supported by computational docking. J Formos Med Assoc 2013; 112(11): 676-90.
[http://dx.doi.org/10.1016/j.jfma.2013.08.003] [PMID: 24344360]

[63] Baur AC, Brandsch C, König B, Hirche F, Stangl GI. Plant oils as potential sources of vitamin D. Front Nutr 2016; 3: 29.
[http://dx.doi.org/10.3389/fnut.2016.00029] [PMID: 27570765]

[64] Mathieu C, Gysemans C, Giulietti A, Bouillon R. Vitamin D and diabetes. Diabetologia 2005; 48(7): 1247-57.
[http://dx.doi.org/10.1007/s00125-005-1802-7] [PMID: 15971062]

[65] Talaei A, Mohamadi M, Adgi Z. The effect of vitamin D on insulin resistance in patients with type 2 diabetes. Diabetol Metab Syndr 2013; 5(1): 8.
[http://dx.doi.org/10.1186/1758-5996-5-8] [PMID: 23443033]

[66] Afkhami-Ardekani M, Shojaoddiny-Ardekani A. Effect of vitamin C on blood glucose, serum lipids & serum insulin in type 2 diabetes patients. Indian J Med Res 2007; 126(5): 471-4.
[PMID: 18160753]

[67] Albarracin CA, Fuqua BC, Evans JL, Goldfine ID. Chromium picolinate and biotin combination improves glucose metabolism in treated, uncontrolled overweight to obese patients with type 2 diabetes. Diabetes Metab Res Rev 2008; 24(1): 41-51.
[http://dx.doi.org/10.1002/dmrr.755] [PMID: 17506119]

[68] Grace MH, Ribnicky DM, Kuhn P, *et al.* Hypoglycemic activity of a novel anthocyanin-rich formulation from lowbush blueberry, Vaccinium angustifolium Aiton. Phytomedicine 2009; 16(5): 406-15.
[http://dx.doi.org/10.1016/j.phymed.2009.02.018] [PMID: 19303751]

[69] Kumar GR, Reddy KP. Reduced nociceptive responses in mice with alloxan induced hyperglycemia after garlic (*Allium sativum* Linn.) treatment. Indian J Exp Biol 1999; 37(7): 662-6.

[70]   Saeed F, Afzaal M, Niaz B, *et al.* Bitter melon (*Momordica charantia*): a natural healthy vegetable. Int J Food Prop 2018; 21(1): 1270-90.
[http://dx.doi.org/10.1080/10942912.2018.1446023]

[71]   Hou CC, Lin SJ, Cheng JT, Hsu FL. Antidiabetic dimeric guianolides and a lignan glycoside from Lactuca indica. J Nat Prod 2003; 66(5): 625-9.
[http://dx.doi.org/10.1021/np0205349] [PMID: 12762795]

[72]   Kadam SU, Prabhasankar P. Marine foods as functional ingredients in bakery and pasta products. Food Res Int 2010; 43(8): 1975-80.
[http://dx.doi.org/10.1016/j.foodres.2010.06.007]

[73]   Sharifuddin Y, Chin YX, Lim PE, Phang SM. Potential bioactive compounds from seaweed for diabetes management. Mar Drugs 2015; 13(8): 5447-91.
[http://dx.doi.org/10.3390/md13085447] [PMID: 26308010]

[74]   Telle-Hansen VH, Gaundal L, Myhrstad MCW. Polyunsaturated fatty acids and glycemic control in type 2 diabetes. Nutrients 2019; 11(5): 1067.
[http://dx.doi.org/10.3390/nu11051067] [PMID: 31091649]

[75]   Min SH, Yoon JH, Hahn S, Cho YM. Efficacy and safety of combination therapy with an α-glucosidase inhibitor and a dipeptidyl peptidase-4 inhibitor in patients with type 2 diabetes mellitus: A systematic review with meta-analysis. J Diabetes Investig 2018; 9(4): 893-902.
[http://dx.doi.org/10.1111/jdi.12754] [PMID: 28950431]

[76]   Hwang PA, Hung YL, Tsai YK, Chien SY, Kong ZL. The brown seaweed Sargassum hemiphyllum exhibits α-amylase and α-glucosidase inhibitory activity and enhances insulin release *in vitro.* Cytotechnology 2015; 67(4): 653-60.
[http://dx.doi.org/10.1007/s10616-014-9745-9] [PMID: 25344877]

[77]   Shehadeh MB, Suaifan GARY, Abu-Odeh AM. Plants Secondary Metabolites as Blood Glucose-Lowering Molecules. Molecules 2021; 26(14): 4333.
[http://dx.doi.org/10.3390/molecules26144333] [PMID: 34299610]

CHAPTER 6

Marine Algal Bioactive Metabolites and their Pharmacological Applications

Neetu Kachhwaha[1], Mukesh Kumar Sharma[2], Renu Khandelwal[1] and Pallavi Kaushik[1,*]

[1] *Department of Zoology, University of Rajasthan, Jaipur-302004, India*

[2] *Department of Zoology, SPC Government College, Ajmer-305001, India*

Abstract: Thousands of bioactive components are derived from various marine macro and microalgae. Such beneficial algae are considered as a renewable and sustainable resource of bioactives with potential use as dietary food supplement, anti-viral, antiinflammatory, anti-cancerous, anti-oxidant, anti-diabetic, anti-bacterial agents which can provide nutritive and health care benefits. The biochemical infrastructure of algae comprises proteins, lipids, polysaccharides, minerals, vitamins *etc.* which can be used as nutritional and dietary sources along with use in therapeutics and cosmetics. The therapeutic and industrial applications of the algal derivatives are primarily due to the secondary metabolites such as astaxanthin, aquamin, alginates, fucoidan, omega-3-fatty acids, polyphenols, fucoxanthin, *etc.* This chapter focuses on various algae derived bioactives and their wide range of applications.

Keywords: Algae, Alginates, Aquamin, Astaxanthin, Bioactive, Fucoidan, Fucoxanthin, Polyphenols, Omega-3- fatty acids, Therapeutics.

INTRODUCTION

Algae is much familiar for their cosmopolitan distribution found anywhere in all kinds of aquatic biotypes from temperate, tropical, extremes of cold and hot regions like oceans, ponds, lakes, and wastewater due to their tremendous capability to tolerate the wide variation in physical factors. There are as many as 12,272 algae classified into red, green, blue green, and brown algae on the basis of the pigment they contain *viz* Cyanobacteria (chlorophyll-a, chlorophyll-d, chlorophyll-f, phycocyanin, phycoerythrin, phycobiliprotein), Glaucophytes (chlorophyll-a, phycobiliprotein), Phaeophyta (chlorophyll-a, chlorophyll-c, β-carotene, fucoxanthin, violaxanthin), Chlorophyta (chlorophyll-a, chlorophyll-b, β-carotene, xanthophyll), and Rhodophyta (phycocyanin, phycoerythrin, carotene,

* **Corresponding author Pallavi Kaushik:** Department of Zoology, University of Rajasthan, Jaipur-302004, India; Tel: +91-98286 96079; E-mail: pallavikaushik512@gmail.com

Mukesh Kumar Sharma and Pallavi Kaushik (Eds.)

xanthophyll) [1]. The algae can also be classified on the basis of multicellularity (macroalgae) and unicellularity (microalgae). Both the algae are photosynthetic and aquatic but macroalgae are plant-like and can be seen by naked eyes therefore, called as seaweeds while the microalgae are smaller in size, can be seen under microscope called as phytoplankton. The seaweeds and phytoplankton's both belong to the basic tropic level (primary producers) in the marine water ecosystem. These are genetically diverse group of organisms that keep balance between the abiotic and biotic factors of oceanic life directly or indirectly [2]. These are the major source of potential minerals, vitamins, lipids, polysaccharides, sterols, proteins, fibres, macro and micronutrients [3]. The ecologist, pharmacologist, researchers and aqua culturist are now more focused on the seaweeds for their tremendous chemical composition and properties. Particularly the aqua culturist started growing the sea weeds with other animal groups to generate integrated and multitrophic groups that provide both sustainability and proper management practices [4]. New era of technological evolution leads to the use of algae in diverse branches like pharmaceuticals, cosmeceuticals, nutraceuticals, therapeutics, metabolomics, biofuel production, biofertilizer production, and generation of new medicinal group because of the presence of their ultimate and distinct bioactive components [5, 6].

The bioactive compounds are primary and secondary metabolites derived from algal sources, and can be purified and isolated by different techniques. The biochemical infrastructure of the macro and microalgae comprises the variable concentration of proteins, lipids, carbohydrates, minerals, vitamins, fatty acids, *etc.*, depending upon the type of the strain and abiotic factors they live in [7]. Microalgal proteins are used as food and food by-products due to their well-defined amino acid profiling [8]; microalgal polysaccharides are used extensively in cosmetic production and hygroscopic agents [9]; their lipids are a source of biodiesel production, nutraceuticals and infant formulation [10]; and microalgal Polyunsaturated fatty acids (PUFAs) are comparable to the fish oil and used in production of high valued commercial products [10]. Other compounds like omega 3-polyunsaturated fatty acids play therapeutic role in treating chronic inflammatory diseases [11]; their carotenoids are used as anti-inflammatory bioactive compounds [12], and sulfated polysaccharides (SPS) are extensively studied in both the macro and microalgal for anti-inflammatory activity [13].

The essential benefits of algae-based metabolites can be obtained from the primary metabolites as various types of lipids, amino acids and proteins, and different carbohydrates which are generally present in various types of algae in variable concentrations. But the specific benefits of various marine macro and microalgae are due to the unique compounds called secondary metabolites. Thousands of such secondary metabolites acting as bioactive components have been extracted and screened for their potential properties such as anti-viral, anti-inflammatory, anti-cancerous, anti-oxidant, anti-diabetic, anti-bacterial, nutritive and health care benefits (Fig. **1**).

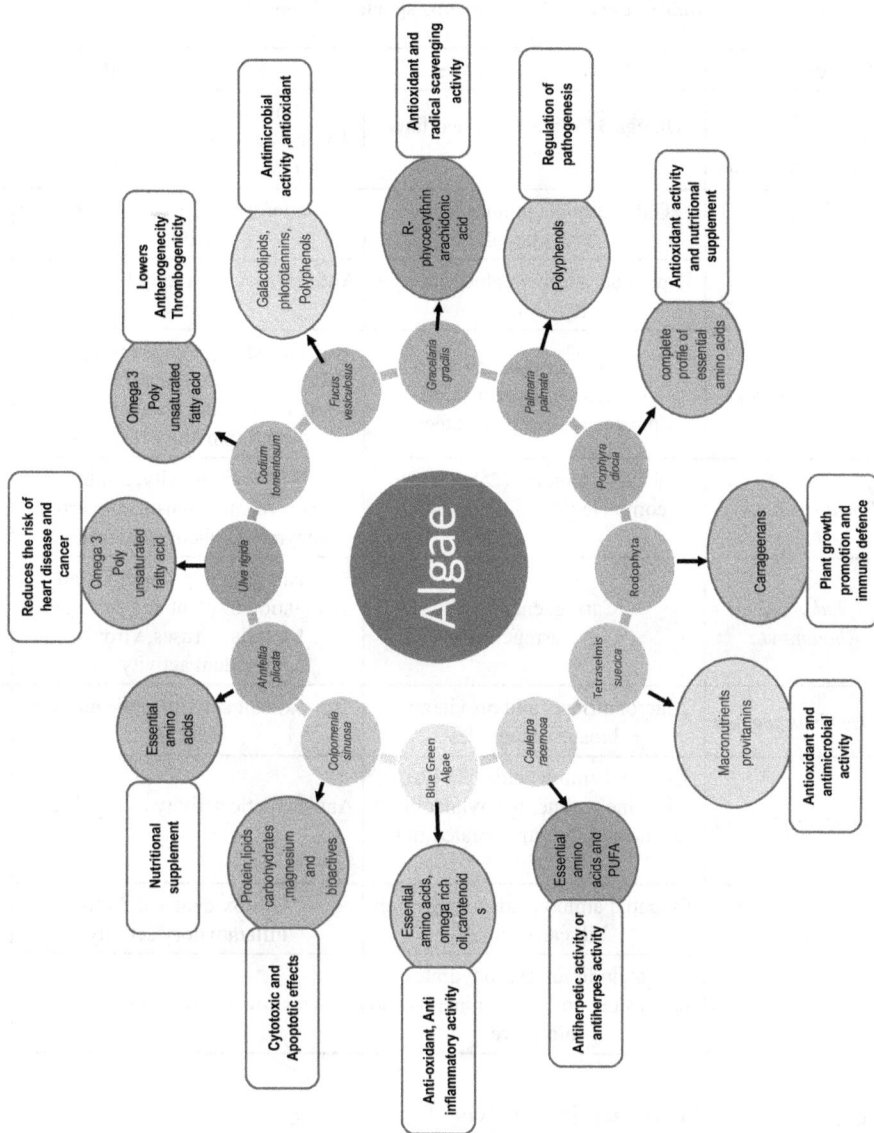

Fig. (1). Represents the Marine algae derived bioactive compounds and their potential uses.

The recent research reports on the most valuable bioactive compounds derived from marine algae are compiled and presented in this chapter (Fig. **5**). Various metabolites derived from multiple species of algae and their bioactivity are shown in Table **1**.

Table 1. Bioactivity of metabolites derived from various species of algae.

S.No.	Species Name	Bioactive Molecules	Activity or Effect	Refs.
1	*Ulva rigida*	Omega 3 Poly unsaturated fatty acids	Lower Antherogenecity, Thrombogenicity, Reduces the risk of heart disease and cancer	[14, 15]
2	*Codium tomentosum*			
3	*Fucus vesiculosus*	Galactolipids, phlorotannins, Polyphenols	Anti-microbial activity, anti-oxidant activity	[16, 17]
4	*Gracelariagracilis*	R-phycoerythrin arachidonic acid (PUFA ω-6),	Anti-oxidant and radical scavenging activity	[18]
5	*Palmaria palmate*	Polyphenols such as 4—hydroxybenzoic acid, Epicatechin, Epigallocatechin	Regulation of pathogenesis related disorder by disruption of neutrophil activation and pro control of proinflammatory response	[19]
6	*Porphyradiocia*	Rich in proteins (25%) with complete profile of essential amino acids	Anti-oxidant activity, inhibitory effects on angiotensin converting enzyme, Diphenypeptidase IV	[20, 21]
7	*Red algae Rhodophyta*	Carrageenans and oligocarrageenans	Plant growth promotion and modulation of plant defense against bacteria, viruses, viroids, antioxidant activity, *etc.*	[22, 23]
8	*Tetraselmis suecica*	Macronutrients and provitamins, bioactive peptides	Anti-oxidant activity, anti-microbial activity	[24-26]
9	*Caulerpa racemosa*	Essential amino acids like lysine, leucine, valine, phenylalanine Mono and Polyunsaturated fatty acid	Anti-herpetic activity or anti-herpes activity	[27]
10	Blue-green algae	Essential amino acids, omega rich oil, carotenoids	Anti-oxidant and Anti-inflammatory activity	[28]
11	*Colpomenia sinuosa*	Protein,lipids carbohydrates, magnesium and other minerals and bioactive	Cytotoxic and Apoptotic effects	[29]

Valuable Bioactive Compounds Derived from Algae

1. Aquamin

Aquamin is a component of red algae *Lithothamnion corallioides* and *L.*

calcareum, which inhabits the muddy or sandy substrates in shallow marine water that contains about 74 kinds of different mineral elements (higher amount of Calcium and Magnesium) [30]. *L.corallioides* is fairly unique among all the red algae as it produces a calcareous skeleton [31]. The algae are very much efficient in absorbing the trace elements from the marine sea water due to the presence of multimineral complex aquamin. Aquamin is found suitable to induce osteogenesis which is enhanced in presence of Vitamin D3 [32]. *In vitro* and *in vivo* trials are in the process to use Aquamin as a pain and stiffness reduction, supplement in knee osteoarthritis patients [33]. Aquamin, along with Vitamin D3, promotes bone regeneration, treats malfunctioning of bone strength, preserves basic bone structure [34], and prevents loss of bone minerals (Fig. **2**) [35]. Aquamin has a complex and unique structure that enables them to enhance the absorption of calcium and hence, suitable for the intake of human due to its brilliant properties like chalk free texture, lower sedimentation, allergen free, thermostable, reduced astringency, 100% seaweed product, and innocuous taste. It is best suited for the fortification of the food products (beverages, chocolates, ice creams, bread, pastas) and supplement products which can be used to manage the lipopolysaccharide induced neuroinflammation by controlling the release of inflammatory factors (TNF-alpha and IL-1 beta) by cortical glial cells, reduce symptoms of osteoarthritis, colitis, liver tumor, and loss of bone mineral density [32, 33, 36, 37].

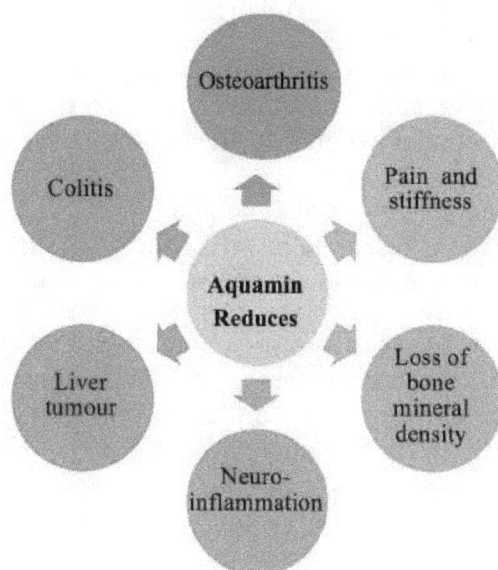

Fig. (2). The Fig. represents the potential therapeutic uses of Aquamin.

2. Fucoidan

Fucoidans complex bio-polysaccharides are composed of complex backbone consisting of molecular masses, branching loci, certain sulfated esters in patterns, monomeric sugars, and many glycosidic linkages. These sulfated minor polysaccharides are mainly composed of fucose with monosaccharides like galactose, glucose, mannose, and xylose, along with uronic acid and certain proteins [38]. Fucoidans are generally found in the cell wall of brown algae [39] such as: *Sargassum thunbergia* [40], *Ascophyllum nodosum* [41], *Chnoospora minima, Sargassum polycystum* [42], *Fucus vesiculosus* [43], and *Laminaria japonica* [38].

This complex polysaccharide has been extensively investigated for its application in therapeutics. The use of fucoidans for anti-cancerous studies is promising as it inhibits the proliferation and induces apoptosis in Human lymphoma cell lines (HS-Sultan cell lines), probably through the caspase and ERK (Extracellular signal regulatory kinase) pathways. The studies on tumour bearing mice models show that the treatment with Fucoidans can increase survival and anti-tumour activity [44] and also inhibit metastasis in lungs [40].

Within the algal group, fucoidan is one of the most effective studied extract with anti-oxidant and anti-coagulant capacities [38]. The Fucoidans extracted from sporophyll of *Undaria pinnatifida* significantly control enveloped viruses and act as an antiviral agents [45].

These marine polymers are multifunctional, with a variety of therapeutic uses including anti-thrombotic, anti-proliferative, anti-inflammatory, and anti-viral (Fig. **3**) [46]. In a study conducted on the effect of high medium and low doses of fucoidans on inflammatory response to arthritic disease showed effective inhibition using low molecular weight fucoidan [47]. The *in vivo* and *in vitro* studies conducted by some researchers [48] show its curative effects in renal failure and injury along with diabetic nephropathy.

The fucoidan extract was found to be efficient in impairing angiogenesis in bone tumour in various co-cultural models that are related to bone vascularization [49]. Furthermore, fucoidans are also incorporated in cosmetic products to enhance anti-wrinkle, anti-freckle, and anti-ageing properties [42].

3. Algal Alginates

Alginate is the biological unbranched polymer found in both bacteria and algae but the difference lies in their chemical composition where algal alginates contain poly guluronate (G) blocks and bacterial alginates contains O-acetylation of the mannuronate residues [50]. These alginates contain monomers blocks of 1,4-β-D-mannuronic acid (M block) and 1,4-α-L- guluronic acid (G block) in the form of homogenous blocks containing either poly G or poly M or in a heterogeneous form containing both the monomer units *i.e* MGblocks. Interestingly, the proportion of these two acids not only varies from species to species but may also vary from parts to parts in a single alga [51].

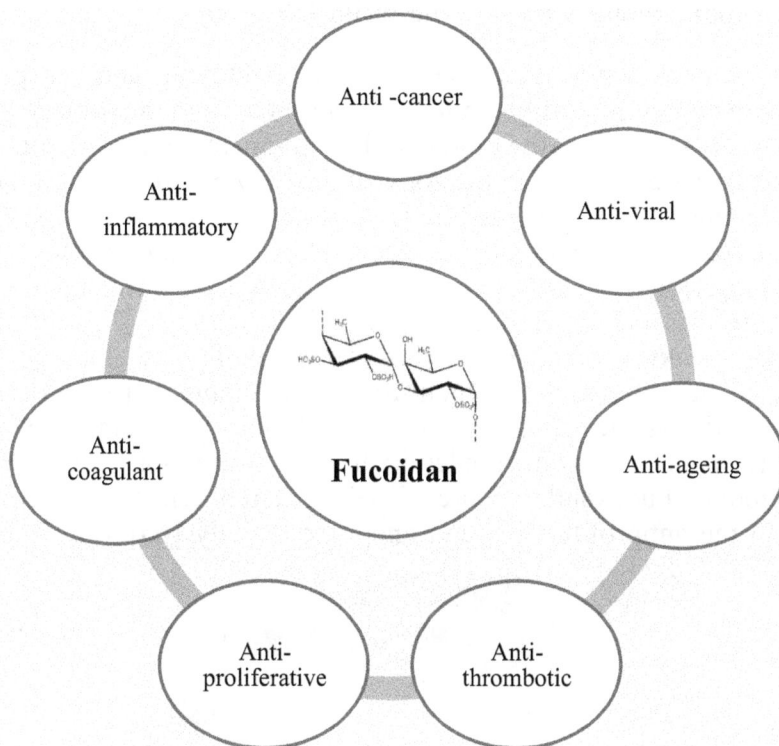

Fig. (3). The Fig. represents the potential therapeutic uses of Fucoidan.

Algal alginates are extracted from a variety of brown algae *viz Laminaria and Lessonia* (dominant species), *Macrocystis, Ascophyllum* [52]. The potential health benefits of algal alginates are because of their high dietary fiber content which makes them suitable as an anti-obesity bioactive agent. These are widely used in commercially prepared food products usually in drinks as it shows satiety effects, reduction in energy consumption, lowering of weight, and keeps a check on blood glucose level. Alginate is a gelling polysaccharide that is highly viscous, indigestible and causes short term effect in the subject thereby, suppresses hunger and is more suitable than the protein drinks [53].

4. Fucoxanthin

Fucoxanthins are carotenoids which are present in chloroplast of marine brown algae/seaweed like *Laminaria japonica* [54], *Sargassum horneri* [55], *Eisenia bicyclis* and *Undaria pinnatifida* [56] *etc.* The molecular structure of fucoxanthin includes a typical allenic bond because of which it is considered as allenic carotenoid. Other structural component includes conjugated double bonds (9 in number),5,6 monoepoxide and functional groups like carboxyl, hydroxyl, carbonyl and epoxy along with polyene chain [57 - 60].

Carotenoids are an essential component of skin lightening and sun protective cosmetics. Skin whitening or lightening's has a special role in cosmeceuticals all around the world. To achieve the motive of hypopigmentation many products are launched every year especially in the Asian markets. The prominent approach to achieve hypopigmentation is the inhibition of tyrosinase enzyme that catalyzes the rate limiting step of pigmentation [61]. Fucoxanthin acts as an efficient tyrosinase inhibitor by suppression of mRNA expression, photoaging protector and UV ray's protector, therefore widely used in cosmetic industries [62]. Additionally, it exhibits a wide variety of other applications as control of blood glucose levels and management of lipid metabolism when used as supplements [56, 63] and thus, considered as anti-diabetic and anti-obesity (Fig. **4**) nutritional additive which also affects hepatic lipogenesis by manipulating the gene expression [64]. Fucoxanthin and its metabolite Fucoxanthinol are also considered effective in controlling cancer due to the antiproliferative and apoptotic activity [65].

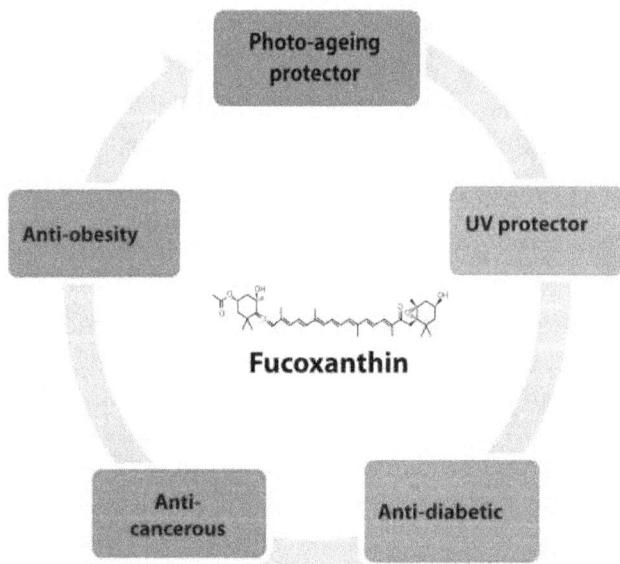

Fig. (4). Representation of chemical structure and beneficial properties of Fucoxanthin.

5. *Astaxanthin*

It is a red pigmented multifunctional carotenoid (xanthophyll) present in many microalgae, macroalgae, and sometimes in other marine animals. Astaxanthin is extracted from the *Haematococcus pluvialis, Chlorococcum* sps., *Chlorella zofingiensis,* and *Neochloris wimmeri* [66].

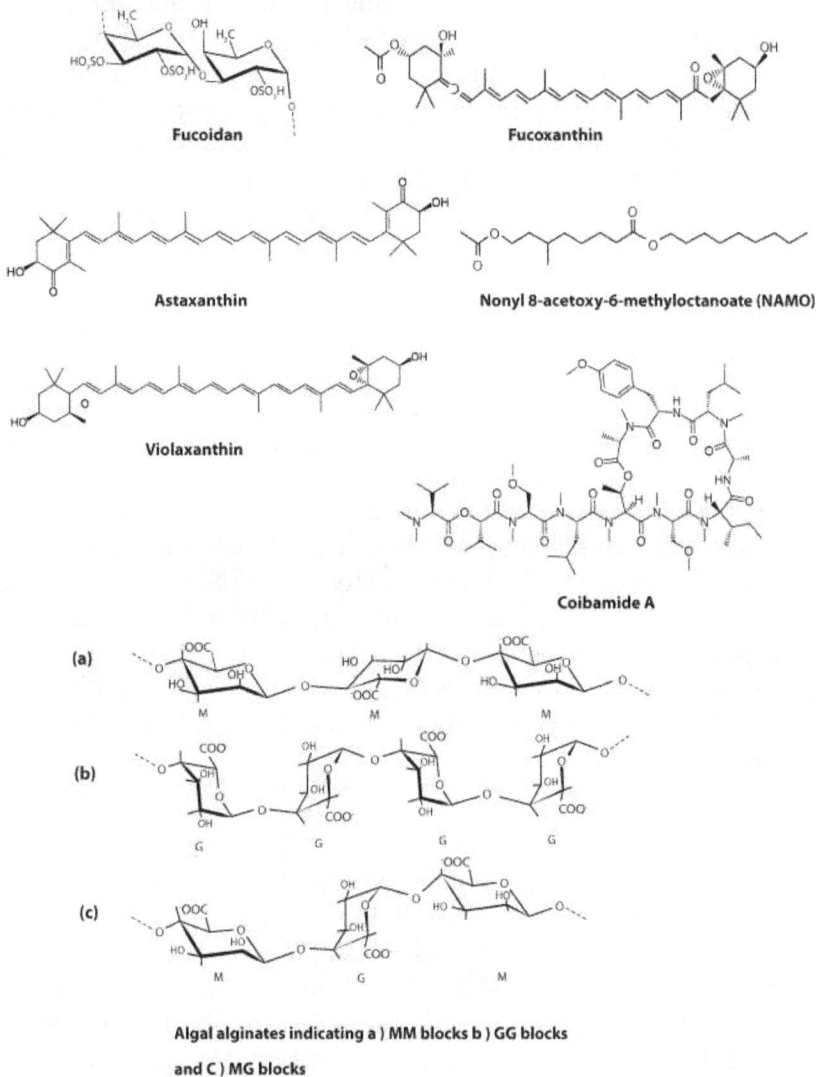

Fig. (5). Molecular structure of bioactive compounds from algal sources.

During the stress condition like high temperature, high light intensity, high salt concentration, nitrogen deficient environment, *etc. Haematococcus pluvialis* accumulates more amount of astaxanthin as reported by Sarada and co-workers [67]. Astaxanthin is a multi-purpose component that exhibits various properties to manage human health. This includes the protection of the body from free radicals and exhibits anti-oxidant property therefore, reported to increase the anti-oxidant enzymes in mice [68]. Due to their ultimate molecular structure, these can be present both inside or outside the plasma membrane and thereby, acting as a protector against peroxidative damage to lipids [69]. Oxidative stress increases glucose level in patients suffering from Diabetes mellitus and astaxanthin protect the beta cells of pancreas by lowering the toxicity occurring due to high glucose levels [70]. Furthermore, protection of skin, anti-inflammatory property, prevention of cardiovascular diseases, anti-cancer activity, inhibition of cell death & cell proliferation, anti-ulcer properties are the additional significance of astaxanthin.

6. Nonyl 8-acetoxy-6-methyloctanoate (NAMO)

The Nonyl 8-acetoxy-6-methyloctanoate (NAMO) is the ester of fatty acid alcohol derived from the marine microalgae or diatom *Phaeodactylum tricornutum*. This microalga is polymorphic depending upon changes in the environmental conditions. It acts as a potential source of energy in microbiota that grows rapidly with stored lipids constituting 20-30% of the dried weight [71]. NAMO exhibit apoptotic anti-cancer activity as per the experimentations on three different cell lines *viz.* a human lung carcinoma (A549), human promyelocytic leukemia (HL-60), and mouse melanoma (B16F10) where HL-60 reported the strongest suppression of cancerous activity. NAMO efficiently condenses the nuclear DNA in G1 sub-phase of interphase to arrest the mechanism of cell division [72].

7. Violaxanthin

Violaxanthin is an extensive carotenoid derived from the microalgae *Chlorella ellipsoidea* and green leafy vegetable spinach. It was illustrated by Soontornchaiboon *et al.* [73] that violaxanthin shows promising results when tested against the RAW 264.7 mouse macrophage cells for their anti-inflammatory activities. Violaxanthin works by inhibiting the nitric oxide and prostaglandin E2 and ultimately results in the cessation of translocation at LPS-mediated nuclear factor-κB (NF-κB) p65 subunit within the nucleus. The carotenoid extracted from *C.ellipsoidea* consists of three xanthin pigments violaxanthin, antheraxanthin and zeaxanthin which have been evaluated by the scientist group [74] for their anti-proliferative effects on human colon cancer cells. The major component is violaxanthin which works by enhancing the fluorescence intensity and inhibiting of cell growth in HCT116 cell population. Violaxanthin has also been extracted from other green algae, *Dunaliella tertiolectaon* and screened for their anti-cancerous properties in many kinds of cell lines specifically MCF-7, MDA-MB-231, A549 and LNCaP [75].

8. Coibamide A

Leptolyngbya cyanobacterium or Cyanophyta and *Leptolyngbya sps.* are the members of blue green algae that contain a bioactive component named as Coibamide A. This is a cyclic depsipeptide having many chains of amino acids in their chemical structure which makes them very complicated. Their structure consists of the large number of methylated N and O groups and alkyl amino groups. Such a complicated structure is known to be effective against NCIH-420 lung cancer cells by showing cytotoxicity [76]. The importance of Coibamide A was realized when National Cancer Institute tested their anti-proliferative properties against NCI-60 tumour cell line panel *in vitro* due to their highly methylated structure [77]. Coibamide A has been also compared to another bioactive component apratoxin A which is a potent cytotoxic marine secondary metabolite derived from cyanobacteria giving similar results. Both bioactive components share a common mechanism of action in utilizing the autophagy for pro death signalling.

CONCLUSION

Marine macroalgae and microalgae are vital and value-added source of nutritive food supplements which can be used as an alternative nourishment source due to their wide range of differential combinations of essential amino acids, polysaccharides, fatty acids, minerals, terpenoids, carotenoids, alkaloids, and vitamins. Concomitantly, the vast variety of algal masses also produces unique metabolites which can possibly be used in pharma and cosmetic industry due to the specific functionalities as per the *in vitro* and *in vivo* studies reported. Such bioactive compounds can be extracted, screened, and further prepared as algal metabolite-based drugs for the treatment of innumerable complicated as well as common diseases such as cancer, diabetes, colitis, bone resorption, osteoporosis, ulcers, cardiovascular diseases, *etc.* Although, large-scale cultivation, proper availability of space, maintenance and biorefining process of the marine algae is another challenge to meet the demands of the world's population. Additionally, the proper screening and clinical trials for long term human health benefits are in the pipeline which need to be examined thoroughly prior to the formulation, development, application, and commercialization of new era bio-drugs.

CONSENT FOR PUBLICATION

Not applicable.

CONFLICT OF INTEREST

The authors declare no conflict of interest, financial or otherwise.

ACKNOWLEDGEMENTS

The authors show a great sense of gratitude towards all the research papers & scientists from which the content was prepared.

REFERENCES

[1]   Barkia I, Saari N, Manning SR. Microalgae for High-Value Products Towards Human Health and Nutrition. Mar Drugs 2019; 17(5): 304.
[http://dx.doi.org/10.3390/md17050304] [PMID: 31137657]

[2]   Nicoletti R, Trincone A. Bioactive Compounds Produced by Strains of Penicillium and Talaromyces of Marine Origin. Mar Drugs 2016; 14(2): 37.
[http://dx.doi.org/10.3390/md14020037] [PMID: 26901206]

[3]   Collins K, Fitzgerald G, Stanton C, Ross R. Looking Beyond the Terrestrial: The Potential of Seaweed Derived Bioactives to Treat Non-Communicable Diseases. Mar Drugs 2016; 14(3): 60.
[http://dx.doi.org/10.3390/md14030060] [PMID: 26999166]

[4]   Largo DB, Diola AG, Marababol MS. Development of an integrated multi-trophic aquaculture (IMTA) system for tropical marine species in southern cebu, Central Philippines. Aquacult Rep 2016; 3: 67-76.
[http://dx.doi.org/10.1016/j.aqrep.2015.12.006]

[5]   Tanna B, Mishra A. Metabolites Unravel Nutraceutical Potential of Edible Seaweeds: An Emerging Source of Functional Food. Compr Rev Food Sci Food Saf 2018; 17(6): 1613-24.
[http://dx.doi.org/10.1111/1541-4337.12396] [PMID: 33350143]

[6]   Nagaraj SR, Osborne JW. Bioactive compounds from Caulerpa racemosa as a potent larvicidal and antibacterial agent 2014.https://agris.fao.org/agris-search/search.do?recordID=US201600025878
[http://dx.doi.org/10.1007/s11515-014-1312-4]

[7]   Tibbetts SM, Milley JE, Lall SP. Chemical composition and nutritional properties of freshwater and marine microalgal biomass cultured in photobioreactors. J Appl Phycol 2015; 27(3): 1109-19.
[http://dx.doi.org/10.1007/s10811-014-0428-x]

[8]   Williams PJB, Laurens LML. Microalgae as biodiesel & biomass feedstocks: Review & analysis of the biochemistry, energetics & economics. Energy Environ Sci 2010; 3(5): 554-90.
[http://dx.doi.org/10.1039/b924978h]

[9]   Raposo M, De Morais R, Bernardo de Morais A. Bioactivity and applications of sulphated polysaccharides from marine microalgae. Mar Drugs 2013; 11(1): 233-52.
[http://dx.doi.org/10.3390/md11010233] [PMID: 23344113]

[10]   Ryckebosch E, Bruneel C, Termote-Verhalle R, Goiris K, Muylaert K, Foubert I. Nutritional evaluation of microalgae oils rich in omega-3 long chain polyunsaturated fatty acids as an alternative for fish oil. Food Chem 2014; 160: 393-400.
[http://dx.doi.org/10.1016/j.foodchem.2014.03.087] [PMID: 24799253]

[11]   Yates CM, Calder PC, Ed Rainger G. Pharmacology and therapeutics of omega-3 polyunsaturated

fatty acids in chronic inflammatory disease. Pharmacol Ther 2014; 141(3): 272-82.
[http://dx.doi.org/10.1016/j.pharmthera.2013.10.010] [PMID: 24201219]

[12]   Ohgami K, Shiratori K, Kotake S, *et al.* Effects of astaxanthin on lipopolysaccharide-induced inflammation *in vitro* and *in vivo.* Invest Ophthalmol Vis Sci 2003; 44(6): 2694-701.
[http://dx.doi.org/10.1167/iovs.02-0822] [PMID: 12766075]

[13]   Matsui MS, Muizzuddin N, Arad S, Marenus K. Sulfated polysaccharides from red microalgae have antiinflammatory properties *in vitro* and *in vivo.* Appl Biochem Biotechnol 2003; 104(1): 13-22.
[http://dx.doi.org/10.1385/ABAB:104:1:13] [PMID: 12495202]

[14]   Lopes D, Melo T, Rey F, *et al.* Valuing Bioactive Lipids from Green, Red and Brown Macroalgae from Aquaculture, to Foster Functionality and Biotechnological Applications. Molecules 2020; 25(17): 3883.
[http://dx.doi.org/10.3390/molecules25173883] [PMID: 32858862]

[15]   Shahidi F, Miraliakbari H. Omega-3 (n-3) fatty acids in health and disease: Part 1--cardiovascular disease and cancer. J Med Food 2004; 7(4): 387-401.
[http://dx.doi.org/10.1089/jmf.2004.7.387] [PMID: 15671680]

[16]   Buedenbender L, Astone FA, Tasdemir D. Bioactive Molecular Networking for Mapping the Antimicrobial Constituents of the Baltic Brown Alga *Fucus vesiculosus.* Mar Drugs 2020; 18(6): 311.
[http://dx.doi.org/10.3390/md18060311] [PMID: 32545808]

[17]   Corsetto PA, Montorfano G, Zava S, *et al.* Characterization of Antioxidant Potential of Seaweed Extracts for Enrichment of Convenience Food. Antioxidants 2020; 9(3): 249.
[http://dx.doi.org/10.3390/antiox9030249] [PMID: 32204441]

[18]   Francavilla M, Franchi M, Monteleone M, Caroppo C. The red seaweed Gracilaria gracilis as a multi products source. Mar Drugs 2013; 11(10): 3754-76.
[http://dx.doi.org/10.3390/md11103754] [PMID: 24084791]

[19]   Millan-Linares MC, Martin ME, Rodriguez NM, *et al.* Nutraceutical Extract from Dulse (*Palmaria palmata* L.) Inhibits Primary Human Neutrophil Activation. Mar Drugs 2019; 17(11): 610.
[http://dx.doi.org/10.3390/md17110610] [PMID: 31731428]

[20]   Pimentel FB, Machado M, Cermeño M, *et al.* Enzyme-Assisted Release of Antioxidant Peptides from *Porphyra dioica* Conchocelis. Antioxidants 2021; 10(2): 249.
[http://dx.doi.org/10.3390/antiox10020249] [PMID: 33562036]

[21]   Cermeño M, Stack J, Tobin PR, *et al.* Peptide identification from a *Porphyra dioica* protein hydrolysate with antioxidant, angiotensin converting enzyme and dipeptidyl peptidase IV inhibitory activities. Food Funct 2019; 10(6): 3421-9.
[http://dx.doi.org/10.1039/C9FO00680J] [PMID: 31134998]

[22]   Shukla PS, Borza T, Critchley AT, Prithiviraj B. Carrageenans. Front Mar Sci 2016; 3: 81.

[23]   Sun T, Tao H, Xie J, Zhang S, Xu X. Degradation and antioxidant J Appl Polym Sci 2010; 117(1): 194-9.

[24]   Guzmán F, Wong G, Román T, *et al.* Identification of Antimicrobial Peptides from the Microalgae *Tetraselmis suecica* (Kylin) Butcher and Bactericidal Activity Improvement. Mar Drugs 2019; 17(8): 453.
[http://dx.doi.org/10.3390/md17080453] [PMID: 31374937]

[25]   Pereira J, Portron S, Dizier B, *et al.* The *in vitro* and *in vivo* effects of a low-molecular-weight fucoidan on the osteogenic capacity of human adipose-derived stromal cells. Tissue Eng Part A 2014; 20(1-2): 275-84.
[http://dx.doi.org/10.1089/ten.tea.2013.0028] [PMID: 24059447]

[26]   Pereira H, Silva J, Santos T, *et al.* Nutritional Potential and Toxicological Evaluation of *Tetraselmis* sp. CTP4 Microalgal Biomass Produced in Industrial Photobioreactors. Molecules 2019; 24(17): 3192.
[http://dx.doi.org/10.3390/molecules24173192] [PMID: 31484299]

[27]   Magdugo RP, Terme N, Lang M, *et al.* An Analysis of the Nutritional and Health Values of *Caulerpa racemosa* (Forsskål) and *Ulva fasciata* (Delile)—Two Chlorophyta Collected from the Philippines. Molecules 2020; 25(12): 2901.
[http://dx.doi.org/10.3390/molecules25122901] [PMID: 32599734]

[28]   Ferrazzano GF, Papa C, Pollio A, Ingenito A, Sangianantoni G, Cantile T. Cyanobacteria and Microalgae as Sources of Functional Foods to Improve Human General and Oral Health. Molecules 2020; 25(21): 5164.
[http://dx.doi.org/10.3390/molecules25215164] [PMID: 33171936]

[29]   Al Monla R, Dassouki Z, Kouzayha A, Salma Y, Gali-Muhtasib H, Mawlawi H. The Cytotoxic and Apoptotic Effects of the Brown Algae *Colpomenia sinuosa* are Mediated by the Generation of Reactive Oxygen Species. Molecules 2020; 25(8): 1993.
[http://dx.doi.org/10.3390/molecules25081993] [PMID: 32344512]

[30]   https://onlinelibrary.wiley.com/doi/abs/10.1002/ptr.3601

[31]   O'Gorman DM, Tierney CM, Brennan O, O'Brien FJ. The marine-derived, multi-mineral formula, Aquamin, enhances mineralisation of osteoblast cells *in vitro*. Phytother Res 2012; 26(3): 375-80.
[http://dx.doi.org/10.1002/ptr.3561] [PMID: 21751268]

[32]   Widaa A, Brennan O, O'Gorman DM, O'Brien FJ. The osteogenic potential of the marine-derived multi-mineral formula aquamin is enhanced by the presence of vitamin D. Phytother Res 2014; 28(5): 678-84.
[http://dx.doi.org/10.1002/ptr.5038] [PMID: 23873476]

[33]   Frestedt JL, Walsh M, Kuskowski MA, Zenk JL. A natural mineral supplement provides relief from knee osteoarthritis symptoms: a randomized controlled pilot trial. Nutr J 2008; 7(1): 9.
[http://dx.doi.org/10.1186/1475-2891-7-9] [PMID: 18279523]

[34]   Green D, Padula M, Santos J, Chou J, Milthorpe B, Ben-Nissan B. A therapeutic potential for marine skeletal proteins in bone regeneration. Mar Drugs 2013; 11(12): 1203-20.
[http://dx.doi.org/10.3390/md11041203] [PMID: 23574983]

[35]   Aslam MN, Bergin I, Naik M, *et al.* A multi-mineral natural product inhibits liver tumor formation in C57BL/6 mice. Biol Trace Elem Res 2012; 147(1-3): 267-74.
[http://dx.doi.org/10.1007/s12011-011-9316-2] [PMID: 22222483]

[36]   Ryan S, O'Gorman DM, Nolan YM. Evidence that the marine-derived multi-mineral aquamin has anti-inflammatory effects on cortical glial-enriched cultures. Phytother Res 2011; 25(5): 765-7.
[http://dx.doi.org/10.1002/ptr.3309] [PMID: 21520469]

[37]   Brennan O, Sweeney J, O'Meara B, *et al.* A Natural, Calcium-Rich Marine Multi-mineral Complex Preserves Bone Structure, Composition and Strength in an Ovariectomised Rat Model of Osteoporosis. Calcif Tissue Int 2017; 101(4): 445-55.
[http://dx.doi.org/10.1007/s00223-017-0299-7] [PMID: 28647775]

[38]   Wang J, Zhang Q, Zhang Z, Song H, Li P. Potential antioxidant and anticoagulant capacity of low molecular weight fucoidan fractions extracted from Laminaria japonica. Int J Biol Macromol 2010; 46(1): 6-12.
[http://dx.doi.org/10.1016/j.ijbiomac.2009.10.015] [PMID: 19883681]

[39]   Vo T-S, Kim S-K. 2014.https://www.sciencedirect.com/science/article/pii/B9780128002681000019

[40]   Itoh H, Noda H, Amano H, Ito H. Immunological analysis of inhibition of lung metastases by fucoidan (GIV-A) prepared from brown seaweed Sargassum thunbergii. Anticancer Res 1995; 15(5B): 1937-47.
[PMID: 8572581]

[41]   Marinval N, Saboural P, Haddad O, *et al.* Identification of a Pro-Angiogenic Potential and Cellular Uptake Mechanism of a LMW Highly Sulfated Fraction of Fucoidan from Ascophyllum nodosum. Mar Drugs 2016; 14(10): 185.
[http://dx.doi.org/10.3390/md14100185] [PMID: 27763505]

[42] Shanura Fernando IP, Asanka Sanjeewa KK, Samarakoon KW, *et al.* The potential of fucoidans from Chnoospora minima and Sargassum polycystum in cosmetics: antioxidant, anti-inflammatory, skin-whitening, and antiwrinkle activities. J Appl Phycol 2018; 30(6): 3223-32.
[http://dx.doi.org/10.1007/s10811-018-1415-4]

[43] Meyers SP, Mulder AM, Baker DG, Robinson SR, Rolfe MI, Brooks L, *et al.* Effects of fucoidan from Fucus vesiculosus in reducing symptoms of osteoarthritis: a randomized placebo-controlled trial. Biol Targets Ther 2016; 10: 81-8.

[44] Azuma K, Ishihara T, Nakamoto H, *et al.* Effects of oral administration of fucoidan extracted from Cladosiphon okamuranus on tumor growth and survival time in a tumor-bearing mouse model. Mar Drugs 2012; 10(12): 2337-48.
[http://dx.doi.org/10.3390/md10102337] [PMID: 23170088]

[45] Hayashi T. [Studies on evaluation of natural products for antiviral effects and their applications]. Yakugaku Zasshi 2008; 128(1): 61-79.
[http://dx.doi.org/10.1248/yakushi.128.61] [PMID: 18176057]

[46] Fitton JH. Therapies from fucoidan; multifunctional marine polymers. Mar Drugs 2011; 9(10): 1731-60.
[http://dx.doi.org/10.3390/md9101731] [PMID: 22072995]

[47] Park SB, Chun KR, Kim JK, Suk K, Jung YM, Lee WH. The differential effect of high and low molecular weight fucoidans on the severity of collagen-induced arthritis in mice. Phytother Res 2010; 24(9): 1384-91.
[http://dx.doi.org/10.1002/ptr.3140] [PMID: 20812282]

[48] Wang J, Geng L, Yue Y, Zhang Q. Use of fucoidan to treat renal diseases: A review of 15 years of clinic studies. Zhang L. Progress in Molecular Biology and Translational Science 2019; 95-111.https://www.sciencedirect.com/science/article/pii/S1877117319300560

[49] Wang F, Schmidt H, Pavleska D, Wermann T, Seekamp A, Fuchs S. Crude Fucoidan. Mar Drugs 2017; 15(6): 186.
[http://dx.doi.org/10.3390/md15060186] [PMID: 28632184]

[50] Fabich HT, Vogt SJ, Sherick ML, *et al.* Microbial and algal alginate gelation characterized by magnetic resonance. J Biotechnol 2012; 161(3): 320-7.
[http://dx.doi.org/10.1016/j.jbiotec.2012.04.016] [PMID: 22728394]

[51] Szekalska M, Puciłowska A, Szymańska E, Ciosek P, Winnicka K. Alginate: Current Use and Future Perspectives in Pharmaceutical and Biomedical Applications. Int J Polym Sci 2016; 2016: 1-17.
[http://dx.doi.org/10.1155/2016/7697031]

[52] Bixler HJ, Porse H. A decade of change in the seaweed hydrocolloids industry. J Appl Phycol 2011; 23(3): 321-35.
[http://dx.doi.org/10.1007/s10811-010-9529-3]

[53] Wan-Loy C, Siew-Moi P. Marine Algae as a Potential Source for Anti-Obesity Agents. Mar Drugs 2016; 14(12): 222.
[http://dx.doi.org/10.3390/md14120222] [PMID: 27941599]

[54] Shimoda H, Tanaka J, Shan SJ, Maoka T. Anti-pigmentary activity of fucoxanthin and its influence on skin mRNA expression of melanogenic molecules. J Pharm Pharmacol 2010; 62(9): 1137-45.
[http://dx.doi.org/10.1111/j.2042-7158.2010.01139.x] [PMID: 20796192]

[55] Terasaki M, Kawagoe C, Ito A, *et al.* Spatial and seasonal variations in the biofunctional lipid substances (fucoxanthin and fucosterol) of the laboratory-grown edible Japanese seaweed (*Sargassum horneri* Turner) cultured in the open sea. Saudi J Biol Sci 2017; 24(7): 1475-82.
[http://dx.doi.org/10.1016/j.sjbs.2016.01.009] [PMID: 30294215]

[56] Maeda H, Hosokawa M, Sashima T, Murakami-Funayama K, Miyashita K. Anti-obesity and anti-diabetic effects of fucoxanthin on diet-induced obesity conditions in a murine model. Mol Med Rep

2009; 2(6): 897-902.
[http://dx.doi.org/10.3892/mmr_00000189] [PMID: 21475918]

[57] Englert G, Bjørnland T, Liaaen-Jensen S. 1D and 2D NMR study of some allenic carotenoids of the fucoxanthin series. Magn Reson Chem 1990; 28(6): 519-28.
[http://dx.doi.org/10.1002/mrc.1260280610]

[58] Kumar S, Hosokawa M, Miyashita K. Fucoxanthin: a marine carotenoid exerting anti-cancer effects by affecting multiple mechanisms. Mar Drugs 2013; 11(12): 5130-47.
[http://dx.doi.org/10.3390/md11125130] [PMID: 24351910]

[59] Sangeetha RK, Bhaskar N, Divakar S, Baskaran V. Bioavailability and metabolism of fucoxanthin in rats: structural characterization of metabolites by LC-MS (APCI). Mol Cell Biochem 2010; 333(1-2): 299-310.
[http://dx.doi.org/10.1007/s11010-009-0231-1] [PMID: 19701609]

[60] Zhang H, Tang Y, Zhang Y, *et al.* Fucoxanthin. Evid Based Complement Alternat Med 2015; 2015: 1-10.
[http://dx.doi.org/10.1155/2015/723515] [PMID: 26106437]

[61] Solano F, Briganti S, Picardo M, Ghanem G. Hypopigmenting agents: an updated review on biological, chemical and clinical aspects. Pigment Cell Res 2006; 19(6): 550-71.
[http://dx.doi.org/10.1111/j.1600-0749.2006.00334.x] [PMID: 17083484]

[62] Thomas N, Kim SK. Beneficial effects of marine algal compounds in cosmeceuticals. Mar Drugs 2013; 11(12): 146-64.
[http://dx.doi.org/10.3390/md11010146] [PMID: 23344156]

[63] Woo MN, Jeon SM, Kim HJ, *et al.* Fucoxanthin supplementation improves plasma and hepatic lipid metabolism and blood glucose concentration in high-fat fed C57BL/6N mice. Chem Biol Interact 2010; 186(3): 316-22.
[http://dx.doi.org/10.1016/j.cbi.2010.05.006] [PMID: 20519145]

[64] Ha AW, Kim WK. The effect of fucoxanthin rich power on the lipid metabolism in rats with a high fat diet. Nutr Res Pract 2013; 7(4): 287-93.
[http://dx.doi.org/10.4162/nrp.2013.7.4.287] [PMID: 23964316]

[65] Martin L. Fucoxanthin. Mar Drugs 2015; 13(8): 4784-98.
[http://dx.doi.org/10.3390/md13084784] [PMID: 26264004]

[66] Ravi S, Ambati RR, Kamath SB, Chandrappa D, Narayanan A, Chauhan VS, *et al.* Influence of Different Culture Conditions on Yield of Biomass and Value Added Products in Microalgae. (2):9.

[67] Sarada R, Tripathi U, Ravishankar GA. Influence of stress on astaxanthin production in Haematococcus pluvialis grown under different culture conditions. Process Biochem 2002; 37(6): 623-7.
[http://dx.doi.org/10.1016/S0032-9592(01)00246-1]

[68] Ranga Rao A, Raghunath Reddy RL, Baskaran V, Sarada R, Ravishankar GA. Characterization of microalgal carotenoids by mass spectrometry and their bioavailability and antioxidant properties elucidated in rat model. J Agric Food Chem 2010; 58(15): 8553-9.
[http://dx.doi.org/10.1021/jf101187k] [PMID: 20681642]

[69] Rao AR, Sindhuja HN, Dharmesh SM, Sankar KU, Sarada R, Ravishankar GA. Effective inhibition of skin cancer, tyrosinase, and antioxidative properties by astaxanthin and astaxanthin esters from the green alga Haematococcus pluvialis. J Agric Food Chem 2013; 61(16): 3842-51.
[http://dx.doi.org/10.1021/jf304609j] [PMID: 23473626]

[70] Uchiyama K, Naito Y, Hasegawa G, Nakamura N, Takahashi J, Yoshikawa T. Astaxanthin protects β-cells against glucose toxicity in diabetic db/db mice. Redox Rep 2002; 7(5): 290-3.
[http://dx.doi.org/10.1179/135100002125000811] [PMID: 12688512]

[71] Chisti Y. Biodiesel from microalgae. Biotechnol Adv 2007; 25(3): 294-306.

[http://dx.doi.org/10.1016/j.biotechadv.2007.02.001] [PMID: 17350212]

[72] Samarakoon KW, Ko JY, Lee JH, Kwon ON, Kim SW, Jeon YJ. Apoptotic anticancer activity of a novel fatty alcohol ester isolated from cultured marine diatom, *Phaeodactylum tricornutum*. J Funct Foods 2014; 6: 231-40.
[http://dx.doi.org/10.1016/j.jff.2013.10.011]

[73] Soontornchaiboon W, Joo SS, Kim SM. Anti-inflammatory effects of violaxanthin isolated from microalga *Chlorella ellipsoidea* in RAW 264.7 macrophages. Biol Pharm Bull 2012; 35(7): 1137-44.
[http://dx.doi.org/10.1248/bpb.b12-00187] [PMID: 22791163]

[74] Cha KH, Koo SY, Lee DU. Antiproliferative effects of carotenoids extracted from *Chlorella ellipsoidea* and Chlorella vulgaris on human colon cancer cells. J Agric Food Chem 2008; 56(22): 10521-6.
[http://dx.doi.org/10.1021/jf802111x] [PMID: 18942838]

[75] Pasquet V, Morisset P, Ihammouine S, *et al.* Antiproliferative activity of violaxanthin isolated from bioguided fractionation of Dunaliella tertiolecta extracts. Mar Drugs 2011; 9(5): 819-31.
[http://dx.doi.org/10.3390/md9050819] [PMID: 21673891]

[76] Soria-Mercado IE, Pereira A, Cao Z, Murray TF, Gerwick WH. Alotamide A, a novel neuropharmacological agent from the marine cyanobacterium Lyngbya bouillonii. Org Lett 2009; 11(20): 4704-7.
[http://dx.doi.org/10.1021/ol901438b] [PMID: 19754100]

[77] Medina RA, Goeger DE, Hills P, *et al.* Coibamide A, a potent antiproliferative cyclic depsipeptide from the Panamanian marine *cyanobacterium Leptolyngbya* sp. J Am Chem Soc 2008; 130(20): 6324-5.
[http://dx.doi.org/10.1021/ja801383f] [PMID: 18444611]

CHAPTER 7

Nutritive Importance and Medicinal Properties of *Foeniculum vulgare* Mill. (Fennel) and *Trachyspermum ammi* L. (Ajwain)

Nandini Goswami[1], Shalini Jain[1] and Sreemoyee Chatterjee[1,*]

[1] *IIS (deemed to be University) Jaipur, Rajasthan, 302020, India*

Abstract: In tropical and sub-tropical countries, spices have a long history in traditional food preparations. Several spices are described to have medicinal effects. Among them are *Foeniculum vulgare* Mill. and *Trachyspermum ammi* L. belonging to the Apiaceae family are the most common spices known for their highly aromatic nature and flavor with culinary and traditional uses. *F. vulgare* seeds increase urine flow, improve the digestive system, promote menstruation and improve milk flow. Various pharmacological activities of *F. vulgare* such as antioxidant, hepatoprotective, antimicrobial, estrogenic, acaricidal, antihirutism, antidiabetic, anti-inflammatory, and antithrombotic, have been reported in the literature. *T. ammi* seeds are used for relieving flatulence, dyspepsia, spasmodic disorders, common cold, acute pharyngitis, sore and congested throat, dipsomania, and hysteria. *T. ammi* seeds are reported to possess antimicrobial, antioxidant, hepatoprotective, nematicidal, antihelmintic, and gastroprotective activities. The review presents an overview of the traditional uses, phytochemical constituents, and pharmacological properties of *F. vulgare* and *T. ammi* seeds.

Keywords: *Foeniculum vulgare* Mill, *Trachyspermum ammi* L, Phytochemical constituents, Anethole, Thymol, Apiaceae family, Estrogenic activity, Antioxidant, Acaricidal, Antibacterial, Antihirutism, Hepatoprotective, Anti-inflammatory, Antifungal, Antithrombotic, Antidiabetic, Antihypertensive, Antilithiasis, Nematicidal, Ameliorative, Antitussive.

INTRODUCTION

Spices are often assumed to be safe based on their traditional use for a long period. As estimated by the World Health Organization, about 80% population of developing countries depends on plant-derived drugs for their primary health care needs [1, 2]. *Foeniculum vulgare* Mill (Fig. **1a**) and *Trachyspermum ammi* L.

---

* **Corresponding author Sreemoyee Chatterjee:** Department of Biotechnology, IIS (deemed to be University) Jaipur, Rajasthan 302020 India; Tel: 9783307311; E-mail: sreemoyee.chatterjee@iisuniv.ac.in

Mukesh Kumar Sharma and Pallavi Kaushik (Eds.)

seeds (Fig. **1b**) are the commonly used spices known for their beneficial effects on humans and animals.

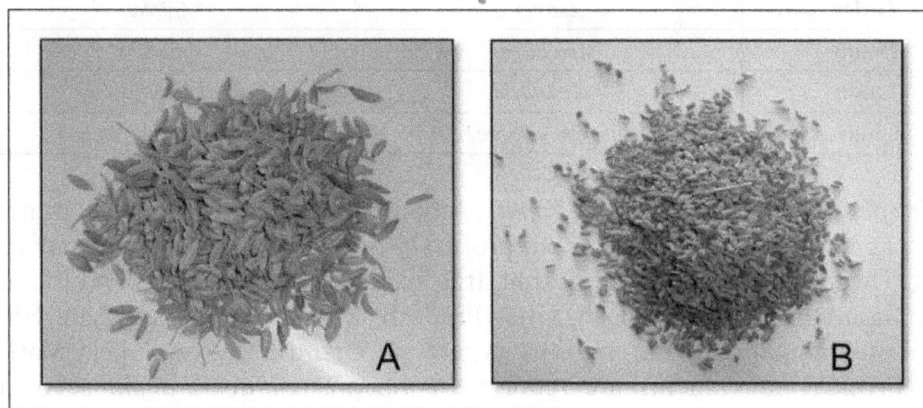

Fig. (1). **a.***Foeniculum vulgare* Mill (Fennel) seeds and **b.** *TrachyspermumammiL.* (Ajwain) seeds.

Foeniculum vulgare Mill or *F. vulgare* (Apiaceae family; Table **1**), commonly known as fennel, is one of the widespread perennials or an annual herb having feathery leaves, yellow flowers, and aromatic odor. Earlier, the Mediterranean region and Southern Europe were native places of *F. vulgare,* but the plant is widely cultivated in the tropical and temperate regions of the world. The plant is about 2.5 m tall with hollow stems [3]. The fruit is a dry seed of 4–10 mm in length containing phenolic glycosides, flavonoids, phytosterols, triterpenes, saponins, and volatile oils (thymol, trans-anethole, fenchone, carvacrol, terpinene, P-thymene and thymol methyl ether) [4]. Fennel seeds are highly aromatic in nature and used as a flavor enhancer in baked foods, ice cream, alcoholic liqueurs, and herbal preparations [5]. Fresh and dried seeds of *F. vulgare* are brown/green in color which gradually turns to grey on the aging of the seeds. Green seeds are best known for cooking. In Kashmiri Pandit and Gujarati cooking, fennel is the most important spice used [6].

Table 1. Bentham and Hooker system of classification of fennel and ajwain.

-	Fennel	Ajwain
Kingdom	*Plantae*	*Plantae*
Subkingdom	*Tracheobionta*	*Tracheobionta*
Superdivision	*Spermatophyta*	*Spermatophyta*
Division	*Magnoliophyta*	*Magnoliophyta*
Class	*Magnoliopsida*	*Magnoliopsida*

(Table 1) cont.....

-	Fennel	Ajwain
Subclass	*Rosidae*	*Rosidae*
Order	*Apiales*	*Apiales*
Family	*Apiaceae*	*Apiaceae*
Genus	*Foeniculum*	*Trachyspermum*
Species	*Foeniculum vulgare* Mill	*Trachyspermum ammi* L.

Trachyspermum ammi L. or *T. ammi* (Apiaceae family; Table **1**), commonly known as Ajwain is a 60-90 cm tall, profusely branched annual herb a native of Egypt. The seeds are cultivated in Iran, Iraq, Pakistan, Afghanistan, and India. In India, Gujarat, Madhya Pradesh, Uttar Pradesh, Maharashtra, Rajasthan, Bihar, and West Bengal are the regions where *T. ammi* is grown [7]. Various phytochemical constituents are reported to be present in *T. ammi* seeds *viz.* glycosides, carbohydrates, phenolic compounds, saponins, volatile oil (γ-terpinene, thymol, para-cymene, and α- and β-pinene), fats, protein, fiber and mineral substance containing phosphorous, calcium, iron and nicotinic acid [8]. It is regarded as a traditionally potential herb known for its curative properties in humans and animals [9]. In the Indian system of medicine, *T. ammi* seeds are administered for various stomach disorders in which a hot and dry fomentation of the seeds is lapped on the chest to cure asthma and a paste of powdered seeds is applied externally for decreasing colic pains [10]. Ajwain-ka-arak (aqueous extract of the seeds) is a popular preparation for diarrhea [11]. *T. ammi* seeds are therapeutically used as stomachic, carminative, expectorant, antiseptic, amoebiasis, and antimicrobial agents. Seeds are also known to prevent abdominal tumors, abdominal pains, and piles [12]. Many ajwain ayurvedic formulations are available which are given to overcome infections with worms [8]. Seeds are also used for relieving flatulence, dyspepsia, spasmodic disorders, common cold, acute pharyngitis, sore and congested throat, dipsomania, and hysteria [13].

The review aims to present the reported knowledge of phytochemical composition, culinary uses, and pharmacological studies of plant-derived extracts of fennel and ajwain seeds.

Phytochemistry of *F. vulgare* and *T. ammi*

F. vulgare seeds have been reported to possess moisture (6.3%), proteins (9.5%), fats (10%), minerals (13.4%), fibers (18.5%), and carbohydrates (42.3%). The minerals such as potassium, calcium, iron, sodium, phosphorus, and vitamins *viz.* riboflavin, thiamine, vitamin C and niacin are also present [14]. Pasirija *et al.* studied that *F. vulgare* seeds constitute 8% volatile oil (about 10-15% fenchone, 50-60%, anethole, and 2-9% estragole and methylchavicol) flavonoids, coumarins (including bergapten), sterols and (E)-9- octadecenoic acid [15]. They also contain methyl chavicol, d-apenine, and camphene (Fig. **2**). Anethole, the major constituent of fennel seed/oil is an active estrogenic agent with less hepatotoxic activity and minimal/no teratogenic effect [16]. In the respiratory tract, it has been shown to have a secretolytic action along with fenchone [14]. The method of extraction and geographical origin are the key factors responsible for the considerable chemodiversity in the essential oil composition of *F. vulgare* seeds [5, 17].

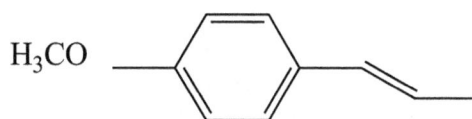

Trans-anethole

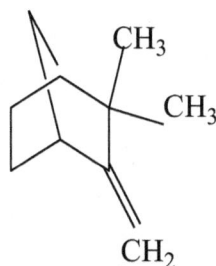

Camphene

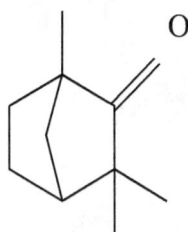

Fenchone

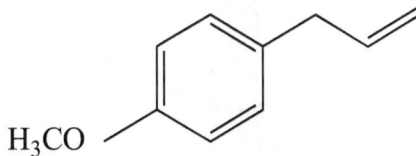

Estragol

Fig. (2). Structures of reported phyto-constituents of fennel.

T. ammi seeds have been reported to possess carbohydrates (38.6%), fibers (11.9%), glycosides, tannins, proteins (15.4%), moisture (8.9%), fats (18.1%), flavones, saponins and mineral matter (7.1%) containing phosphorous, calcium, iron and nicotinic acid [18]. *T. ammi* seeds yield 2-4% essential oil, with carvone (46%), limonene (3 8%), dillapiole (9%) [19, 20] and thymol (35-60%) [21] as major constituents. Para-cymene, γ-terpenine, α- and β-pinenes, dipentene, α-terpinene, and carvacrol constitute the nonthymol fraction (thymene) (Fig. **3**) [22]. Some amount of myrcene, camphene, and α-3-carene are also present in the seeds [23, 24]. Table **2** represents the essential oil description of fennel and ajwain seeds.

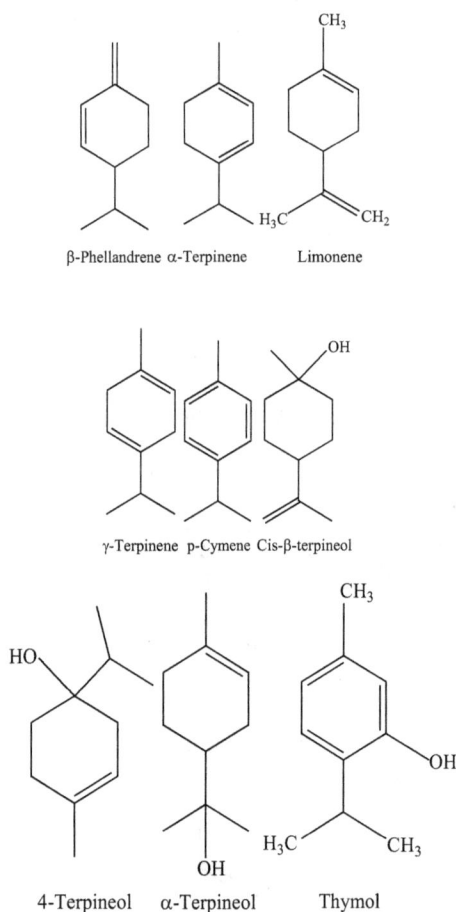

Fig. (3). Structures of reported Phytoconstituents of ajwain.

Table 2. Essential oil description of fennel [25, 26] and ajwain seeds [27, 28].

S.No.	Characteristics	Fennel	Ajwain
1.	Botanical Name	*Foeniculum vulgare*	*Trachyspermum ammi*
2.	Family	Apiaceae	Apiaceae
3.	Parts Used	Fruit	Fruit
4.	Origin	Southern Europe and the Mediterranean region	Egypt
5.	Mode of Extraction of oil	Steam Distillation	Steam Distillation
6.	Main Constituents	Anethole, estragole, fenchone	Thymol, p-cymene, gamma-terpene
7.	Description	Clear Transparent Liquid	Clear Transparent Liquid
8.	Refractive index at 20 °C	1.5280-1.5380	1.498- 1.504
9.	Specific Gravity at 20 °C	0.953-0.973	0.910-0.930
10.	Appearance	Colorless to Pale yellow liquid	Colorless to pale yellow liquid
11.	Solubility	Slightly soluble in water; soluble in 1 volume 90% or 8 volumes 80% alcohol; very soluble in ether, chloroform	Insoluble in water; soluble in organic solvents

Organoleptic Properties

Kumar *et al.* reported the detailed organoleptic characteristics of ajwain seed powder [29]. These properties help in the identification as well as standardization of the various attributes and purity of the seeds. Table **3** represents the various organoleptic properties of fennel [30] and ajwain seed powder.

Table 3. Organoleptic properties of fennel and ajwain seed powder.

S.No.	Appearance	Seed Powder	
		Fennel [30]	Ajwain [31]
1.	Color	Grayish-brown to grayish-yellow	Light brown
2.	Taste	Sweet to bitter.	Pleasant
3.	Odor	Characteristic, aromatic in nature.	Characteristic
4.	Foreign organic matter	1.5% peduncles and not more than 1.5% foreign matter	2.4%
5.	Total ash	$\geq 1.5\%$	8.6%
6.	Acid insoluble ash	$\geq 1.5\%$	0.49%
7.	Water-soluble extractive	$\geq 20\%$	42%
8.	Alcohol soluble extractive	$\geq 11\%$	17.9%

(Table 3) cont.....

S.No.	Appearance	Seed Powder	
		Fennel [30]	**Ajwain [31]**
9.	Moisture content	$\geq 8\%$	-

Pharmacological Activities

T. ammi and *F. vulgare* seeds are known for their characteristic aromatic smell and taste and have widespread use as a traditional medicine [32]. These seeds are used as preservatives, as flavoring agents, in medicine, and for the preparation of essential oil in perfumery [33]. Various pharmacological properties of fennel and ajwain seeds have been listed in Tables **4** and **5**, respectively.

Table 4. Reported pharmacological properties of fennel seeds.

S.No.	Properties	References
1.	Estrogenic activity	[19]
2.	Antioxidant activity	[34-36]
3.	Effect on uterine contraction	[37]
4.	Acaricidal activity	[38]
5.	Antibacterial activity	[39-42]
6.	Antihirustism activity	[43]
7.	Hepatoprotective activity	[6, 44]
8.	Anti-inflammatory activity	[45]
9.	Antifungal activity	[46-49]
10.	Antithrombotic activity	[50]
11.	Antimutagenic and chemopreventive activity	[51]
12.	Antidiabetic activity	[52, 53]

Table 5. Reported pharmacological properties of ajwain seeds.

S.No.	Properties	References
1.	Antihypertensive, antispasmodic, and broncho-dilating activity	[61]
2.	Hepatoprotective activity	[61]
3.	Antilithiasis and diuretic activity	[62]
4.	Antiplatelet-aggregatory	[63]
5.	Anti-inflammatory potential	[64]
6.	Antitussive effects	[65]
7.	Antifilarial activity	[66]

(Table 5) cont.....

8.	Gastroprotective activity	[67]
9.	Detoxification of aflatoxins	[68]
10.	Antioxidant effect	[69]
11.	Antimicrobial actions *in vitro*	[23, 70, 71]
12.	Hypolipidemic action *in vivo*	[72]
13.	Digestive stimulant actions *in vivo* and *in vitro*	[73, 74]
14.	Nematicidal activity	[48, 75-79]
15.	Anthelmintic activity	[80-83]

Fennel (F.vulgare)

Estrogenic Activity

Since time immemorial, *F. vulgare* is known for its estrogenic activity, increasing milk secretion, promoting menstruation, and facilitating birth. The active estrogenic agent of fennel seed oil was found to be anethole [54]. Some other studies have suggested that dianethole and photoanethole (polymers of anethole) are the actual pharmacologically active agents [19].

Antioxidant Activity

The Antioxidant activity assays of *F. vulgare* were carried out using its acetonic seed extract and essential oil which showed strong free radical scavenging activity with BHT (butylated hydroxytoluene) and BHA (butylated hydroxyanisole) as standard antioxidants [55]. In the linoleic acid system, the inhibitory action of acetone extract and essential oil of *F. vulgare* seeds was observed by an accumulation of peroxide in the emulsion. The moderate antioxidant ability of n-BuOH extract of the *F. vulgare* seeds was seen in lipid peroxidation assay and it has been increased with an increase in concentration. The antioxidant power of pure compounds isolated from *F. vulgare* seeds was higher than the crude extracts [56]. Aqueous and ethanolic extracts of *F. vulgare* seeds have also been studied for their antioxidant activity. In the linoleic acid system, both the extracts (100 µg) exhibited 77.5% and 99.1% inhibition of peroxidation, respectively which was higher than the same dose of α-tocopherol (36.1%).

Effect on Uterine Contraction

The reported studies have supported the protective effects of *F. vulgare* essential oil against uterine contraction in rats. On administration of different doses of fennel essential oil (25 and 50 µg/ml for oxytocin and 10 and 20 µg/ml for PGE_2 respectively), there was a significant reduction in the intensity of contractions induced by oxytocin and prostaglandin $E_2(PGE_2)$. The contraction frequency induced by PGE_2 was also reduced but the same result was not observed in contractions induced by oxytocin. The estimated LD_{50} value obtained in female rats was 1326 mg/kg. Besides, the vital organs of the dead animals were not affected by the treatment [37].

Acaricidal Activity

Direct contact application of essential oil of *F. vulgare* seeds showed significant acaricidal activity against two species of house dust mite i.e.*Dermatophagoides farina* and *Dermatophagoides pteronyssinus* when used in comparison with the commercially available repellent, benzyl benzoate. Also, the methanolic seed extract of *F. vulgare* exhibited mosquito repellent activity against female *Aedes aegypti* [38].

Antibacterial Activity

Mohsenzadeh [42] reported the antibacterial activity of *F. vulgare* seed oil against *Escherichia* coli, *Bacillus megateriumde,* and *Staphylococcus aureus.* The essential oil of *F. vulgare* seeds was also effective against human pathogenic bacteria. The multidrug-resistant *Acinetobacter baumannii* infections have also been controlled by antimicrobial agents such as a phenyl propanoid derivative – Dillapional and a coumarin -Scopoletin, isolated from *F. vulgare* [40]. Ethanolic and aqueous extracts of *F. vulgare* seeds displayed antibacterial activity against *Campylobacter jejuni* and *Helicobacter pylori* [39, 41].

Antihirutism Activity

The ethanolic extract of *F. vulgare* seeds exhibited antihirutism activity. The creams containing 1% and 2% of fennel seed extract and placebo were used to treat patients in a double-blind study. The study concluded that the cream containing 2% fennel seed extract displayed better results as compared with 1% fennel seed extract cream [43].

Hepatoprotective Activity

The hepatoprotective activity of *F. vulgare* essential oil was studied in rats. The essential oil inhibited the hepatotoxicity induced by acute CCl_4 administration. The study revealed decreased levels of Alanine Amino Transferase (ALT), serum Aspartate Amino Transferase (AST), Bilirubin, and Alkaline Phosphatase (ALP) [57].

Anti-Inflammatory Activity

Oral administration of methanolic extract of *F. vulgare* seeds (200 mg/kg) in male, Sprague-Dawley rats, and Swiss Albino mice displayed protective effects against type IV allergic reactions and acute and sub-acute inflammatory diseases [45].

Antifungal Activity

The essential oil, seed, and bark extracts of *F. vulgare* have shown inhibitory effects against Mycobacteria and *Candida sp* [46, 47]. *F. vulgare* essential oil reduced the mycelial growth and germination of *Sclerotinia sclerotiorum*. The seeds could serve as bio fungicides- an alternative to synthetic fungicides against phytopathogenic fungi [49]. A complete zone of inhibition was observed against *Aspergillum niger* van, *Aspergillum* flavus, Fusarium *graminearum,* and *Fusarium moniliforme* at a 6 µl dose of the essential oil of *F. vulgare* seeds [48].

Antithrombotic Activity

The *F. vulgare* essential oil has been proved to possess safe antithrombotic activity. The seeds are protective against destabilizing clots, and display vasorelaxant action and antiplatelet activity [58, 59]. Anethole has been tested in guinea pig plasma showing inhibition against aggregation induced by arachidonic acid and collagen-ADP. Anethole at similar concentrations of fennel oil also prevented thrombin-induced clot reaction. Comparable NO-independent vasorelaxant activity was observed by administration of *F. vulgare* essential oil and anethole in rat aorta. Significant protection was also seen against gastric lesions induced by ethanol in rats after oral administration of both essential oil and anethole at a 100 mg/kg dose level [50].

Antimutagenic and Chemopreventive Potential

The hot water crude extract of *F. vulgare* seeds was evaluated for its antimutagenic and cancer chemopreventive potentialities in Swiss albino mice and Drosophila. There was an insignificant effect of *F. vulgare* extract on mitosis rate during chromosomal aberration assay in bone marrow cells of mice while mitomycin C-induced chromosomal aberration was significantly reduced [51].

Antidiabetic Activity

The essential oil of *F. vulgare* seeds has been reported to possess hypoglycemic activity in Streptozotocin-treated diabetic rats. When the rats were orally administered with essential oil of *F. vulgare*, hyperglycemia improved from 162.5± 3.19 mg/dl to 81.97± 1.97 mg/dl and serum glutathione peroxidase activity was also enhanced on essential oil administration from 59.72±2.78 U/g Hb to 99.60± 6.38 U/g Hb. The study supported the effective use of *F. vulgare* seed essential oil as an antidiabetic agent [60].

Ajwain (T.ammi)

Antihypertensive, Antispasmodic, and Broncho-Dilating Activity

In vivo antihypertensive effect and *in vitro* antispasmodic and broncho-dilating actions of *T. ammi* seeds were investigated, which stated that calcium channel blockage was responsible to mediate the spasmolytic effects of *T. ammi* seeds. The study strongly supported that hyperactive disease states of the gut *viz.* diarrhea as well as hypertension can be cured by *T. ammi* seeds [61].

Hepatoprotective Activity

The hepatoprotective effect of *T. ammi* seeds against paracetamol-induced toxicity was determined in Swiss Albino mice. The results stated that *T. ammi* seeds were 80% effective against a 1g/kg normal-lethal dose of paracetamol. The prolongation of pentobarbital sleeping time induced by CCl_4 in mice was also inhibited by *T. ammi* seeds and high serum levels of liver enzymes in mice were also normalized [61].

Antioxidant Activity

Effects of *T. ammi* extract on oxidative stress and toxicity induced by hexachlorocyclohexane (HCH) in rats were investigated. Pre-feeding of *T. ammi* *extract* resulted in enhanced levels of GSH-peroxidase, GSH, SOD, G-6-PDH, glutathione S-transferase (GST), and catalase activities and lowering of hepatic levels of lipid peroxides. It was concluded that hepatic free radical stress caused by HCH administration, hence, causing toxicity, was compensated by the dietary *T. ammi* extract [69].

Antilithiasis and Diuretic Activity

T. ammi seeds were investigated for *in vivo* anti-lithiasis and diuretic actions which inhibited oxalate urolithiasis induced in rats. Further studies revealed that *T. ammi* seeds were not effective in increasing the 24h urine production. Even the experimental evidence did not support the use of *T. ammi* seeds in the treatment of kidney stones [62].

Antiplatelet-Aggregatory Potential

Administration of dried etheral extract of *T. ammi* seeds inhibited the arachidonic acid, collagen, and epinephrine-induced aggregation of platelets in humans. The study also supported the effective use of *T. ammi* seeds in women post-parturition [63].

Anti-Inflammatory Potential

TAE and TAQ seed extracts of the *T. ammi* were tested for their anti-inflammatory potential in which both the extracts at 100mg/kg dose displayed significant ($P<0.001$) anti-inflammatory effect in rat models. The weight of the adrenal glands of rats was significantly increased after the administration of TAE and TAQ extracts [64].

Antitussive Effects

By counting the number of coughs, different concentrations of aqueous and crude extracts of *T. ammi* seeds in the form of aerosols were tested for their antitussive effects in guinea pigs. Carvacrol, codeine, and saline were also used. The number of coughs was significantly reduced in the presence of *T. ammi* seed extract ($P< 0.001$) and codeine ($P< 0.01$) [65].

Antifilarial Activity

In vitro antifilarial activity of *T. ammi* methanolic seed extract has been studied against *Setaria digitata* worms by both worm motility and MTT [3-(4, 5-dimethylthiazol-2-yl)-2, 5- diphenyltetrazolium bromide] reduction assays. *In vivo,* antifilarial activity of *T. ammi* was carried out against the human filarial worm *Brugia malayi* in *Mastomys coucha,* which resulted in female worm sterility and macrofilaricidal activity [66]. The active principle behind this effect was phenolic monoterpenes.

Gastro Protective Activity

T. ammi seeds were tested for their antiulcer activity by using different ulcer models. Animals were pre-treated with ethanolic extract and displayed a significant decrease in percentage ulcer protection and ulcer index in all models. The study concluded that the *T. ammi* seed extract was significantly protective (p<0.001) by lowering the ulcerative lesions when compared with the animals of the control group [67].

Detoxification of Aflatoxins

The *T. ammi* seed extract displayed the maximum degradation of aflatoxin G1 (AFG1). Boiling of seed extract significantly reduced its ability to detoxify aflatoxins. Dialyzed seed extract also significantly degraded the levels of other aflatoxins *viz.*, AFB1, AFG2, and AFB2.78% degradation of AFG1was seen within the time of 6 h and there was more than 91% degradation at 24 h after incubation [68].

Antimicrobial Actions in vitro

The antimicrobial action of *T. ammi* seeds was investigated for the protection of foodstuffs against microbial spoilage and its use as an antimicrobial agent in humans [84]. Carvacrol and thymol are the active principle components of *T. ammi* seeds which are thought to be responsible for their antimicrobial potential [85].

Thymol kills the microbial pathogens resistant to multidrug treatment and bacteria which could resist even prevalent antibiotics belonging to the third generation. This proves the plant to be based on IV generation herbal drug formulation [70].

Hypolipidemic action *in vivo*

Anti-hyperlipidemic actions of *T. ammi* seeds have been observed in Albino rabbits. It was reported that *T. ammi* seed powder and its methanolic extract at a dose rate of 2 g/kg body weight were significantly active in lipid-lowering action by decreasing LDL-cholesterol, total cholesterol, total lipids, and triglycerides [72].

Digestive Stimulant Actions in vivo and in vitro

The incorporation of *T. ammi* seeds in the infusion increased the amount of gastric acid nearly four-fold. In experimental rats, the food transit time was decreased on the incorporation of *T. ammi* seeds into the diet and also caused more secretion of bile acids and enhanced the activity of digestive enzymes [73, 74].

Nematicidal Activity

Bursaphelenchus xylophilus, Nickle, and pinewood nematode (PWN) are the major cause of Pine Wilt disease. *T. ammi* essential oil constituents (camphene, pinene, myrcene, limonene, terpinene, terpinen-4-ol, thymol, and carvacrol) act against PWN [86]. PWN bodies were treated with morantel tartrate and levamisole hydrochloride which acted as muscle activity blockers [79]. In nematodes, methyl isothiocyanate targets amino and hydroxyl groups [87]. The study confirmed that thymol and carvacrol were protective against PWN [88]. The nematicidal potential of *T. ammi* essential oil was reported to be 0.431 mg/ml (LC_{50} value) [82].

Antihelmintic Activity

T. ammi seeds displayed an antihelmintic effect on particular helminths, *e.g. Haemonchus contortus* in sheep and *Ascaris lumbricoides* in humans [82]. Kostyukovsky *et. al.* reported the anthelmintic potential of *T. ammi* seeds in which the seeds interfere with the energy metabolism of these parasites and lead to decreased energy reserves [81]. The plant also displayed cholinergic activity with peristaltic movements of the gut and helped in the removal of intestinal parasites which could be an additional factor to its anthelmintic activity [80, 83].

CONCLUSION

Foeniculum vulgare Mill and *Trachyspermum ammi* have been used as traditional medicines for a very long time. The seeds of these plants are used as preservatives, as flavoring agents, and for the preparation of essential oil in perfumery. These are flavorful spices with high aromatic odor and culinary uses. *F. vulgare* seeds cure indigestion, provide relief in menstrual cramps, improve milk flow, reduce inflammation and even show promising anticancer effects. On the other hand, *T. ammi* seeds have been used traditionally as an important remedial agent for diarrhea, abdominal pains & tumors, bronchial issues, lack of appetite & asthma. Both the plants are even reported to act as antioxidant, anti-inflammatory, hepatoprotective, antibacterial, and antifungal agents. In this review article, an attempt has been made to aggregate all the reported information about the traditional and pharmacological properties of *F. vulgare* and *T. ammi* seeds. This review can provide enormous opportunities for planning and conducting high-level research activities related to various aspects of these spices. Moreover, shortly, the seed extract of these plants could even be explored further as a source of several useful phytochemicals which could play a beneficial role in the modern medicine system.

CONSENT FOR PUBLICATION

Not applicable.

CONFLICT OF INTEREST

The authors declare no conflict of interest, financial or otherwise.

ACKNOWLEDGEMENTS

Declared none.

REFERENCES

[1]   Gabhe SY, Tatke PA, Khan TA. Evaluation of the immunomodulatory activity of the methanol extract of *Ficus benghalensis* roots in rats. Indian J Pharmacol 2006; 38(4): 271-5.
[http://dx.doi.org/10.4103/0253-7613.27024]

[2]   Premanathan M, Rajendran S, Ramanathan T, Kathiresan K, Nakashima H, Yamamoto N. A survey of some Indian medicinal plants for anti-human immunodeficiency virus (HIV) activity. Indian J Med Res 2000; 112: 73-7.
[PMID: 11094851]

[3]   Singh SP. A Comprehensive Review on Pharmacological Activity of *Foeniculum vulgare*. Pharm Sci: 5.

[4]   PhEur. Pharmacopoea Europaea. 5th ed., 2005.

[5]   Díaz-Maroto MC, Díaz-Maroto Hidalgo IJ, Sánchez-Palomo E, Pérez-Coello MS. Volatile components and key odorants of fennel (*Foeniculum vulgare* Mill.) and thyme (*Thymus vulgaris* L.) oil extracts obtained by simultaneous distillation-extraction and supercritical fluid extraction. J Agric Food Chem 2005; 53(13): 5385-9.
[http://dx.doi.org/10.1021/jf050340+] [PMID: 15969523]

[6]   Rather MA, Dar BA, Sofi SN, Bhat BA, Qurishi MA. *Foeniculum vulgare*: A comprehensive review of its traditional use, phytochemistry, pharmacology, and safety. Arab J Chem 2016; 9: S1574-83.
[http://dx.doi.org/10.1016/j.arabjc.2012.04.011]

[7]   Part 1. Ayurvedic Pharmacopoeia India 2011; 1: 170-1.

[8]   Ranjan B, Manmohan S, Singh S, Singh R. Medicinal Uses of *Trachyspermum ammi*: A Review. Pharm Res 2011; 5(2): 247-58.

[9]   Khan N, Jamila N, Ejaz R, Nishan U, Kim KS. Volatile Oil, Phytochemical, and Biological Activities Evaluation of *Trachyspermum ammi* Seeds by Chromatographic and Spectroscopic Methods. Anal Lett 2020; 53(6): 984-1001.
[http://dx.doi.org/10.1080/00032719.2019.1688825]

[10]   Singh VK, Govil J, Arunachalam C. Recent Progress in Medicinal Plants. 2007.

[11]   Dahake PT, Dadpe MV, Dhore SV, Kale Y, Kendre S, Siddiqui A. Evaluation of antimicrobial efficacy of *Trachyspermum ammi* (Ajwain) oil and chlorhexidine against oral bacteria: An *in vitro* study. J Indian Soc Pedod Prev Dent 2018; 36(4): 357-63.
[http://dx.doi.org/10.4103/JISPPD.JISPPD_65_18] [PMID: 30324925]

[12]   Shivapriya K, Prabha ML, Issac R. Health benefits of bishop's weed (AJWAIN). Drug Invent Today 2019; 12(7): 3.

[13]   Asif HM, Sultana S, Akhtar N. A panoramic view on phytochemical, nutritional, ethanobotanical uses and pharmacological values of *Trachyspermum ammi* Linn. Asian Pac J Trop Biomed 2014; 4: S545-53.
[http://dx.doi.org/10.12980/APJTB.4.2014APJTB-2014-0242]

[14]   Pasrija A, Singh R, Katiyar C. Standardization of Fennel (*Foeniculum vulgare*), Its Oleoresin and Marketed Ayurvedic Dosage Forms. Intenational J Pharm Sci Drug Res 2011; 3(3): 265-9.

[15]   Akbar S. Fennel (*Foeniculum vulgare* Mill.): A Common Spice with Unique Medicinal Properties. 2018;1(1):9.

[16]   Anka ZM, Gimba SN, Nanda A, Salisu L. Phytochemistry and Pharmacological Activities of

Foeniculum vulgare. IOSR J Pharm 2020; 10(1): 1-10.

[17] Gross M, Lewinsohn E, Tadmor Y, *et al.* The inheritance of volatile phenylpropenes in bitter fennel (*Foeniculum vulgare* Mill. var. *vulgare*, Apiaceae) chemotypes and their distribution within the plant. Biochem Syst Ecol 2009; 37(4): 308-16.
[http://dx.doi.org/10.1016/j.bse.2009.05.007]

[18] Pruthi JS. Spices and Condiments. 4th ed. National Book trust, New Delhi; 1992.

[19] Albert-Puleo M. Fennel and anise as estrogenic agents. J Ethnopharmacol 1980; 2(4): 337-44.
[http://dx.doi.org/10.1016/S0378-8741(80)81015-4] [PMID: 6999244]

[20] Choudhury S, Ahmed R, Kanjilal PB, Leclercq PA. Composition of the seed oil of *Trachyspermum ammi* (L.) Sprague from northeast India. J Essent Oil Res 1998; 10(5): 588-90.
[http://dx.doi.org/10.1080/10412905.1998.9700979]

[21] Anonymous . The Wealth of India, A Dictionary of Indian Raw Materials and Industrial Products Publications and Information Directorate. New Delhi CSIR 2003; 10: 267-72.

[22] Mohagheghzadeh A, Faridi P, Ghasemi Y. Carum copticum Benth. & Hook., essential oil chemotypes. Food Chem 2007; 100(3): 1217-9.
[http://dx.doi.org/10.1016/j.foodchem.2005.12.002]

[23] Bashyal S, Guha A. Evaluation of *Trachyspermum ammi* seeds for antimicrobial. Asian J Pharm Clin Res 2018; 11(5): 274-7.
[http://dx.doi.org/10.22159/ajpcr.2018.v11i5.24430]

[24] Bilal M, Ahmad S, Rehman T, Abbasi WM, Ghauri AO, Arshad MA. Effects of *Trachyspermum ammi* L. (Apiaceae) on serum, urine and hepatic uric acid levels in oxonate-induced rats and *in vitro* xanthine oxidase inhibition assay. IJTK 2019; 18(1): 52-7.

[25] Masoodi KZ, Amin I, Mansoor S, Ahmed N, Altay V, Ozturk M. Botanicals from the Himalayas with anticancer. In: Ozturk M, Egamberdieva D, Pešić M, Eds. Biodiversity and Biomedicine. Academic Press 2020; pp. 189-234. https://www.sciencedirect.com/ science/article/pii/B9780128195413000116
[http://dx.doi.org/10.1016/B978-0-12-819541-3.00011-6]

[26] Diao WR, Hu QP, Zhang H, Xu JG. Chemical composition, antibacterial activity and mechanism of action of essential oil from seeds of fennel (*Foeniculum vulgare* Mill.). Food Control 2014; 35(1): 109-16.
[http://dx.doi.org/10.1016/j.foodcont.2013.06.056]

[27] Asangi H, Saxena SN, Kattimani KN, *et al.* Genetic Variation in Essential Oil Constituents of Ajwain (*Trachyspermum ammi* L. Sprague) Varieties at Varying Nitrogen Levels under Semiarid Tropics of Northern Karnataka, India. J Essent Oil-Bear Plants 2020; 23(6): 1324-33.
[http://dx.doi.org/10.1080/0972060X.2020.1871075]

[28] Chung I-M, Khanh TD, Lee O-K, Ahmad A. Chemical Constitutents from Ajwain Seeds (*Trachyspermum ammi*) and Inhibitory Activity of Thymol, Lupeol Asian J Chem 2007; 19(2): 11.

[29] Kumar H, Sahoo L, Patel J. Pharmacognostic studies on *Trachyspermum ammi* Linn, A powder analysis. Int J Res Ayurveda Pharm 2011; 2(4): 1272-7.

[30] WHO monographs on selected medicinal plants. Vol. 3. World Health Organization; 2001. 136–138.

[31] Jeet K, Devi N, Narender T, Sunil T, Lalit S, Thakur R. *Trachyspermum ammi*: A comprehensive review. Int Res J Pharm 2012; 3: 6.

[32] Mahmood RT, Shamim A, Ahsan F, Parveen S, Shariq M. *Foeniculum vulgare*, Solanum nigrum and *Cichorium intybus*: A collectanea of pharmacological and clinical uses. Res J Pharm Technol 2021; 14(1): 555-61.
[http://dx.doi.org/10.5958/0974-360X.2021.00101.3]

[33] Goswami N, Chatterjee S. Assessment of free radical scavenging potential and oxidative DNA damage preventive activity of *Trachyspermum ammi* L. (carom) and *Foeniculum vulgare* Mill. (fennel) seed

extracts. BioMed Res Int 2014; 2014: 1-8.
[http://dx.doi.org/10.1155/2014/582767] [PMID: 25143939]

[34] Ahmed AF, Shi M, Liu C, Kang W. Comparative analysis of antioxidant activities of essential oils and extracts of fennel (*Foeniculum vulgare* Mill.) seeds from Egypt and China. Food Sci Hum Wellness 2019; 8(1): 67-72.
[http://dx.doi.org/10.1016/j.fshw.2019.03.004]

[35] Chang S, Mohammadi Nafchi A, Karim AA. Chemical composition, antioxidant activity and antimicrobial properties of three selected varieties of Iranian fennel seeds. J Essent Oil Res 2016; 28(4): 357-63.
[http://dx.doi.org/10.1080/10412905.2016.1146169]

[36] Faudale M, Viladomat F, Bastida J, Poli F, Codina C. Antioxidant activity and phenolic composition of wild, edible, and medicinal fennel from different Mediterranean countries. J Agric Food Chem 2008; 56(6): 1912-20.
[http://dx.doi.org/10.1021/jf073083c] [PMID: 18303817]

[37] Ostad SN, Soodi M, Shariffzadeh M, Khorshidi N, Marzban H. The effect of fennel essential oil on uterine contraction as a model for dysmenorrhea, pharmacology and toxicology study. J Ethnopharmacol 2001; 76(3): 299-304.
[http://dx.doi.org/10.1016/S0378-8741(01)00249-5] [PMID: 11448553]

[38] Kim DH, Kim SI, Chang KS, Ahn YJ. Repellent activity of constituents identified in *Foeniculum vulgare* fruit against *Aedes aegypti* (Diptera: Culicidae). J Agric Food Chem 2002; 50(24): 6993-6.
[http://dx.doi.org/10.1021/jf020504b] [PMID: 12428949]

[39] Kaur GJ, Arora DS. *In vitro* antibacterial activity of three plants belonging to the family Umbelliferae. Int J Antimicrob Agents 2008; 31(4): 393-5.
[http://dx.doi.org/10.1016/j.ijantimicag.2007.11.007] [PMID: 18191549]

[40] Kwon YS, Choi WG, Kim WJ, *et al.* Antimicrobial constituents of *Foeniculum vulgare*. Arch Pharm Res 2002; 25(2): 154-7.
[http://dx.doi.org/10.1007/BF02976556] [PMID: 12009028]

[41] Mahady GB, Pendland SL, Stoia A, *et al. In Vitro* susceptibility of*Helicobacter pylori* to botanical extracts used traditionally for the treatment of gastrointestinal disorders. Phytother Res 2005; 19(11): 988-91.
[http://dx.doi.org/10.1002/ptr.1776] [PMID: 16317658]

[42] Mohammad Mohsenzadeh . Evaluation of antibacterial activity of selected Iranian essential oils against *Staphylococcus aureus* and *Escherichia coli* in nutrient broth medium. Pak J Biol Sci 2007; 10(20): 3693-7.
[http://dx.doi.org/10.3923/pjbs.2007.3693.3697] [PMID: 19093484]

[43] Javidnia K, Dastgheib L, Mohammadi Samani S, Nasiri A. Antihirsutism activity of Fennel (fruits of *Foeniculum vulgare*) extract – A double-blind placebo controlled study. Phytomedicine 2003; 10(6-7): 455-8.
[http://dx.doi.org/10.1078/094471103322331386] [PMID: 13678227]

[44] Samadi-Noshahr Z, Hadjzadeh MAR, Moradi-Marjaneh R, Khajavi-Rad A. The hepatoprotective effects of fennel seeds extract and *trans*-Anethole in streptozotocin-induced liver injury in rats. Food Sci Nutr 2021; 9(2): 1121-31.
[http://dx.doi.org/10.1002/fsn3.2090] [PMID: 33598196]

[45] Choi E, Hwang J. Anti-inflammatory, analgesic and antioxidant. Fitoterapia 2004; 75(6): 557-65.
[http://dx.doi.org/10.1016/j.fitote.2004.05.005] [PMID: 15351109]

[46] Abed K. Antimicrobial activity of essential oils of some medicinal plants from Saudi Arabia. Saudi J Biol Sci 2007; 14(1): 53-60.

[47] Pai MB, Prashant GM, Murlikrishna KS, Shivakumar KM, Chandu GN. Antifungal efficacy of *Punica*

granatum, Acacia nilotica, Cuminum cyminum and *Foeniculum vulgare* on *Candida albicans*: an *in vitro* study. J Dent Res 2010; 21(3): 334-6.
[PMID: 20930339]

[48]   Singh G, Maurya S, de Lampasona MP, Catalan C. Chemical constituents, antifungal and antioxidative potential of *Foeniculum vulgare* volatile oil and its acetone extract. Food Control 2006; 17(9): 745-52.
[http://dx.doi.org/10.1016/j.foodcont.2005.03.010]

[49]   Soylu S, Yigitbas H, Soylu EM, Kurt Ş. Antifungal effects of essential oils from oregano and fennel on *Sclerotinia sclerotiorum*. J Appl Microbiol 2007; 103(4): 1021-30.
[http://dx.doi.org/10.1111/j.1365-2672.2007.03310.x] [PMID: 17897206]

[50]   Tognolini M, Ballabeni V, Bertoni S, Bruni R, Impicciatore M, Barocelli E. Protective effect of *Foeniculum vulgare* essential oil and anethole in an experimental model of thrombosis. Pharmacol Res 2007; 56(3): 254-60.
[http://dx.doi.org/10.1016/j.phrs.2007.07.002] [PMID: 17709257]

[51]   Naglaa M, Halima S, Hoda F, Sherifa H, Ekram S. Antimutagenic. J Am Sci 2010; 6(9): 831-42.

[52]   Pereira ASP, Banegas-Luna AJ, Peña-García J, Pérez-Sánchez H, Apostolides Z. Evaluation of the Anti-Diabetic Activity of Some Common Herbs and Spices: Providing New Insights with Inverse Virtual Screening. Molecules 2019; 24(22): 4030.
[http://dx.doi.org/10.3390/molecules24224030] [PMID: 31703341]

[53]   Shabbir R. Assessment and Effectiveness of Fennel Powder Extract Based Cookies in Hyperglycemic Subjects 2020; 2: 5.

[54]   Sadeghpour N, Khaki A, Najafpour A, Dolatkhah H, Montaseri A. Study of *Foeniculum vulgare* (Fennel) Seed Extract Effects on Serum Level of Estrogen, Progesterone and Prolactin in Mouse. Crescent J Med Biol Sci 2015; 2: 23-7.

[55]   Ruberto G, Baratta MT, Deans SG, Dorman HJD. Antioxidant and antimicrobial activity of *Foeniculum vulgare* and *Crithmum maritimum* essential oils. Planta Med 2000; 66(8): 687-93.
[http://dx.doi.org/10.1055/s-2000-9773] [PMID: 11199122]

[56]   De Marino S, Gala F, Borbone N, *et al.* Phenolic glycosides from *Foeniculum vulgare* fruit and evaluation of antioxidative activity. Phytochemistry 2007; 68(13): 1805-12.
[http://dx.doi.org/10.1016/j.phytochem.2007.03.029] [PMID: 17498761]

[57]   Özbek H, Uğraş S, Dülger H, *et al.* Hepatoprotective effect of *Foeniculum vulgare* essential oil. Fitoterapia 2003; 74(3): 317-9.
[http://dx.doi.org/10.1016/S0367-326X(03)00028-5] [PMID: 12727504]

[58]   Badgujar SB, Patel VV, Bandivdekar AH. *Foeniculum vulgare* Mill: a review of its botany, phytochemistry, pharmacology, contemporary application, and toxicology. BioMed Res Int 2014; 2014: 1-32.
[http://dx.doi.org/10.1155/2014/842674] [PMID: 25162032]

[59]   Mehra N, Tamta G, Nand V. A review on nutritional value, phytochemical and pharmacological attributes of *Foeniculum vulgare* Mill. J Pharmacogn Phytochem 2021; 10(2): 1255-63.
[http://dx.doi.org/10.22271/phyto.2021.v10.i2q.13983]

[60]   El-Soud N, El-Laithy N, El-Saeed G, Wahby M, Khalil MM, Shaffie N. Antidiabetic activities of *Foeniculum vulgare* Mill. Essential oil in Streptozotocin-induced diabetic rats. Maced J Med Sci 2011; 4(2): 139-46.

[61]   Gilani AH, Jabeen Q, Ghayur MN, Janbaz KH, Akhtar MS. Studies on the antihypertensive, antispasmodic, bronchodilator and hepatoprotective activities of the *Carum copticum* seed extract. J Ethnopharmacol 2005; 98(1-2): 127-35.
[http://dx.doi.org/10.1016/j.jep.2005.01.017] [PMID: 15763373]

[62]   Ahsan S, Shah A, Tanira M, Ahmad M, Tariq M, Ageel A. Studies on some herbal drugs used against kidney stones in Saudi folk medicine. Fitoterapia 1990; 61(5): 435-8.

[63]   Srivastava KC. Extract of a spice — Omum (*Trachyspermum ammi*)-shows antiaggregatory effects and alters arachidonic acid metabolism in human platelets. Prostaglandins Leukot Essent Fatty Acids 1988; 33(1): 1-6.
[http://dx.doi.org/10.1016/0952-3278(88)90115-9] [PMID: 3141935]

[64]   Thangam C, Dhananjayan R. Anti-inflammatory Potential of The Seeds of *Carum copticum* Linn. Indian J Pharmacol 2003; 35(6): 388-91.

[65]   Boskabady MH, Jandaghi P, Kiani S, Hasanzadeh L. Antitussive effect of *Carum copticum* in guinea pigs. J Ethnopharmacol 2005; 97(1): 79-82.
[http://dx.doi.org/10.1016/j.jep.2004.10.016] [PMID: 15652279]

[66]   Mathew N, Misra-Bhattacharya S, Perumal V, Muthuswamy K. Antifilarial lead molecules isolated from *Trachyspermum ammi*. Molecules 2008; 13(9): 2156-68.
[http://dx.doi.org/10.3390/molecules13092156] [PMID: 18830147]

[67]   Ramaswamy S, Sengottuvelu S, Sherief S. HajaJaikumar S, Saravanan R, Prasadkumar C. Gastroprotective Activity of Ethanolic Extract of *Trachyspermum ammi* Fruit. Int J Pharma Bio Sci 2010; 1(1): 1-15.

[68]   Velazhahan R, Vijayanandraj S, Vijayasamundeeswari A, *et al.* Detoxification of aflatoxins by seed extracts of the medicinal plant, *Trachyspermum ammi* (L.) Sprague ex Turrill – Structural analysis and biological toxicity of degradation product of aflatoxin G1. Food Control 2010; 21(5): 719-25.
[http://dx.doi.org/10.1016/j.foodcont.2009.10.014]

[69]   Anilakumar KR, Saritha V, Khanum F, Bawa AS. Ameliorative effect of ajwain extract on hexachlorocyclohexane-induced lipid peroxidation in rat liver. Food Chem Toxicol 2009; 47(2): 279-82.
[http://dx.doi.org/10.1016/j.fct.2008.09.061] [PMID: 18940228]

[70]   Khanuja SPS, Srivastava S, Shasney AK, Darokar MP, Kumar TRS, Agarwal KK, *et al.* Formulation comprising thymol useful in the treatment of drug-resistant bacterial infections [Internet]. US6514541B2, 2003 [cited 2021 Aug 17]. https://patents.google.com/patent/US6514541B2/en

[71]   Caccioni DRL, Guizzardi M, Biondi DM. Agatino Renda, Ruberto G. Relationship between volatile components of citrus fruit essential oils and antimicrobial. Int J Food Microbiol 1998; 43(1): 73-9.
[http://dx.doi.org/10.1016/S0168-1605(98)00099-3] [PMID: 9761340]

[72]   Javed I, Akhtar T, Khaliq M, Khan G, Muhammad M. Antihyperlipidaemic effect of *Trachyspermum ammi* (Ajwain) in rabbits. Proc 33rd Pak Sci Conf Univ Agric. 80-1.

[73]   Platel K, Srinivasan K. Studies on the influence of dietary spices on food transit time in experimental rats. Nutr Res 2001; 21(9): 1309-14.
[http://dx.doi.org/10.1016/S0271-5317(01)00331-1]

[74]   Vasudevan K, Vembar S, Veeraraghavan K, Haranath PS. Influence of intragastric perfusion of aqueous spice extracts on acid secretion in anesthetized albino rats. Indian J Gastroenterol 2000; 19(2): 53-6.
[PMID: 10812814]

[75]   Sikora RA, Hartwig J. Mode-of-action of the carbamate nematicides cloethocarb, aldicarb and carbofuran on Heterodera schachtii 2. Systemic Activity: 6.

[76]   Kong JO, Lee SM, Moon YS, Lee SG, Ahn YJ. Nematicidal Activity. J Asia Pac Entomol 2006; 9(2): 173-8.
[http://dx.doi.org/10.1016/S1226-8615(08)60289-7]

[77]   Shin S-C, Park I-K, Choi I-H. Nematicidal activity of onion (*Allium cepa*) oil and its components against the pine wood nematode (Bursaphelenchus xylophilus). Nematology 2007; 9(2): 231-5.
[http://dx.doi.org/10.1163/156854107780739018]

[78]   Kwon H-R, Son S-W, Han H-R, Choi G-J, Jang K-S, Choi Y-H, *et al.* Nematicidal Activity Plant

Pathol J 2007; 23.

[79]   Murthy P, Borse B, Khanum H, Srinivas P. Inhibitory effects of Ajwain (*Trachyspermum ammi*) ethanolic extract on *A. ochraceus* growth and ochratoxin production. Turk J Biol 2009; 33: 211-7.

[80]   Jabbar A, Iqbal Z, Khan M. *In vitro* anthelmintic activity of *Trachyspermum ammi* seeds. Pharmacogn Mag 2006; 2(6): 126-9.

[81]   Kostyukovsky M, Rafaeli A, Gileadi C, Demchenko N, Shaaya E. Activation of octopaminergic receptors by essential oil constituents isolated from aromatic plants: possible mode of action against insect pests. Pest Manag Sci 2002; 58(11): 1101-6.
[http://dx.doi.org/10.1002/ps.548] [PMID: 12449528]

[82]   Park IK, Kim J, Lee SG, Shin SC. Nematicidal Activity. J Nematol 2007; 39(3): 275-9.
[PMID: 19259498]

[83]   Tamura T, Iwamoto H. Thymol: a classical small-molecule compound that has a dual effect (potentiating and inhibitory) on myosin. Biochem Biophys Res Commun 2004; 318(3): 786-91.
[http://dx.doi.org/10.1016/j.bbrc.2004.04.085] [PMID: 15144906]

[84]   Ardestani MM, Aliahmadi A, Toliat T, Dalimi A, Momeni Z, Rahimi R. Evaluation of Antimicrobial Activity of *Trachyspermum ammi* (L.) Sprague Essential Oil and Its Active Constituent, Thymol, against Vaginal Pathogens. Tradit Integr Med. 2020 Jun 27;49–58.

[85]   Saxena A, Vyas K. Antimicrobial activity of seeds of some ethnomedicinal plants. J Econ Taxon Bot 1986; 8: 291-300.

[86]   Pelczar MJ, Chan EC, Krieg N. Microbiology, Control of microorganism by physical agents. Mcgraw Hill International, New York; 1988. 469–509.

[87]   Singh G, Maurya S, Catalan C. Chemical, antifungal, antioxidative studies of Ajwain oil and its acetone extract. J Agric Food Chem 2004; 52(11): 3292-6.
[http://dx.doi.org/10.1021/jf035211c] [PMID: 15161185]

[88]   Wright DJ. Nematicides: Mode of action and new approaches to chemical control. BM Zuckerman RA Rohde Eds Plant-Parasit Nematodes Lond N Y Acad Press. 1981;421–4.

CHAPTER 8

New Insights into Biological and Pharmaceutical Properties of Bioactive Compounds in Various Diseases of Farm Animals

Sneha Keelka[1], Pallavi Kaushik[1,*] and Mukesh Kumar Sharma[2]

[1] *Department of Zoology, University of Rajasthan, Jaipur-302004, Rajasthan, India*

[2] *Department of Zoology, SPC Government College, Ajmer-305001, Rajasthan, India*

Abstract: Farm animals have a crucial role in producing sources of protein and other nutritive products for humans. However, these animals are confronting diverse challenging ailments and subsequent oxidative stress, which reduces the efficiency of production and impairs animal welfare. Bioactive compounds obtained from plants and other natural provenances have now been accredited as the crucial steppingstone against the numerous persistent diseases encountered by farm animals. Bioactive compounds possess remarkable molecular diversity and modulate numerous metabolic processes with high precedence goals, low toxicity, exhibiting high efficacy with low cost, easy availability with less or no side effects.

In this context, the chapter addresses recently observed bioactive compounds for the treatment of various livestock diseases. Moreover, an attempt to consolidate information on numerous bioactive compounds has been made which brings aid in unrelenting research into potential use.

Keywords: Bioactive compounds, Coccidiosis, Livestock disease, Phytochemicals, Poultry.

INTRODUCTION

Livestock animals play a crucial role in the economic and socio-cultural lifestyle population residing in developing and developed countries' rural and urban areas. These contribute to the food supply, source of earning, source of employment, and sustainable agriculture production [1]. Animal waste is used to manure soil and as a source of biofuel. Farm animals and their products are an economical source of high-quality protein and another energy source for human consumption. Thus, the

---

* **Corresponding author Pallavi Kaushik:** Department of Zoology, University of Rajasthan, Jaipur-302004, Rajasthan, India; Tel: +91-98286 96079; E-mail: pallavikaushik512@gmail.com

Mukesh Kumar Sharma and Pallavi Kaushik (Eds.)

well-being of livestock seems essential for an uninterrupted supply of aforesaid benefits which can be achieved through good husbandry and proper hygiene.

The production of farm animals has been challenged by environmental issues and consumers' attitudes as well as diseases. Farm animals are prone to some diseases, such as foot and mouth disease that affect all cloven-footed animals, Coccidiosis which affects poultry animals, Anthrax, and various other diseases caused by protozoans, bacteria, and other parasites [2 - 4].

A range of feed additives such as antibiotics, phytobiotics, probiotics, and prebiotics have been used to improve the health and production of farm animals. The livestock production system and welfare standards are continuously changing for farm animals. Their production in developed countries relies on several synthetic compounds to maintain the health of animals and to increase production. However, a few terrible consequences and outcomes of these practices are rising, so there is a requirement of some natural alternative methods to cope with healthy animal production [5].

In livestock, antibiotics are used as therapeutic agents to treat disease. The excessive use of these antibiotics has led to an increase in antibiotic resistance in pathogens. Therefore, there is an imperative need for devising castigating interventions with broad exploration and novel health promising strategies comprising naturally occurring bioactive compounds. Bioactive compounds extracted from plants and other sources can be a milestone in farm animal management [6 - 9].

There is worldwide interest in utilizing the bioactive properties of plants as a less costly, easily available alternative to chemical and synthetic food products and drugs. Medicinal plants have been exploited by developing countries for centuries to treat animals. Various medicinal plants from traditional phytotherapy are used for animal health care and food supplements. These supplements are also referred to as phytobiotics or phytogenics, which are derived from plants and are incorporated into animal feed and medicines to increase the immunity and productivity of animals [6]. Plant secondary metabolites (*e.g.* tannins, essential oils, and saponins) have the ability to manipulate rumen fermentation to improve the ruminant production system and also provide health benefits to livestock [2, 4].

Marine-derived bioactive compounds, on the other hand, are a subset, having only been exploited since the 1970s, but hold an auspicious source, as their chemical ingenuity and diversity outweigh that of terrestrial founts [10]. Marine weeds, sponges, and other organisms have also been reported as potential bioactive compounds containing sources. These bioactive compounds isolated from marine sources exhibit various bioactivities such as antimicrobial, anti-inflammatory, and antioxidative effects on humans, aquaculture, and veterinary commodities (*e.g.* cattle and poultry farming) [7 - 9].

Plant-based Bioactive Compound for the Treatment of Livestock Diseases and their Mechanism of Action

Among an enormous miscellany of functional bioactive compounds, phytochemicals have engrossed broad recognition for their extensive bioactivities linked with antioxidant and immune-stimulating applications impacting health and wellness. Numerous findings have highlighted that therapeutic plant-derived compounds can augment the effectiveness of various farm animal disease remedial treatments. Some of the significant bioactive compounds with prospective use in the treatment of livestock diseases are described in the following text:

Natural Phenolic Compounds

These are the bioactive compounds that are derived from secondary metabolites of plant tissue [11]. They are classified based on carbon chain length, side groups, distribution in nature, and part of the plant from which they are derived [12]. Herbs, vegetables, and spices have abundant phenolic compounds [13, 14]. These compounds have the capability to control oxidative stress in animal cells and act as an immune booster. In the remnants, polyphenols perform the following role:

a. Interact with rumen microbiota, affecting various biochemical processes such as protein degradation, lipid metabolism, and carbohydrate fermentation. Inhibitory effects of these compounds have also been reported on some fibrolytic bacteria and protozoa [12, 15].
b. Enhance the production of livestock products such as meat production [12].

Few phenolic compounds with their uses in the treatment of livestock are mentioned in the following text:-

Tannins

Tannins are defined as polyphenolic compounds. Tannins exist in fruits (*e.g.* berries, pears, and apples), foraged legumes, nuts, *etc* [16, 17]. The antimicrobial effects of tannins in chicken have been reported by various investigators. One of the most common parasitic ailments in poultry farm animals is coccidiosis, which is induced by *Eimeria* species of protozoan family [18]. Coccidiosis can result in reduced growth, and cause various digestive disorders and oxidative stress [19]. Tannins (hydrolyzable tannins, condensed tannins) and their derivatives with other compounds such as essential oils, organic acid has been reported as potent anticoccidial bioactive compounds as these can form complex with parasitic enzymes and metal ion which are essential for protozoan to survive, this, in turn, enhances the immunity of host against protozoan and attenuate effects of oxidative stress [17, 20, 21]. The advantageous effect of tannins has also been reported in cattle as they help to maintain a healthy gut environment by reducing the adverse effects of nematodes [22].

Flavonoids

Flavonoids are a benzo-pyrone derivative of phenolic compounds which have a 15-C skeleton that consists of two phenyl rings and a heterocyclic ring. It constitutes the largest subcategory of natural phenolic compounds (*e.g.* flavanols, flavones, anthocyanin) [12]. Flavonoids exist in herbs, fruits (berries, citrus fruits, and tropical fruits), vegetables, nuts, and certain beverages [23 - 25]. These have antimicrobial and anti-oxidative properties; therefore, these are useful in treating various diseases in farm animals, such as mastitis, influenza, and oxidative stress caused by various parasites and other factors [25, 26]. Flavones activate the immune system by increasing the activity of hydroxy derivatives of flavones in case of mastitis [27]. Hydroxyl group of flavonoids mediate their antioxidant properties by chelating metal ions and by interrupting free radical chain reactions [23].

Phenolic Acids

These compounds consist of a benzene ring bonded to a carboxylic group. Phenolic acids such as caffeic acid, gallic acid, ferulic acid, coumaric acid, and hydroxytyrosol and its derivatives found in various plants such as coffee, olive, cabbage, apples, dried ginger, *etc.* and agriculture by-products play a crucial role in maintaining the reproductive health of farm animals and increase antioxidant properties of cells [28, 29]. Gallic acid plays an important role in decreasing the concentration of free radicals by directly combining with these radicals [29].

Saponin

Saponins are a diverse group of secondary metabolites present in plants that contain either tetracyclic steroidal or pentacyclic triterpenoid aglycone which are connected to sugar moieties [30]. The word *sapo* is Latin in origin that means foam which indicates that saponin exhibits foaming properties [31]. Saponin has been reported as a potential compound to improve the health and production of poultry farm animals. It acts as an anticoccidial agent, immunostimulant, growth promoter, cholesterol-reducing agent, antifungal agent, and antioxidant in nature for poultry farm animals [30 - 34]. Saponin binds to the outer membrane of protozoa that in turn causes lysis of protozoa. It promotes antioxidant activities to scavenge free radicals and prevent the action of lipid peroxidation by increasing glutathione peroxidase and superoxide dismutase activity [35].

Essential Oils

Essential oils are a group of plant secondary metabolites. The composition of essential oils depends on various factors such as season of harvesting, type of plant part, and environmental conditions. Essential oils have been reported as potential antibacterial, antifungal agents in poultry and cattle farm diseases [36, 37]. Thymol, eugenol, and carvacrol have been reported as potent antimicrobial agents against disease conditions arising due to *Escherichia coli* and *Salmonella* sp. in poultry [36, 38] Clove and Cinnamon essential oils have evidenced good antibacterial activities as they damage the inner cell materials of *E.coli*. These oils can function in combination as well as solely [37, 39].

Terpenes

It is a class of unsaturated hydrocarbons which are produced predominantly by plants. Ursolic acid, linalool, geniposide, and ginsenosides are the major compounds available in various herbs and shrubs. These compounds have been reported as potential bioactive compounds against virus infection in foot and mouth disease (FMD). These might inhibit the viral infection either by viral particle uncoating or by blocking the translation of viral proteins and by reducing viral capsid protein expression [40 - 44].

Vitamins

Vitamin E is a fat-soluble antioxidant that protects animals against oxidative stress and also acts as an immunomodulator. Vitamin E supplementation has been also reported as a potential supplement against Newcastle disease virus titer and lymphocyte proliferation with increased egg production in poultry farm animals [45].

Vitamin D has various functions in the organism, from calcium homeostasis to modulation of the immune system. It promotes optimal innate and adaptive immune function of cattle and other animals. Vitamin D in feed can be either of plant origin or animal origin as cattle can synthesize their own vitamin D (cholecalciferol) [46].

Other important bioactive compounds that retain inherent characteristics to act in opposition to assorted livestock diseases from the explicit medicinal plants are mentioned in Table **1** and the chemical structure of bioactive compounds is mentioned in Fig. (**1**).

Table 1. A Compilation of Important Phytochemicals Against Various Farm Animal Diseases.

S.No.	Name	Source	Disease	Therapeutic Attributes/Mechanism of Action	Refs.
1	Artemisinin	Sweet wormwood	Coccidiosis	Inhibit sporulation *Eimeria tenella*	[47, 48]
2	Catechin and Epicatechin (Flavonoids)	Green tea	Influenza in chicken and mastitis in cow	Antibacterial effect (inhibit quorum sensing) on *S. aureus*	[25]
3	Allicin	Garlic	Coccidiosis	Inhibit sporulation in *Eimeria tenella*	[49]
4	Papain	Papaya leaves	Coccidiosis	Proteolytic destruction of protozoa(*Eimeria* sp)	[48, 50]
5	Maslinic acid	Leaves and fruits of the olive tree	Coccidiosis	Anticoccidial activity	[48, 51]
6	Proanthocyanidin (polyphenol)	Grape seed	Coccidiosis	Downregulation of oxidative stress	[48]
7	Arabinoxylan	Wheat bran	Coccidiosis	Immuno-stimulation against protozoan	[52]
8	Curcumin	Turmeric	Coccidiosis	Destroy sporozoites of *Eimeria tenella*, immune-stimulation	[48, 53, 54]
9	Gallic acid	Herbs	Brucellosis	Antipyretic activities	[55]
10	Tea tree essential oil compounds(terpinene,α-pinene)	Tea tree	Mycoplasma	Antioxidant and anti-inflammatory	[56]
11	Alkaloids, Tannins	*Cymodoceaserrulata* root, herbs, vegetables	*E. coli* infection and Salmonellosis	Antimicrobial (direct interaction with the cell wall and alter the permeability of membrane) and anti-inflammatory	[57]
12	Carvacrol (Essential oil)	Oregano	Campylobacteriosis (*Campylobacter sp.*)	Antimicrobial (alter the morphology of cell of the microbe and decrease the activity of enzymes) activities	[58]
13	Allicin, terpenoids, steroids	Garlic	Tick-borne diseases	Acaricidal activity	[59, 60]

(Table 1) cont.....

S.No.	Name	Source	Disease	Therapeutic Attributes/Mechanism of Action	Refs.
14	Tannic acid	Gallnut	Coccidiosis Salmonellosis	Antioxidant and antimicrobial (inhibit quorum sensing, biofilm production of bacteria)	[3, 17]
15	Alkaloids	Garlic	Mastitis	Antibacterial, anti-inflammatory	[61]
16	Gallotannin	Tasmanian pepper berry	Anthrax	Anti-inflammatory, antioxidant	[62]
17	α-tocopherol and selenium	Green leafy vegetables, grains	Mastitis in cow	Antioxidant, Anti-inflammatory	[63]
18	Baicalein (Flavones) and Morin (Flavonol)	Guava, apple, onion, almond, herbs, citrus fruits	Mastitis	Anti-inflammatory	[63, 64]
19	Terpenes and terpenoids	*Annona squamosa,* fruits, vegetables	Infection due to nematodes	Nematocidal effect	[63]

Bioactive Compounds Isolated From Other Sources

Marine acquired natural products have been accredited as another promising source of bioactive substances with vast pharmacological potential. These metabolites generally belong to peptides, phenols, sulfated polysaccharides, carotenoids, and their derivatives. The chemical structures of bioactive compounds are mentioned below in Fig. (**1**).

Some of the important ones are described below:

Polysaccharides

Seaweeds contain various types of polysaccharides, among them, sulfated polysaccharides inhibit the activity of several bacterial as well as viral species that infect humans and animals. Among different algal polysaccharides, the most important are laminarian, galactans, fucoidan and alginates.

Sulfated galactans

Sulfated galactans are present in the cell wall and intercellular matrix of green seaweed. It contains disaccharide based repeating units and possesses anti-tumor and antiviral properties [65, 66].

Fucoidan

Fucoidan is a sulfated polysaccharide found in various species of brown seaweed such as *Laminaria and Sargassum sp.* The chemical composition of this compound depends on the algal source and harvesting time. It has anti-inflammatory, antiviral, and antioxidative properties. It can serve as an antibiotic for farm animals [67 - 70].

Laminarin

Laminarin is a major class of polysaccharides found in brown alga such as *Laminaria*. It is a dietary fiber and can act as a prebiotic compound and is antioxidant by nature. It can serve as an alternative to in-feed antibiotics for farm animals and also enhance the intestinal health of animals [67 - 71]. Alginates are also extracted from brown seaweeds and are absent in terrestrial plants. They have antibacterial and anti-inflammatory properties [66].

Polyphenol

Many polyphenols have been reported to possess antimicrobial, strong anti-oxidative and anti-inflammatory properties. Some of the important ones are described briefly in the following text.

Phlorotannins

Phlorotannins isolated from brown seaweed act as a prebiotic for poultry and pigs and increase the anti-oxidative status of the animals [72].

Bromophenols

Bromophenols isolated from brown and green seaweed have anti-oxidative and antimicrobial activity against bacterial species such as *Staphylococcus aureus* and *Pseudomonas* sp [72].

Flavonoids

Flavonoids such as catechin, flavones, isoflavones, and flavonols isolated green, red and brown seaweeds have immunomodulatory effects on humans and other animals [72].

Phenolic terpenoids

Phenolic terpenoids have been detected and characterized in brown and red seaweed. Terpenoids are characterized as meroditerpenoids, diterpenes and sesquiterpenes which are antioxidant and immunomodulatory in nature [72, 73].

Carotenoids

Carotenoids are organic pigments which are present in chloroplast and chromoplasts and are produced by marine algae, plants, and by a few bacteria. The most crucial carotenoids are β- carotene, fucoxanthin and tocopherol. These are essential for farm animals and humans for growth and healthy life [66]. Carotenoids are anti-inflammatory, anti-oxidative, and immunomodulatory in nature so they are used in poultry and cattle feed [74].

Phycobiliproteins

Phycobiliproteins are water-soluble pigment isolated from red algae that contain anti-inflammatory, antiviral and antioxidative properties [66].

Peptides

Bioactive peptides isolated from marine sponges contain amino acids which are either absent or rare in terrestrial plant-based peptides and microbial peptides [9]. Antimicrobial peptides can be used as an alternative to antibiotics or can be used with a combination of existing antibiotics [75]. These peptides exhibit antifungal and anti-inflammatory properties [9].

Briefings about other bioactive compounds isolated from marine or other sources along with their therapeutic attributes are compiled in Table **2**.

Table 2. Bioactive compounds against various farm animal diseases.

S.No.	Name	Source	Disease and Pathogen	Mechanism of Action	Refs.
1	Floridoside with antibiotic (tetracycline)	Red seaweed	Salmonellosis (*Salmonella enteritidis*) in poultry	Inhibition of quorum sensing and efflux related genes of a pathogen such as marA, arcB, ramA	[76]
2	Phenolic compounds and polysaccharides	*Chondrus crispus* and *Sarcodio the cagaudichaudii* (Red seaweed)	Clostridial enteritis (*Clostridium perfringens*) in poultry	Increase humoral immune response	[77, 78]
3	Fructo-oligosaccharide with extract(essential oil, polyphenol)	*Chondrus crispus* (Red seaweed)	*Pseudomonas aeruginosa* infection	Inhibition of quorum sensing and virulence factors	[79]

(Table 2) cont.....

S.No.	Name	Source	Disease and Pathogen	Mechanism of Action	Refs.
4	Xylan, sulfated galactans and porphyrins	*Chondrus crispus* (Red seaweed)	Salmonellosis (*Salmonella enteritidis*) in poultry	Inhibition of quorum sensing and efflux related genes and colonization of pathogen by attenuation of virulence factors	[78, 80, 81]
5	MT.X+®, Olmix	Commercial algal clay	Mycotoxicosis	Increase antibody production to overcome the negative effect of fungus	[82]
6	Phlorotanin	Brown seaweed	Salmonellosis (*Salmonella agona*), Streptococcosis	Antioxidant and Antimicrobial effect by reducing quorum sensing	[83]
7	Lambda- carrageenans (Polysaccaride)	Red seaweed	Bovine herpesvirus	Antiviral activity by directly interacting virion	[84]
8	NOR- Batzelladine L	*Monanchora* sp.(marine sponge)	Avian metapneumovirus	Antiviral activity	[85]
9	Phorioadenine A	*Phoriospongia* sp.(marine sponge)	Nematode infection	Anti-parasitic effect against larval development	[9]

Uses of Bioactive Compounds

Antibiotics have been used for years to prevent infection and also as growth-promoting factors in humans and animals [76]. Due to the continuous use of antibiotics microbes have developed resistance to them. This unfortunate situation has resulted in the uncontrolled division of disease-causing microbes such as *Salmonella* and *Clostridium* that in turn can cause harmful effects on host animals [86]. So to overcome this situation the use of antibiotics is reduced and they are combined with natural bioactive extracts isolated from plants and other sources which have antimicrobial active compounds such as peptides, essential oils, *etc* [76, 87]. Functional extracts of brown seaweed *Laminaria japonica* and red seaweed have been mixed with clarithromycin and this combination inhibited the activity of the efflux pump [88]. Reduced consumption of antibiotics is highly desired, and this can be achieved by various natural products which can easily be available and are less expensive as compared to antibiotics.

Some seaweeds are commercialized as poultry feed and additive by various companies which are natural sources of bioactive compounds for healthy and efficient production by farm animals [7, 76]. A few of these are mentioned below:

a. MT.X+, Mfeed, Algimun, Searup by Olmix group – They are helpful against mycotoxin and improve the feed efficiency of poultry and pigs.
b. Brown seaweed meal containing mineral macro elements by Algea, The Arctic Company- This product is helpful in animal metabolism and performance.
c. *Asparagopsis* seaweed based diet by Future Feed Australia- This product have antibacterial properties and is helpful in methane reduction in livestock during fermentation.

CHEMICAL STRUCTURE OF BIOACTIVE COMPOUNDS

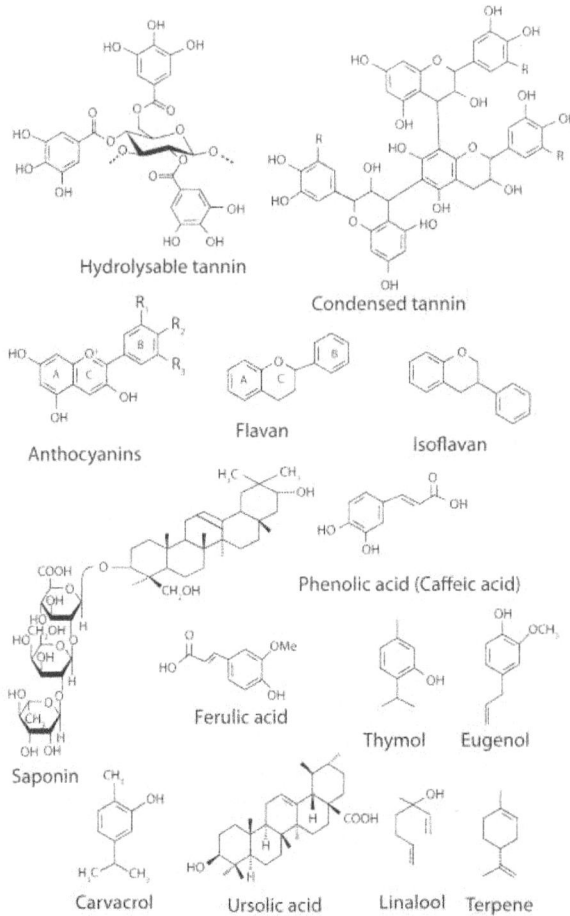

Fig. (1a). Chemical structure of bioactive compounds effective against farm animal diseases.

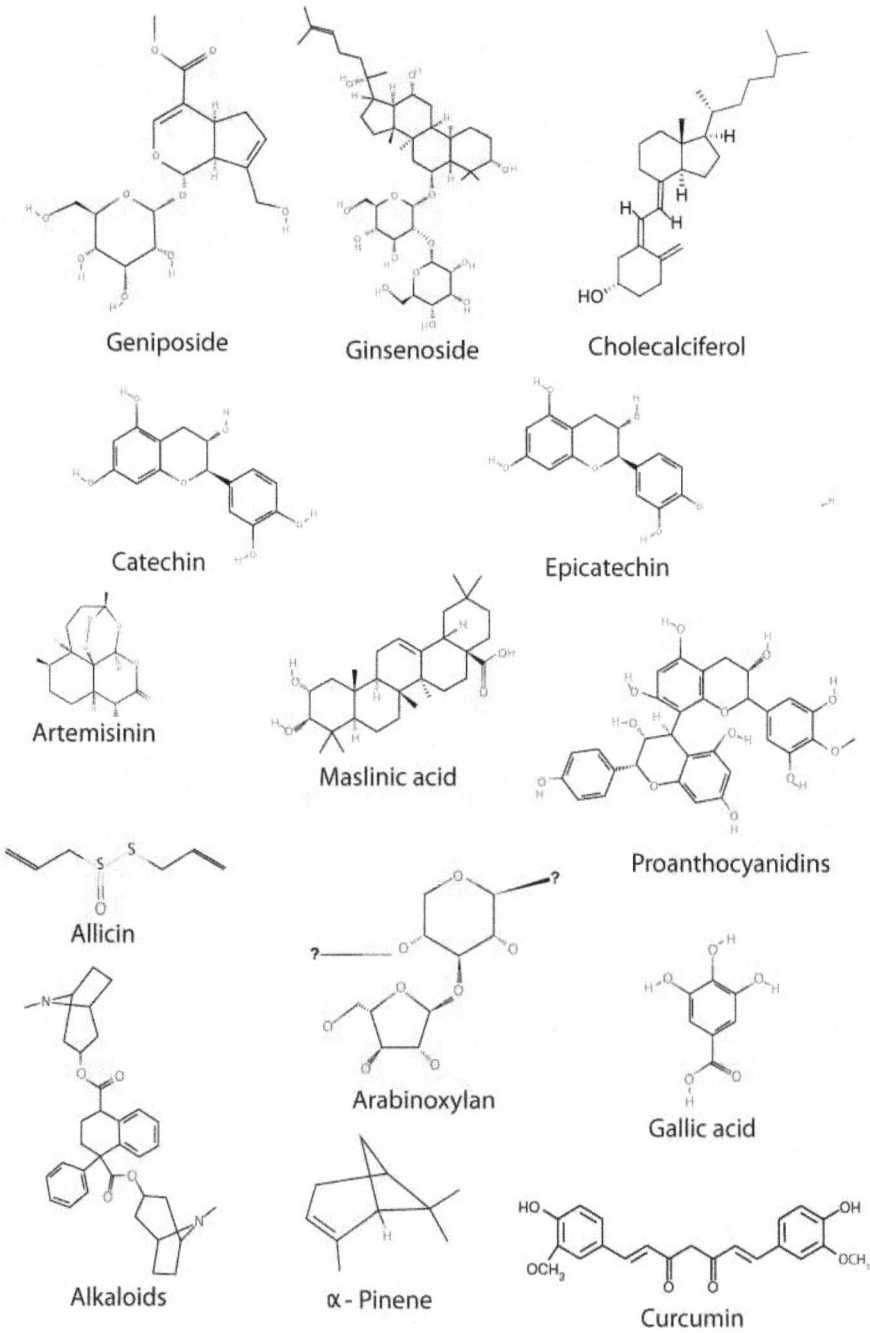

Geniposide

Ginsenoside

Cholecalciferol

Catechin

Epicatechin

Artemisinin

Maslinic acid

Proanthocyanidins

Allicin

Arabinoxylan

Gallic acid

Alkaloids

α - Pinene

Curcumin

Fig. (1b). Chemical structure of bioactive compounds effective against farm animal diseases.

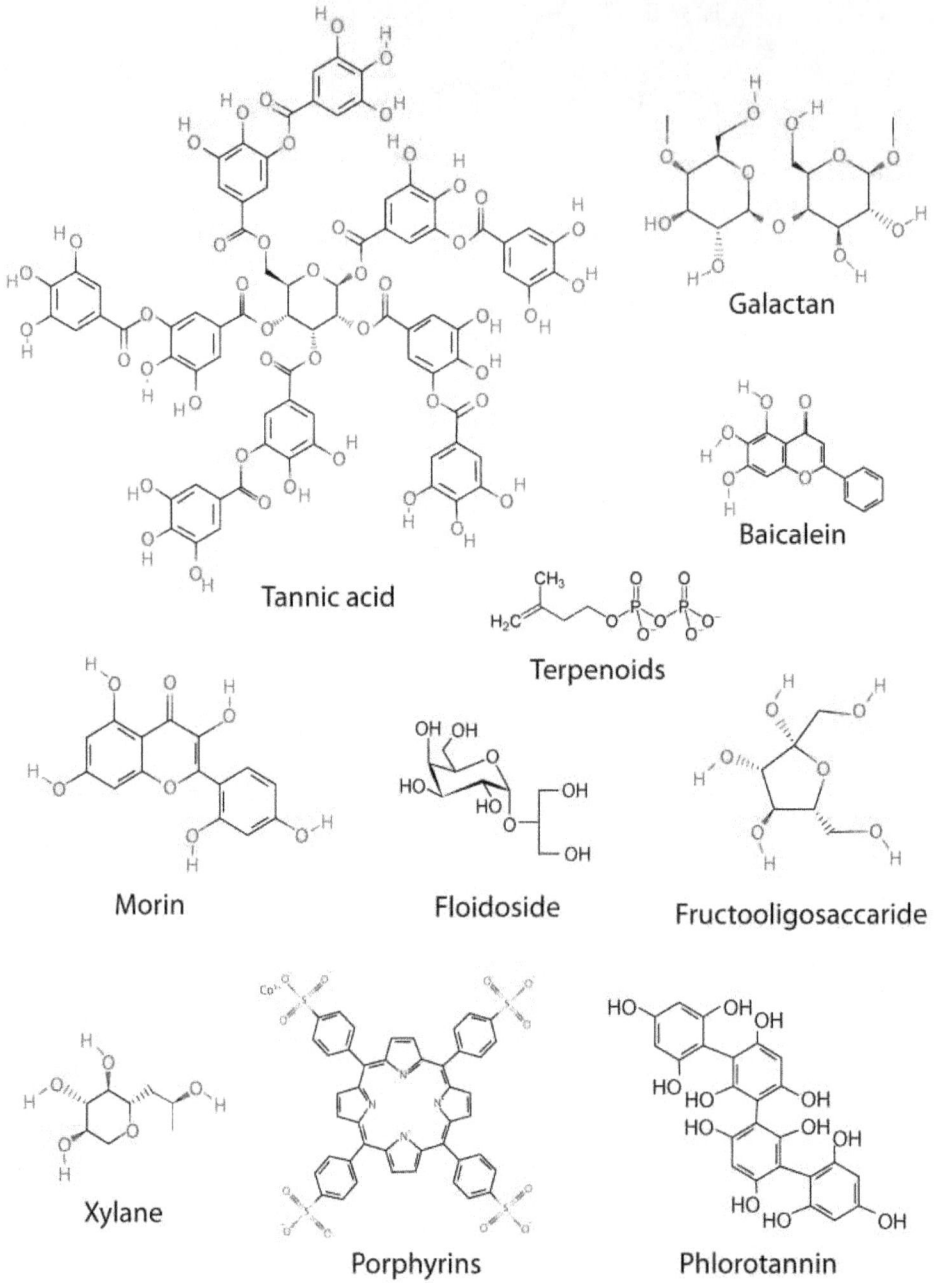

Fig. (1c). Chemical structure of bioactive compounds effective against farm animal diseases.

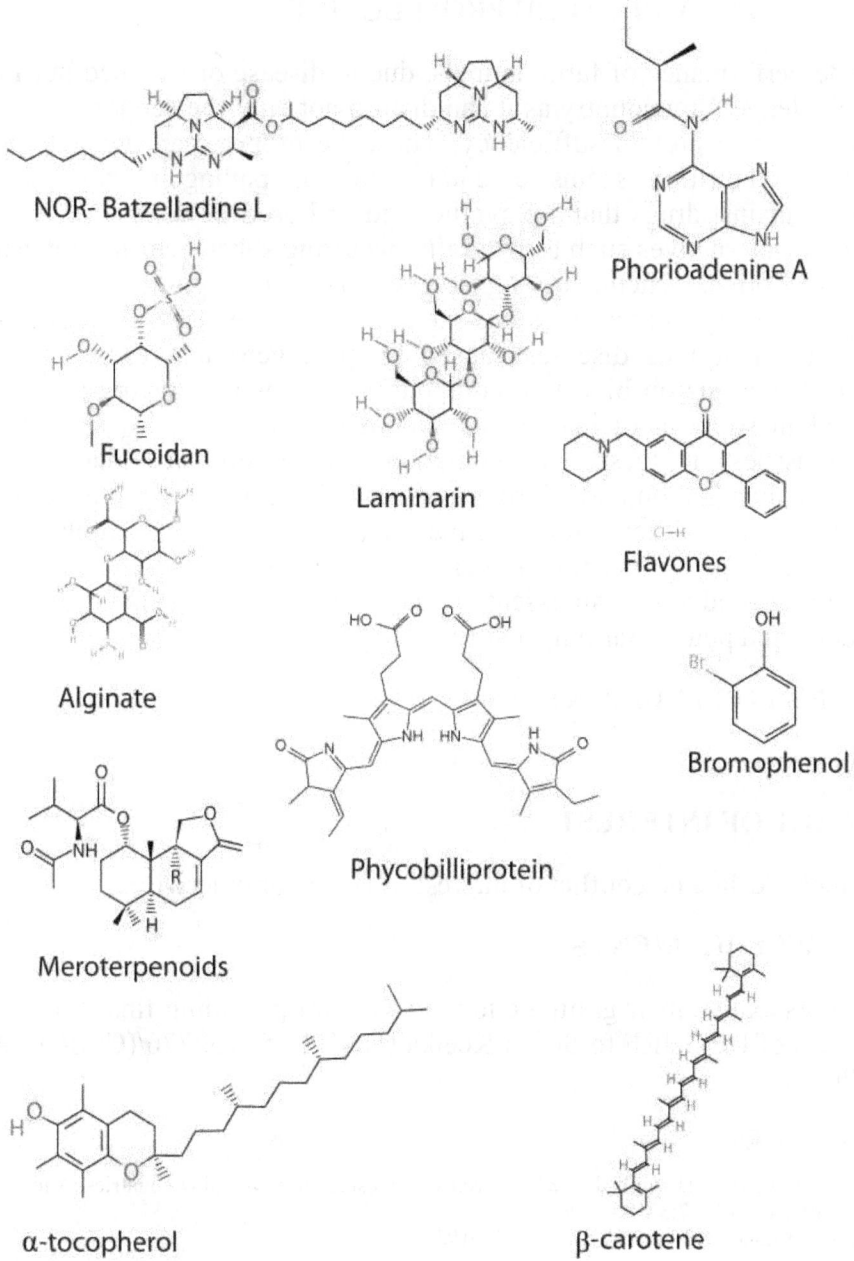

NOR- Batzelladine L

Phorioadenine A

Fucoidan

Laminarin

Flavones

Alginate

Phycobilliprotein

Bromophenol

Meroterpenoids

α-tocopherol

β-carotene

Fig. (1d). Chemical structure of bioactive compounds effective against farm animal diseases.

CONCLUSION AND FUTURE PROSPECTIVES

The underperformance of farm animals, due to disease or subdued nutrition is a major challenge for a country as it can disturb not only the economic growth but also compromise protein sufficiency. Thus, the proper management of animal disease and nutrition seems essential. Various pathogens have developed resistance against drugs that are synthesized and used in treatment. As a result, demand for alternatives such as naturally occurring substances has intensified as these are novel chemical signatures that are quite productive and pharmacologically active. In sum, we discussed the use of natural organic ingredients in various diseases caused by pathogens and their effects, with particular emphasis on bioactive compounds and their derivatives ubiquitously expressed in some medicinal plants and other sources. However, one of the important issues with these active compounds is their low bioavailability because of probable dilapidation under a rigorous gastro-intestinal environment, diffusion, absorption, or interaction with other nutrients could impede research progress in drug formulations. Further research and development in this field are required to make natural products as an essential part of disease management protocols for better dairy and poultry farming, cattle, *etc.*

CONSENT FOR PUBLICATION

Not applicable.

CONFLICT OF INTEREST

The authors declare no conflict of interest, financial or otherwise.

ACKNOWLEDGEMENTS

The authors extend their gratitude to the UGC, for providing financial assistance in the form of UGC-JRF to Sneha Keelka (UGC Ref. No.:776/(CSIR-UGC NET DEC. 2018).

REFERENCES

[1]   Herrero M, Grace D, Njuki J, *et al.* The roles of livestock in developing countries. Animal : an Int J AnimBiosci. 2013; 7:3–18.
[http://dx.doi.org/10.1017/S1751731112001954]

[2]   Pavarini DP, Pavarini SP, Niehues M, Lopes NP. Exogenous influences on plant secondary metabolite levels. Anim Feed Sci Technol 2012; 176(1-4): 5-16.
[http://dx.doi.org/10.1016/j.anifeedsci.2012.07.002]

[3]   Sivasankar C, Jha NK, Ghosh R, Shetty PH. Anti quorum sensing and anti virulence activity of tannic acid and it's potential to breach resistance in Salmonella enterica Typhi / Paratyphi A clinical isolates. Microb Pathog 2020; 138103813
[http://dx.doi.org/10.1016/j.micpath.2019.103813] [PMID: 31654777]

[4]   Mahfuz S, Shang Q, Piao X. Phenolic compounds as natural feed additives in poultry and swine diets: a review. J Anim Sci Biotechnol 2021; 12(1): 48.
[http://dx.doi.org/10.1186/s40104-021-00565-3] [PMID: 33823919]

[5]   Durmic Z, Blache D. Bioactive plants and plant products: Effects on animal function, health and welfare. Anim Feed Sci Technol 2012; 176(1-4): 150-62.
[http://dx.doi.org/10.1016/j.anifeedsci.2012.07.018]

[6]   Lillehoj H, Liu Y, Calsamiglia S, *et al.* Phytochemicals as antibiotic alternatives to promote growth and enhance host health. Vet Res 2018; 49(1): 76.
[http://dx.doi.org/10.1186/s13567-018-0562-6] [PMID: 30060764]

[7]   Kulshreshtha G, Hincke MT, Prithiviraj B, Critchley A. A review of varied uses of Macroalgae as dietry supplements in selected poultry with special reference to laying hen and broiler chicken. J Mar Sci Eng 2020; 8(7): 536.
[http://dx.doi.org/10.3390/jmse8070536]

[8]   Michalak I, Mahrose K. Seaweed intact and processed, as a valuable component of poultry feeds. J Mar Sci Eng 2020; 8(8): 620.
[http://dx.doi.org/10.3390/jmse8080620]

[9]   Varijakzhan D, Loh JY, Yap WS, *et al.* Bioactive compounds and marine sponges: Fundamentals and Application. Mar Drugs 2021; 19(5): 246.
[http://dx.doi.org/10.3390/md19050246] [PMID: 33925365]

[10]   Khalifa SAM, Elias N, Farag MA, *et al.* Marine natural products: A source of novel anticancer drugs. J. Mar Drugs 2019; 17(9): 491.
[http://dx.doi.org/10.3390/md17090491] [PMID: 31443597]

[11]   Veneziani G, Novelli E, Esposto S, *et al.* Applications of recovered bioactive compounds in foodproducts In olive mill waste: Recent advances for sustainable management. London, UK: Academic Press 2017; pp. 231-5.

[12]   Kalogianni AI, Lazou T, Bossis I, Gelasakis AI. Natural phenolic compounds for the control of oxidation, bacterial spoilage and foodborn pathogen in meat. Foods 2020; 9(6): 794.
[http://dx.doi.org/10.3390/foods9060794] [PMID: 32560249]

[13]   Brewer MS. Natural antioxidants: Sources, compounds, mechanism of action and potential application. Compr Rev Food Sci Food Saf 2011; 10(4): 221-47.
[http://dx.doi.org/10.1111/j.1541-4337.2011.00156.x]

[14]   Fernandes RDP, Tridade MD, De Melo MP. Natural antioxidants and food applications: Healthy perspectives. In: Grumezescu AM, Ed. Handbook of Food Bioengineering, Alternative and Replacement Foods, Holban, AM. London, UK: Academic Press 2018; pp. 31-64.
[http://dx.doi.org/10.1016/B978-0-12-811446-9.00002-2]

[15]   Vasta V, Daghio M, Cappucci A, *et al.* Invited review: Plant polyphenols and rumen microbiota responsible for fatty acid biohydrogenation, fiber digestion, and methane emission: Experimental evidence and methodological approaches. J Dairy Sci 2019; 102(5): 3781-804.
[http://dx.doi.org/10.3168/jds.2018-14985] [PMID: 30904293]

[16]   Martinez KB, Mackert JD, McIntosh MK. Polyphenols and intestinal health. Nutrition and Functional Foods for Healthy Aging. Amsterdam, The Netherlands: Elsevier 2017; pp. 191-210.
[http://dx.doi.org/10.1016/B978-0-12-805376-8.00018-6]

[17]   Choi J, Kim WK. Dietary Application of Tannins as a Potential Mitigation Strategy for Current Challenges in Poultry Production: A Review Animals. open access journal from MDPI 2020; 10(12): 2389.
[http://dx.doi.org/10.3390/ani10122389]

[18]   Grilli G, Borgonovo F, Tullo E, Fontana I, Guarino M, Ferrante V. A pilot study to detect coccidiosis in poultry farms at early stage from air analysis. Biosyst Eng 2018; 173: 64-70.

[http://dx.doi.org/10.1016/j.biosystemseng.2018.02.004]

[19]   Abbas R, Iqbal Z, Mansoor M. Role of natural antioxidants for the control of coccidiosis in poultry. Pak Vet J 2013; 33: 401-7.

[20]   Min B, Hart S. Tannins for suppression of internal parasites. J Anim Sci 2003; 81: 102-9.
[http://dx.doi.org/10.2527/2003.8114_suppl_2E102x]

[21]   Yang R, Hui Q, Jiang Q, *et al.* Effect of Manitoba-grown red-osier dogwood extracts on recovering Caco-2 cells from H2O2-induced oxidative damage. Antioxidants 2019; 8(8): 250.
[http://dx.doi.org/10.3390/antiox8080250] [PMID: 31357693]

[22]   Attia YA, Al-Harthi MA, El-Shafey AS, Rehab YA, Kim WK. Enhancing tolerance of broiler chickens to heat stress by supplementation with vitamin E, vitamin C and/or probiotics. Ann Anim Sci 2017; 17(4): 1155-69.
[http://dx.doi.org/10.1515/aoas-2017-0012]

[23]   Kumar S, Pandey AK. Chemistry and biological activities of flavonoids: an overview. ScientificWorldJournal 2013; 2013: 1-16.
[http://dx.doi.org/10.1155/2013/162750] [PMID: 24470791]

[24]   Xiao J, Kai G, Yamamoto K, Chen X. Advance in dietary polyphenols as α-glucosidases inhibitors: a review on structure-activity relationship aspect. Crit Rev Food Sci Nutr 2013; 53(8): 818-36.
[http://dx.doi.org/10.1080/10408398.2011.561379] [PMID: 23768145]

[25]   M K. The Importance of Flavonoids in Ruminant Nutrition. Archives of Animal Husbandry & Dairy Science 2018; 1(1)
[http://dx.doi.org/10.33552/AAHDS.2018.01.000504]

[26]   Iwaya T, Isogai E, Ide A, *et al.* Beneficial effects of green tea catechin on veterinary sciences and bacterial infections, Approaches in poultry. Dairy Vet Sci 2017.
[http://dx.doi.org/10.31031/APDV.2017.02.000532]

[27]   Adamczak A, Ożarowski M, Karpiński TM. Antibacterial activity of some flavonoids and organic acids widely distributed in plants. J Clin Med 2019; 9(1): 109.
[http://dx.doi.org/10.3390/jcm9010109] [PMID: 31906141]

[28]   Hashem NM, Gonzalez-Bulnes A, Simal-Gandara J. Polyphenols in farm animal: Source of reproductive gain or waste? Antioxidants. 2020; 9: 1023.
[http://dx.doi.org/10.3390/antiox9101023]

[29]   Serra V, Salvatori G, Pastorelli G. Dietery polyphenol supplementation in food producing animals: Effects on the quality of derived products. Anim 2021; 11: 40.
[http://dx.doi.org/10.3390/ani11102401]

[30]   Wina E, Pasaribu T, Rakhmani SIW, *et al.* The role of saponin as feed additive for sustainable poultry production. Indonesian Bulletin of Animal and Veterinary Sciences 2018; 27(3): 117-24.
[http://dx.doi.org/10.14334/wartazoa.v27i3.1588]

[31]   Chaudhary SK, Rokade JJ, Aderao GN, *et al.* Saponin in poultry and monogastric animals: A Review. Int J Curr Microbiol Appl Sci 2018; 7(7): 3218-25.
[http://dx.doi.org/10.20546/ijcmas.2018.707.375]

[32]   Cho J, Choi H, Lee J, Kim MS, Sohn HY, Lee DG. The antifungal activity and membrane-disruptive action of dioscin extracted from *Dioscorea nipponica.* Biochim Biophys Acta Biomembr 2013; 1828(3): 1153-8.
[http://dx.doi.org/10.1016/j.bbamem.2012.12.010] [PMID: 23262192]

[33]   Zhang H. Tyrosinase inhibitory effects and antioxidant activities of saponins from Xanthocerassorbifolia nutshell. 2013.

[34]   Gaurav AK. Studies on supplementation of chlorophytum root and camellia seed as feed additives in broiler ration. MVSc Thesis, Deemed Uni, Indian Vet Res Institute, Izatnagar 2015; 50-61.

[35] Shi YH, Wang J, Guo R, *et al.* Effects of alfalfa saponin extract on growth performance and some antioxidant indices of weaned piglets. Livest Sci 2014; 167: 257-62.
[http://dx.doi.org/10.1016/j.livsci.2014.05.032]

[36] Zhai H, Liu H, Wang S, Wu J, Kluenter AM. Potential of essential oils for poultry and pigs. Anim Nutr 2018; 4(2): 179-86.
[http://dx.doi.org/10.1016/j.aninu.2018.01.005] [PMID: 30140757]

[37] Ebani VV, Mancianti F. Use of essential oils in veterinary medicine to combat bacterial and fungal infections'. Vet Sci 2020; 7(4): 193.
[http://dx.doi.org/10.3390/vetsci7040193] [PMID: 33266079]

[38] Hippenstiel F Abdel-Wareth A, Kehraus S, *et al.* Effects of selected herbs and essential oils and their active compounds on feed intake and performance of broilers- a review. Arch Geflugelkd 2011; 75: 226-34.

[39] Zhang Y, Gong J, Yu H, *et al.* Alginate-whey protein dry powder optimized for target delivery of essential oils to the intestine of chickens. Poult Sci 2014; 93(10): 2514-25.
[http://dx.doi.org/10.3382/ps.2013-03843] [PMID: 25085933]

[40] Chiang LC, Ng LT, Cheng PW, Chiang W, Lin CC. Antiviral activities of extracts and selected pure constituents of *Ocimum basilicum.* Clin Exp Pharmacol Physiol 2005; 32(10): 811-6.
[http://dx.doi.org/10.1111/j.1440-1681.2005.04270.x] [PMID: 16173941]

[41] Choi HJ, Lim CH, Song JH, Baek SH, Kwon DH. Antiviral activity of raoulic acid from Raoulia australis against Picornaviruses. Phytomedicine 2009; 16(1): 35-9.
[http://dx.doi.org/10.1016/j.phymed.2008.10.012] [PMID: 19097770]

[42] Lin YJ, Lai CC, Lai CH, *et al.* Inhibition of enterovirus 71 infections and viral IRES activity by Fructus gardeniae and geniposide. Eur J Med Chem 2013; 62: 206-13.
[http://dx.doi.org/10.1016/j.ejmech.2012.12.038] [PMID: 23353754]

[43] Song J, Yeo SG, Hong EH, *et al.* Antiviral activity of hederasaponin B from hedera helix against enterovirus 71 subgenotypes C3 and C4a. Biomol Ther (Seoul) 2014; 22(1): 41-6.
[http://dx.doi.org/10.4062/biomolther.2013.108] [PMID: 24596620]

[44] Wang M, Tao L, Xu H. Chinese herbal medicines as a source of molecules with anti-enterovirus 71 activity. Chin Med 2016; 11(1): 2.
[http://dx.doi.org/10.1186/s13020-016-0074-0] [PMID: 26834824]

[45] Bobeck EA. Nutrition and health: companion animal applications: Functional nutrition in livestock and companion animals to modulate the immune response. J Anim Sci 2020; 98(3): skaa035.
[http://dx.doi.org/10.1093/jas/skaa035] [PMID: 32026938]

[46] Hodnik JJ, Ježek J, Starič J. A review of vitamin D and its importance to the health of dairy cattle. J Dairy Res 2020; 87(S1): 84-7.
[http://dx.doi.org/10.1017/S0022029920000424] [PMID: 33213577]

[47] Brisbin JT, Gong J, Sharif S. Interactions between commensal bacteria and the gut-associated immune system of the chicken. Anim Health Res Rev 2008; 9(1): 101-10.
[http://dx.doi.org/10.1017/S146625230800145X] [PMID: 18541076]

[48] Yang W-C, Yang W-C, Muthamilselvan T, *et al.* Herbal remedies for cocoidiosis control: A review of plant, compounds and anticoccidial actions 2016.
[http://dx.doi.org/10.1155/2016/2657981]

[49] Alnassan AA, Thabet A, Daugschies A, Bangoura B. *In vitro* efficacy of allicin on chicken Eimeria tenella sporozoites. Parasitol Res 2015; 114(10): 3913-5.
[http://dx.doi.org/10.1007/s00436-015-4637-2] [PMID: 26264230]

[50] Nghonjuyi NW, Tiambo CK, Kimbi HK. Efficacy of ethanolic extract of *Carica papaya* leaves as a substitute of sulphanomide for the control of coccidiosis in KABIR chickens in Cameroon. Journal of

Animal Health and Production 2015; 3(1): 21-7.
[http://dx.doi.org/10.14737/journal.jahp/2015/3.1.21.27]

[51]   De Pablos LM, dos Santos MFB, Montero E, Garcia-Granados A, Parra A, Osuna A. Anticoccidial activity of maslinic acid against infection with *Eimeria tenella* in chickens. Parasitol Res 2010; 107(3): 601-4.
[http://dx.doi.org/10.1007/s00436-010-1901-3] [PMID: 20499099]

[52]   Akhtar M, Tariq AF, Awais MM, *et al.* Studies on wheat bran Arabinoxylan for its immunostimulatory and protective effects against avian coccidiosis. Carbohydr Polym 2012; 90(1): 333-9.
[http://dx.doi.org/10.1016/j.carbpol.2012.05.048] [PMID: 24751049]

[53]   Khalafalla RE, Müller U, Shahiduzzaman M, *et al.* Effects of curcumin (diferuloylmethane) on Eimeria tenella sporozoites *in vitro*. Parasitol Res 2011; 108(4): 879-86.
[http://dx.doi.org/10.1007/s00436-010-2129-y]

[54]   Kim DK, Lillehoj HS, Lee SH, Jang SI, Lillehoj EP, Bravo D. Dietary *Curcuma longa* enhances resistance against Eimeria maxima and Eimeria tenella infections in chickens. Poult Sci 2013; 92(10): 2635-43.
[http://dx.doi.org/10.3382/ps.2013-03095] [PMID: 24046410]

[55]   Rafieian-Kopaei M, Alizadeh M, Safarzadeh A, *et al.* Brucellosis: Pathophysiology and new promising treatments with medicinal plants and natural antioxidants. Asian Pac J Trop Med 2018; 11(11): 597-608.https://www.apjtm.org/text.asp?2018/11/11/597/246336
[http://dx.doi.org/10.4103/1995-7645.246336]

[56]   Puvača N, Lika E, Tufarelli V, *et al.* Influence of Different Tetracycline Antimicrobial Therapy of Mycoplasma (*Mycoplasma synoviae*) in Laying Hens Compared to Tea Tree Essential Oil on Table Egg Quality and Antibiotic Residues. Foods 2020; 9(5): 612.
[http://dx.doi.org/10.3390/foods9050612] [PMID: 32403221]

[57]   Ravikumar S, Ali MS, Anandh P, *et al.* Antibacterial activity of *Cymodoceaserrulata* root extract against chosen poultry pathogen. Ind J Sci Technol 2011; 4: 2.

[58]   Navarro M, Stanley R, Cusack A, Sultanbawa Y. Combinations of plant-derived compounds against *Campylobacterin vitro*. J Appl Poult Res 2015; 24(3): 352-63.
[http://dx.doi.org/10.3382/japr/pfv035]

[59]   Shyma KP, Gupta JP, Ghosh S, Patel KK, Singh V. Acaricidal effect of herbal extracts against cattle tick Rhipicephalus (Boophilus) microplus using *in vitro* studies. Parasitol Res 2014; 113(5): 1919-26.
[http://dx.doi.org/10.1007/s00436-014-3839-3] [PMID: 24633906]

[60]   Adenubi OT, Fasina FO, McGaw LJ, Eloff JN, Naidoo V. Plant extracts to control ticks of veterinary and medical importance: A review. S Afr J Bot 2016; 105: 178-93.
[http://dx.doi.org/10.1016/j.sajb.2016.03.010]

[61]   Amber R, Adnan M, Tariq A, *et al.* Antibacterial activity of selected medicinal plants of northwest Pakistan traditionally used against mastitis in livestock. Saudi J Biol Sci 2018; 25(1): 154-61.
[http://dx.doi.org/10.1016/j.sjbs.2017.02.008] [PMID: 29379373]

[62]   Lee CJ, Wright MH, Greene AC, Aldosary H, Cock IE. Preliminary evaluation of the antibacterial activity of *Tasmannia lanceolata* against *Bacillus anthracis*: Natural Resource probing to prevent Anthrax'. Pharmacogn Commun 2019; 9(4): 124-9.
[http://dx.doi.org/10.5530/pc.2019.4.26]

[63]   Jaiswal L, Isamil H, Worku MA. Review of the effects of plant derived bioactive substances on the inflammatory response of ruminants(sheep, cattle, goat). Int J Vet Anim Med 2020; 3(2): 130.

[64]   Wang J, Guo C, Wei Z, *et al.* Morin suppresses inflammatory cytokine expression by downregulation of nuclear factor-κB and mitogen-activated protein kinase (MAPK) signaling pathways in lipopolysaccharide-stimulated primary bovine mammary epithelial cells. J Dairy Sci 2016; 99(4):

3016-22.
[http://dx.doi.org/10.3168/jds.2015-10330] [PMID: 26851851]

[65]   Ferreira LG, Noseda MD, Gonçalves AG, Ducatti DRB, Fujii MT, Duarte MER. Chemical structure of
the complex pyruvylated and sulfated agaran from the red seaweed Palisada flagellifera (Ceramiales,
Rhodophyta). Carbohydr Res 2012; 347(1): 83-94.
[http://dx.doi.org/10.1016/j.carres.2011.10.007] [PMID: 22055816]

[66]   Chojnacka K, Saeid A, Witkowska Z, *et al.* Biologically active compounds in seaweed extracts- the
prospects for the application. Open Conf Proc J 2012; 3(1): 20-8.
[http://dx.doi.org/10.2174/1876326X01203020020]

[67]   Lynch MB, Sweeney T, Callan JJ, O'Sullivan JT, O'Doherty JV. The effect of dietary Laminaria-
derived laminarin and fucoidan on nutrient digestibility, nitrogen utilisation, intestinal microflora and
volatile fatty acid concentration in pigs. J Sci Food Agric 2009; 90(3)
[http://dx.doi.org/10.1002/jsfa.3834] [PMID: 20355064]

[68]   McDonnell P, Figat S, O' Doherty JV. The effect of dietary laminarin and fucoidan in the diet of the
weanling piglet on performance, selected faecal microbial populations and volatile fatty acid
concentrations. Animal: an Int J AnimBiosci 2010; 4(4): 579-85.
[http://dx.doi.org/10.1017/S1751731109991376]

[69]   O'Shea CJ, McAlpine P, Sweeney T, Varley PF, O'Doherty JV. Effect of the interaction of seaweed
extracts containing laminarin and fucoidan with zinc oxide on the growth performance, digestibility
and faecal characteristics of growing piglets. Br J Nutr 2014; 111(5): 798-807.
[http://dx.doi.org/10.1017/S0007114513003280] [PMID: 24131869]

[70]   Øverland M, Mydland LT, Skrede A. Marine macroalgae as sources of protein and bioactive
compounds in feed for monogastric animals. J Sci Food Agric 2019; 99(1): 13-24.
[http://dx.doi.org/10.1002/jsfa.9143] [PMID: 29797494]

[71]   O'Doherty JV, Dillon S, Figat S, Callan JJ, Sweeney T. The effects of lactose inclusion and seaweed
extract derived from Laminaria spp. on performance, digestibility of diet components and microbial
populations in newly weaned pigs. Anim Feed Sci Technol 2010; 157(3-4): 173-80.
[http://dx.doi.org/10.1016/j.anifeedsci.2010.03.004]

[72]   Cotas J, Leandro A, Monteiro P, *et al.* Seaweed Phenolics: From Extraction to Applications. Mar
Drugs 2020; 18(8): 384.
[http://dx.doi.org/10.3390/md18080384] [PMID: 32722220]

[73]   Stengel DB, Connan S, Popper ZA. Algal chemodiversity and bioactivity: sources of natural
variability and implications for commercial application. Biotechnol Ad 2011; pp. 483-501.
[http://dx.doi.org/10.1016/j.biotechadv.2011.05.016]

[74]   Nabi F, Arain MA, Rajput N, *et al.* Health benefits of carotenoids and potential application in poultry
industry: A review. J Anim Physiol Anim Nutr (Berl) 2020; 104(6): 1809-18.
[http://dx.doi.org/10.1111/jpn.13375] [PMID: 32333620]

[75]   Vitali A. Antimicrobial peptides derived from marine sponges. J Clin Microbiol Antimicrobe 2018; 1:
1006.

[76]   Kulshreshtha G, Critchley A, Rathgeber B, *et al.* Antimicrobial effects of selected, cultivated red
seaweeds and their components in combination with tetracycline, against poultry pathogen *Salmonella
enteridis.* J Mar Sci Eng 2020; 8(7): 511.
[http://dx.doi.org/10.3390/jmse8070511]

[77]   Kulshreshtha G, Rathgeber B, Stratton G, *et al.* Feed supplementation with red seaweeds, *Chondrus
crispus* and *Sarcodiotheca gaudichaudii,* affects performance, egg quality, and gut microbiota of layer
hens. Poult Sci 2014; 93(12): 2991-3001.
[http://dx.doi.org/10.3382/ps.2014-04200] [PMID: 25352682]

[78]   Kulshreshtha G, Rathgeber B, MacIsaac J, *et al.* Feed supplementation with red seaweeds, *Chondrus*

crispus and *Sarcodiothecagaudichaudii*, reduce *Salmonella enteritidis* in laying hens. Front Microbiol 2017; 8: 567.
[http://dx.doi.org/10.3389/fmicb.2017.00567] [PMID: 28443073]

[79] Cornish ML, Monagail MM, Critchley AT. The animal kingdom, Agriculture and seaweeds. J Mar Sci Eng 2020; 8(8): 574.
[http://dx.doi.org/10.3390/jmse8080574]

[80] Tellez G, Pixley C, Wolfenden RE, Layton SL, Hargis BM. Probiotics/direct fed microbials for Salmonella control in poultry. Food Res Int 2012; 45(2): 628-33.
[http://dx.doi.org/10.1016/j.foodres.2011.03.047]

[81] Morais T, Inácio A, Coutinho T, *et al.* Seaweed Potential in the Animal Feed: A Review. J Mar Sci Eng 2020; 8(8): 559.
[http://dx.doi.org/10.3390/jmse8080559]

[82] Suarez MG, Gallissot M, Cierpinski P. Effect of an algae-clay mix on the use by broiler chickens of a diet containing corn DDGS. proceedings of the 4th International Poultry Meat Congress. Antalya, Turkey. 2017; pp. 26-30.

[83] Ford L, Stratakos AC, Theodoridou K, *et al.* Polyphenols from brown seaweeds as a potential antimicrobial agent in animal feeds. ACS Omega 2020; 5(16): 9093-103.
[http://dx.doi.org/10.1021/acsomega.9b03687] [PMID: 32363261]

[84] Diogo JV, Novo SG, González MJ, Ciancia M, Bratanich AC. Antiviral activity of lambda-carrageenan prepared from red seaweed (Gigartina skottsbergii) against BoHV-1 and SuHV-1. Res Vet Sci 2015; 98: 142-4.
[http://dx.doi.org/10.1016/j.rvsc.2014.11.010] [PMID: 25435342]

[85] El-Demerdash A, Atanasov A, Bishayee A, Abdel-Mogib M, Hooper J, Al-Mourabit A. Highly prolific marine sponge genera yielding compounds with potential applications for cancer and other therapeutic areas. Nutrients 2018; 10(1): 33.
[http://dx.doi.org/10.3390/nu10010033] [PMID: 29301302]

[86] Pickard JM, Zeng MY, Caruso R, Núñez G. Gut microbiota: Role in pathogen colonization, immune responses, and inflammatory disease. Immunol Rev 2017; 279(1): 70-89.
[http://dx.doi.org/10.1111/imr.12567] [PMID: 28856738]

[87] Hussin WA, El-Sayed WM. Synergetic interaction between selected botanical extracts and tetracycline against gram positive and gram negative bacteria. J Biosci 2011; 11: 433-41.

[88] Lu W-J, Lin H-J, Hsu P-H, *et al.* Brown and red seaweeds serve as potential efflux pump inhibitors for drug resistant *Escherichia coli*. 2019.
[http://dx.doi.org/10.1155/2019/1836982]

Bioactive Constituents and Anti-diabetic Activity of the Indian Medicinal Plant *Hemidesmus indicus* R. Br.: An Overview

Amit Kumar Dixit[1,*], **Avijit Banerji**[1,2], **Julie Banerji**[2], **Deepti Dixit**[3], **Parvathy G. Nair**[4] and **Damodar Gupta**[5]

[1] *Central Ayurveda Research Institute-CCRAS, Ministry of Ayush, Kolkata, India*

[2] *Formerly of Chemistry Department, University of Calcutta, Kolkata, India*

[3] *School of Biochemistry, Devi Ahilya University, Khandwa Road, Indore, Madhya Pradesh, India*

[4] *National Ayurveda Research Institute for Panchakarma, Cheruthuruthy, Thrissur, Kerala, India*

[5] *Institute for Nuclear Medicine and Allied Sciences, DRDO, New Delhi, India*

Abstract: *Hemidesmus indicus* R. Br. is a laticiferous, slender, and twining shrub, which is found over almost every part of India. Its roots (*Anantmul* - Sanskrit meaning: endless root) are particularly used extensively as a single drug and in formulations with other plants to treat several ailments. In view of the wide range of medicinal properties claimed in traditional medicine, significant efforts have been made to determine the efficacy of *Hemidesmus indicus* through pharmacological experiments *in vitro* and *in vivo* models. These include analgesic, anti-inflammatory, antipyretic, antioxidant, antiarthritic, hepatoprotective, antiepileptic, anticonvulsant, antiulcer, antivenom, antiacne, and antipsychotic activities. Recent studies have also established anti-diabetic, anti-carcinogenic, anti-venom, and wound healing activities. Extensive phytochemical investigations have been carried out by several research groups. The present review provides an overview of the bioactive compounds of this Indian medicinal plant. Several classes of compounds, *viz.* triterpenoids, steroids, steroid glycosides, coumarin-lignoids, flavonoids in addition to many simpler compounds, have been isolated and characterised from different parts of *H. indicus*. These are listed, along with brief write-ups on isolation procedures, spectroscopical and chemical characterization, and their biological properties. Particular emphasis is given to the anti-diabetic properties associated with it, *indicus* root extracts, and the factors contributing to these properties.

Keywords: Anti-diabetic, Ayurvedic drugs, Coumarino-lignoids, *Hemidesmus indicus*, Indian sarsaparilla, Phytochemistry, Terpenoids, Volatile constituents.

---

* **Corresponding author Amit Kumar Dixit:** Central Ayurveda Research Institute, CCRAS, Ministry of AYUSH, Government of India, Kolkata, India; Tel: +91-89205 74307; E-mail: deepdixit20@gmail.com

Mukesh Kumar Sharma and Pallavi Kaushik (Eds.)

INTRODUCTION

Hemidesmus indicus R. Br. (Fam. Periplocaceae), also known as Indian sarsaparilla, is one of the important medicinal plants in the Indian Ayurvedic system [1 - 14]. It also finds use in the Siddha and Unani schools of traditional medicine. *H. indicus* R. Br. (*Sariva, Anantamul,* Indian *sarsaparilla*) (Fig. **1**) is a slender, laticiferous, and twining shrub, that grows throughout India. It grows wild and is also common in hedges. Its root bark and roots are extensively used in the Indian traditional healthcare system. Some of its vernacular names are *Anantamul-* Bengali, Hindi, Punjabi, Marathi; *Onontomulo, Suguddimalo-* Odiya; Sariva, Swet-sariva - Sanskrit; *Sugandhipala* - Telugu; *Namdaberu, Sogadaberu-* Kannada; *Nannari* - Tamil, Malayalam, Gujrati; *Zaiyana* – Arabic; *Ushbanidi* - Persian.

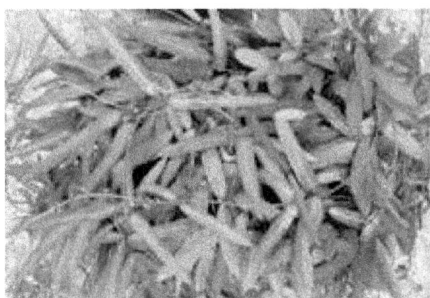

Fig. (1). *Hemidesmus indicus*cultivated in flower-pot at CARI.

The use of *H. indicus* in various traditional and ethnomedical practices [2 - 6] is recorded in different states in India - Bengal, Odisha, Madhya Pradesh, Assam, Goa, Uttar Pradesh, Gujarat, Kerala, Maharashtra, Karnataka, Andhra, Tamilnadu and Telangana. The plant is also found in local schools of traditional medicine in Iran (Persia), Pakistan, Bangladesh, and the Arabic Middle East. Its roots and root bark (*Anantmul* - Sanskrit literally meaning: endless root) are used extensively as a single drug and in formulations with other plants to treat several ailments. It has been reported that *Anantamul* is used as an ingredient in nearly 46 Ayurvedic preparations, as single or in combination with other drugs [10]. *H. indicus*, which was formerly under the family Asclepiadaceae, has been now placed in Periplocaceae family on the basis of the pollinical characters [6]. Genetic fingerprinting has also been used to identify this plant [6]. However, several recent publications still continue to place the plant under Asclepiadaceae.

Detailed phytopharmacognostic studies have already been carried out on the roots of *Anatamul* [15]. *H. indicus* is distinguished by its brown slender, sparsely branched, rigid, tortuous, elongated, cylindrical roots with the rough and wavy outer surface, externally dark tortuous with transversely cracked and longitudinally fissured bark, and internally as yellowish-brown. Rootlets are thin and wiry, the cork is thin and separates easily, peeling off in flakes. Its root and root bark possess a pleasant mild aroma. The leaves are opposite to one another, firm, shiny and smooth varying in shape and size according to age. Flowers are small in size, green externally and deep purple internally.

The therapeutic properties of Sariva summed up in a Sanskrit *sloka*, is quoted in the Treatise of Indian Medicinal Plants, Vol. 4 [2]. It is mentioned that this plant is snigdha (cool), svādu (sweet), spermatopoietic, anti-dyspnoeic, dyspepsia, anorexia, cough, cures vitiated tridosha, fever menorrhagia and diarrhoea, invigorating diuretic and rejuvenating; a remedy for rheumatoid arthritis, skin diseases, gout and gonorrhea and mercury poisoning [2]. The source books [2, 3] also report that root and root-bark of *H. indicus* are diaphoretic, demulcent, diuretic which can be prescribed in fever, chronic cough, anorexia, leucorrhoea, dyspepsia, skin disease, chronic rheumatism and ulcerations, constitutional debility, kidney trouble, and diarrhea.

Other pharmacological properties reported on *H. indicus* include analgesic, antioxidant, antiarthritic, anti-inflammatory, antipyretic, anticonvulsant, hepatoprotective, antiepileptic, cytotoxic, antiulcer, antiacne, antipsychotic activities, antibacterial, antinociceptive, *etc*.

Roots of *H. indicus* are used to cure various skin diseases, anorectal diseases asthma, dysentery, bronchitis, leucorrhoea, syphilis, paralysis and various types of urinary disorders. Recent studies have also established anti-diabetic, anti-cancer, anti-snake venom and wound-healing activities [2 - 14]. In view of the wide range of medicinal properties claimed in traditional medicine, considerable efforts have been made to establish the efficacy of *H. indicus* through pharmacological studies both *in vitro* and *in vivo* models. The growing demand of Anantamool, in view of its widespread use, is resulting in heavy strain on the existing resources causing and depleting its supplies; in fact, its very existence may become endangered. Substitutes and adulterants often used are roots of the following four species- *Cryptolepis buchanani* Roem and Schult., *Decalepis hamiltonii* Wight, *Ichnocarpus frutescens* R. Br., and Arn and *Utleria salicifolia* Bedd. ex Hook. f [6].

Anantamul, introduced to the European healthcare system in 1831 [16], is now receiving attention as an Ayurvedic product in Europe as well as the USA. Weissner in a review entitled 'Anantamul, a review of biomedical studies and US products' [17] has given a useful overview of the usage of this drug in the USA in recent times. She also pointed out the lacunae of available data on it, which limits

its investigations to cardioprotective, anti-hyperlipidemic, diuretic, anti-oxidant, and anti-cancer activities.

One of the co-authors (AB) was involved in early investigations of the antidiabetic potential of the roots extract of *H. indicus* [18]. This work triggered a spate of publications on this aspect.

This chapter mainly focuses on the bioactive constituents and anti-diabetic activity of *H. indicus* extractives and phytoconstituents. The phytoconstituents of *H. indicus* are listed in this chapter. These include the simpler aliphatic and aromatic compounds as well as the more complex compounds (Triterpenoids, Sesterterpenoids, Coumarino-lignoids, phenylpropanoid, Diterpenoids, Steroids, flavonoids). Structural representations of basic skeleta and representative compounds are presented here.

PHYTOCHEMICAL INVESTIGATIONS ON *H. INDICUS*

Various aspects of the *H.indicus* plant, collected from different locations in India have been investigated by several research groups. In this connection, many publications have appeared on phytochemicals present - detection, isolation, and characterisation of the chemical constituents. The spectroscopical properties and chemistry of these constituents have been explored, and certain biological properties investigated. Most of the work has been done on the roots, also on the stems and twigs. Less work has been done on the leaves and very little on the flowers. Extraction procedures have differed from group to group - extracts were prepared with water, ethanol, and methanol and with other organic solvents.

A thorough search of the literature revealed several publications which described the detection and quantification of the simpler aromatic and aliphatic molecules present in *H. indicus*. An aspect, which warrants detailed phytopharmacognostic studies and HPTLC finger-printing and validation, is to differentiate H. indicus extractives from those of the roots of four substitutes and adulterants, *viz. Ichnocarpus frutescens*, *Cryptolepis buchanani*, *Decalepis hamiltonii* and *Utleria salicifolia*.

It should be noted that most of the biological activity reported resides in aqueous, ethanolic, aqueous ethanolic, and methanolic extracts. Bio-assay directed fractionations and screening of the fractions for biological activities are usually lacking.

Preliminary Phytochemical Screening Of Phytochemicals In Extracts

Several publications, reporting preliminary screening of *H. indicus* have described the use of standard colour tests to detect broad classes of active constituents in extracts. These tests are indicative, rather than confirmatory. The available data in this domain is compiled and presented in Table **1**.

Table 1. Chemical constituents reported in root of *H. indicus* collected from different locations on preliminary screening.

Part/Extract Studied	Place of Collection	Findings	Reference
Ethanolic extract of petrol-defatted root material	Tirunelvali, Tamilnadu	Presence of flavonoids, glycosides, phenols, saponins, alkaloids, terpenoids. tannins, phytosterols, Absence of anthraquinones	[19]
Cold ethanolic root extract	Maruthamalai Hills, Coimbatore district, Tamilnadu	Presence of alkaloids phenols, terpenoids, resins, proteins flavonoids, glycosides, saponins, tannins, steroids. Absence of carbohydrates.	[20]
Leaf extracted by cold maceration with ethanol	Cuddalore, Tamilnadu	Presence of flavonoids, glycosides, saponins, phenols, alkaloids, tannins, steroids, lignins. Absence of coumarins, proteins, and fixed oils gums, free amino acids and mucilage.	[21]
Ethanolic root extract	Thanjavur district, Tamil Nadu	Presence of phenolic compounds, volatile oils, proteins, saponins, tannins, glycosides, amino acids, phytosterols. Absence of alkaloids, fixed oils flavonoids, lignins, carbohydrates, fats, gums mucilage, *etc*. Their reports are different from other reports.	[22]
Whole plant methanolic extract	Hyderabad	Presence of phenolic compounds, lignans, tannins, flavonoids, glycosides, carbohydrates, proteins. Absence of terpenoids, alkaloids, saponins.	[23]
Root extracts by successive extractions with different solvents	Bhopal, Madhya Pradesh	Petroleum ether extract - steroids and triterpenoids only Ethanol extract - alkaloids, polyphenols, carbohydrates, glycosides, saponins Aqueous extracts - glycosides, polyphenols, carbohydrates and saponin TLC of ethanol and aqueous extracts have been performed without constituents identification.	[24]

(Table 1) cont.....

Cold root extracts with petroleum ether, chloroform, ethyl alcohol, water	Kolkata, West Bengal	Alkaloids, saponins, tannins – all extracts Flavonoids, polyphenols – all extracts other than petroleum ether extract. Terpenoids and steroids– all extracts other than aqueous extract. Glycosides – ethanol and aqueous extracts. HPTLC finger-printing of these extracts have been reported.	[15]
The methanolic root bark extract	Ahmadabad, Gujarat	TLC analysis and phytochemical estimation indicated the abundant presence of phenols, tannins, and the absence of alkaloids and anthraquinones.	[25]

Simple Aliphatic And Aromatic Compounds; Volatile Constituents

Several simpler compounds – both aliphatic and aromatic, have been detected in extracts of different parts of *H.indicus*. Several of these have been detected by GC- MS analysis of the volatiles present in *H. indicus* roots. Many of these compounds have been isolated - spectroscopic analyses carried out, and in certain cases their biological properties investigated. A study used steam-distillation techniques with *H. indicus* roots to obtain the volatile components. Silica-gel column chromatography of the steam-distillate furnished 2-hydroxy-4-methoxy benzaldehyde (HMBLD, 91% yield) and the terpenoid ledol (4.5% yield). A total of 40 constituents even many in minute amounts were shown to be present by GC-MS analysis which includes camphor, borneol, salicylaldehyde, dihydrocarvyl acetate, nerolidol, linalyl acetate, iso- caryophyllene, 1,8-cineol, terpinyl acetate, hexadecanoic acid, and dodecanoic acid, *etc* [26]. Another study determined considerable amounts of HMBA both in roots of H. indicus and *Decalepis hamiltonii* [27]. Production of HMBLD using root cultures of *H. indicus* was also reported [28, 29]. HPTLC quantification of HMBA and HMBLD in *H. indicus* root powder extract has been carried out [30, 31]. HMBA has shown anti-diabetic (see Section on anti-diabetic activity) and anti-venom properties [32]. GC-MS analysis of the essential oil of *H. indicus* roots collected from South India has reported HMBLD (major component, 95.8%), vanillin, salicylic acid derivatives, and (E, Z)-nonadienal [33]. The steam-distillates of the dried powdered roots of *H. indicus* and *Decalepsis hamiltonii* were extracted with ether and subjected to comparative GC-MS analysis: HMBLD was the major component identified in both plants (98% and 95%, respectively). GC-MS analysis detected six minor components in H. indicus (< 1% each; anisaldehyde, octanoic acid, isobutyl anilide, decanoic acid, thymol, octadecanoic acid), and four (thymol, decanoic acid, palmitic acid, m-guaiacol) in *Decalepsis hamiltonii* [34]. HPLC analysis of methanolic extracts of *H. indicus* root from seven ecotypes exhibited variation in peak number as compared to HMBLD and its concentration was more in ecotype 6 and less in ecotype 3 [35]. Another study has also shown how the Shikimate pathway attenuates the elicitor-stimulated accumulation of fragrant HMBLD in *H. indicus* roots [36]. The consolidated lists of simpler compounds detected/obtained from different parts of *H. indicus* are given in Table **2**.

Table 2. Simpler compounds isolated and identified from different parts of *H. indicus*.

Class of Compound	Name of Compound	Reference
Aromatic aldehydes	2-hydroxy-4-methoxybenzaldehyde (HMBLD) Salicylaldehyde 4-hydroxy-3-methoxy-benzaldehyde (vanillin) 3-hydroxy-4-methoxy-benzaldehyde(*iso*-vanillin) Anisaldehyde 4-hydroxybenzaldehyde	[26-40, 48] [26, 48] [26, 33, 38, 42, 48, 53] [38-40, 48, 53] [34] [38]
Aromatic acids	2-hydroxy-4-methoxy benzoic acid (HMBA) Vanillic acid Ferulic acid Gallic acid, Cinnamic acid,*p*-coumaric acid, Syringic acid, Caffeic acid Gentisic acid, Protocatechuic acid	[26, 32, 38-41, 48] [38, 41] [41, 44] [41]
Aliphatic compounds	Hexatriacontane Octanoic acid Decanoic acid Dodecanoic acid Palmitic acid (hexadecanoic acid) triacontane	[35, 50] [34] [26, 27, 34] [26] [26, 34, 35, 53] [36]
Aromatic compounds	Thymol, isobutyl anilide salicylic acid derivatives, (E, Z)-2,--nonadienal	[33, 34]

Chromatographic Studies and Quantification of Components in *H.indicus*

Petroleum ether and hexane extracts of roots were used to quantify lupeol octacosanoate and HMBLD by HPTLC. The amount of HMBLD determined in hexane extract was higher than in dry powder. It was proposed that lupeol octacosanoate can be used as one of the marker compounds for the quality control of *H. indicus*. HMBLD was found in trace amounts in the common adulterants of the plant. Therefore, the detection of HMBLD as a marker may serve as a tool for the quality control of this plant [30, 37].

The secondary metabolites *i.e.* vanillin, lupeol and rutin isolated from in-vitro and in-vivo grown root and shoot of *H. indicus* were determined by a validated HPTLC method [38]. In plants derived by tissue culture, roots from the parent plants were having rutin, the same was not present in the shoots. HPLC revealed the presence HMBLD, HMBA, isovanillin, vanillic acid, and 4-hydroxy-benzaldehyde. HPTLC fingerprinting method was also studied with different mobile phases to quantify the occurrence of three major marker compounds *viz.* HMBLD, HMBA, and isovanillin from the *H. indicus* roots [39, 40]. HPLC analysis has been employed to identify phenolic acid components of the roots. Phenolics were isolated and quantified as gallic acid equivalent (GAE) using a spectrophotometer following the Folin-Ciocalteu method. The identified phenolic and acid components were – HMBA, gallic acid, ferulic acid, p-coumaric acid, syringic acid cinnamic acid, vanillic acid, caffeic acid, protocatechuic acid, and gentisic acid [41].

Lupeol was found in comparatively higher amounts in shoot and leaf-derived callus cultures compared to that of shoots. Shoot cultures have shown high amount of vanillin [42]. It was also reported that Higher amounts of phenolics and flavonoids were present in Callus and *in-vitro* grown plants compared to the *in-situ* grown plants which supports the notion of modulation of secondary metabolite associated biological activity under different culture conditions and growth processes [43].

Ferulic acid in *H. indicus* roots extract has been determined through validated HPTLC [44]. In view of adulterants and substitutes for *Hemidesmus indicus*, it is important to carry out an analysis of phytochemicals present in the latter and compare them with those present in *Hemidesmus indicus*. In this regard, few studies have been carried out with *Decalepis hamiltonii* [45 - 47]. These were studies carried out many years ago and need to be supplemented now. Comparative studies of the volatile components of these two plants have been reported [28, 34].

Qualitative and quantitative analysis phytomarkers in pharmaceutical preparations of *H. indicus* roots by using Micellar Electrokinetic chromatography and HPLC-mass spectrometry have also been performed. These phytocomponents were HMBA, HMBLD, 3-hydroxy-4- methoxybenzaldehyde, vanillin, and salicylaldehyde [48].

The mineral content of methanolic root extract has been estimated after digesting with a mixture of perchloric acid: HNO_3: H_2SO_4 (11:6:3) - copper 8.2 ppm, zinc 27.5 ppm, iron 108.9 ppm, and manganese 11.4 ppm [49].

Terpenoids – *Triterpenoids*, Sesterterpenoids, Diterpenoids, Sesquiterpenoids, Monoterpenoids

Monoterpenoids and Sesquiterpenoids

Volatile components analysis of *H. indicus* identified several lower terpenoids, as already given in the previous section, under volatile constituents.

Monoterpenoids

Camphor [26], borneol [26], linalyl acetate [26], dihydrocarvyl acetate [26], (E)-nerolidol [26], 1,8-cineol (eucalyptol) [26], α-terpinyl acetate [26].

Sesquiterpenoids

Iso-caryophyllene [26].

Triterpenoids

Triterpenoids c a fairly abundant group of compounds isolated from *H. indicus*. Most of these are pentacyclic triterpenoids based on one of the following basic skeleta *i.e.* Ursane (I), Oleanane (II), and Lupane (III). These components have been listed in Table **3**, with representative structures collected in Chart I.

Table 3. Phytochemicals isolated from *Hemidesmus indicus*.

Sl. No.	Constituents	Part of Plant
	Pentacyclic Triterpenoids	
1.	α-Amyrin (IV)	Roots
2.	α-Amyrin acetate (IVa)	Roots
3.	β-Amyrin (V)	Roots
4.	β-Amyrin acetate (Va)	Roots
5.	β-Amyrin palmitate (Vb)	Roots
6.	Lupeol (VIII)	Roots; *in-vivo* and *in-vitro* grown root and shoot culture
7.	Lupeol acetate (VIIIa)	Roots
8.	Lupeol octacosanoate (VIIIb)	Roots
9.	Taraxasteryl acetate (VII)	Roots

(Table 3) cont.....

10.	Hemidesterpene$\Delta^{12,13}$-dehydro-taraxesteryl acetate (VIII)	Roots
11.	3-Keto-lup-12-ene-21→28-olide (IX)	Stems
12.	Lupanone (X)	Stems
13.	Δ^{12}-Dehydrolupeol acetate (XI)	Stems
14.	Δ^{12}-Dehydrolupanyl-3β -acetate (XII)	Stems
15.	Olean-12-en-21β-yl acetate	Roots
16.	Olean-12-en-3α-yl acetate (XIII)	Roots
17.	16(17)-*seco*-Urs-12,20(30)-dien-18α H-3β-yl acetate	Roots
18.	16(17)-*seco*-Urs-12,20(30)-dien-18 α H-3β-ol	Roots
19.	Urs-20(30)-en-18β H-3β -yl acetate	Roots
20.	Lup-1,12-diene-3-on-21-ol (XIV)	Roots
20.	Hemidesmusoic acid (XV): 2, 6, 10, 14, 18, 22-hexamethyltetracosoi-1-oic acid	Roots
21.	*n*-Non-2'-en-1'-yl-13(15, 19, 19-trimethyl-cyclohex-14, 16- dienyl)- 2,6,10- trimethyl-tetradec-6-ol-13-on-1-oate (XVII)	Roots
22.	3-((3*E*,7*E*)-4,8-dimethyl-10-(2,6,6-trimethylcyclohex-1-enyl)deca-3,7-dienyl)-furan-2(5*H*)-one (XVIII)	Roots
Diterpenoid		
23.	Octyl hemidesdisterpenoate (XVI): *n*-octyl-2, 6, 10, 14-tetramethyl-hexadec-7-ol-10-en-13-on-1-octanoate	Roots
Steroids		
24.	β–Sitosterol	Roots, Stem, Leaves
25.	β–sitosterol glucuronate	Roots
26.	Cholesterol	Stem, Leaves, Roots
27.	Campesterol	Stem, Leaves, Roots
28.	16-dehydropregnenolone (XIX)	Stem, Leaves, Roots
Steroid glycosides		
29.	Desinine: *11-Ac, 3-O-[β-D-Oleandropyranosyl-(1→4)-β-D- oleandropyranoside] on 3,11,12,14-tetrahydroxypregn-5-en-20-one*	Stems and twigs

(Table 3) cont.....

30.	Medidesmine: sarcostin-3-*O*-*a*-D-glucopyranosyl(1→4)-O-*β*-D-digitoxopyranosyl(1→4)-*O*-*β*-D-oleandropyranoside;	Stems and twigs
31.	Hemidescine: 20-O-acetyl calogenin 3-*O*-*β*- D-digitoxopyranosyl(1→4)- *O*-*β*-D-oleandropyranoside.	Stems and twigs
32.	Emidine: calogenin-3-*O*-*β*- D-digitoxopyranosyl (1→4)- *O*-*β*-D-digitoxopyranosyl (1→4)-O− *β* -D-digitoxopyranoside	Stems and twigs
33.	Indicine: calogenin-3-*O*-*β*- D-digitoxopyranoside	Stems and twigs
34.	Hemidine: calogenin-3-*O*-*β*- D-boivinopyranoside	-
35.	Hemisine: calogenin-3-*O*-*β*-D-cymaropyranosyl(1→4)-*O*-(3-*O*-methyl)-*β*-D-glucopyranosyl(1→4)- *O*-*β*-D- glucopyranosyl(1→4)-*O*-*β*-D-cymaropyranoside	Stems and twigs
36.	Desmisine: calogenin-3-*O*-*β*-D-xylopyranosyl(1→4)- *O*-*β*-D-digitoxopyranosyl(1→4)-*O*-*β*-D-xylopyranosyl(1→4)- *O*-*β*-D-digitoxopyranoside)	Stems and twigs
37.	Denicunine: calogenin 3-*O*-3-*O*-methyl-*β*-D-fucopyranosyl-(1→4)- *O*-*β*-D-oleandropyranoside	Stems and twigs
38.	Heminine: calogenin 3-*O*-*β*-D- digitoxopyranoside	Stems and twigs
39.	Indicusin: 11*α*, 12*β*-di-O-acetyl-orgogenin-3-O-*β*-D-cymaropyranosyl-(1→4)-*O*-*β*--cymaropyranosyl-(1→4)-*O*-*β*-D-cymaropyranoside	Stems
40.	Hindicusine: 20-O-benzoyl calogenin-3-O-*β*-D-digitoxopyranoside	Stems
41.	Hemidesimoside A: 3*β*,16α-dihydroxypreg-5-en-20-one 3-*O*-*β*-D-(2″,4″-di-*O*-acetyl-*β*-D-digitalopyranosyl) (1″→4′) cymaropyranoside,16-*O*-*β*-D-glucopyranosyl(1″″″→2″″)-*O*-*β*-D-glucopyranosyl (1″″″→6″″)-*O*-*β*-D-glucopyranoside	Roots
42.	Hemidesimoside B: 3*β*,16α-dihydroxypreg-5-en-20-one 3-*β*-D(2″,4′ -di-*O*-acetyl-*β*−D-digitalopyranosyl)(1″→4′)cymaropyranoside 16-*O*-*β*-D-glucopyranosyl(1″″″→2″″)-*O*-*β*-D-glucopyranosyl, (1″″″→6″″)-*O*-*β*--glucopyranosyl(1″″″→6″″)-*O*-*β*-D-glucopyranoside	Roots
43.	Hemidesimoside C: 3β,16α-dihydroxypreg-5-en-20-one 3-*O*-*β*-D-(*β*-D-oleandropyranosyl)(1″→4′) cymaropyranoside, 16-*O*-*β*-D-glucopyranosyl(1″″″→ 2″″)-*O*-*β*-D-glucopyranosyl(1″″″→ 6″″)-*β*-D-glucopyranoside	Roots
44.	Plocoside A	Roots
Coumarinolignoids		
46.	Hemidesminin(XXIV)	Roots
47.	Hemidesmin - 1 (XXV)	Roots

(Table 3) cont.....

49.	Hemidesmin - 2 (XXVI)	Roots
Phenylpropanoid		
50.	Phenylpropanoid glucoside(XXVII)	Roots
Flavonoids		
51.	Hyperoxide	Flowers, leaves
52.	Isoquercitin	Flowers
53.	Rutin	Leaves, flowers, Roots;*in-vivo* and *in-vitro* grown shoot and root culture.

Chart I

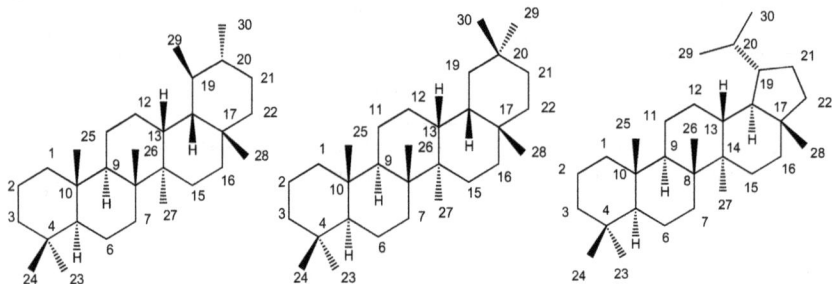

Ursane (I)   Oleanane (II)   Lupane (III)

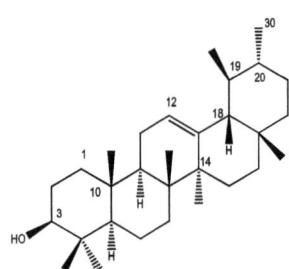
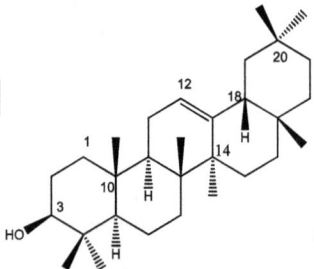
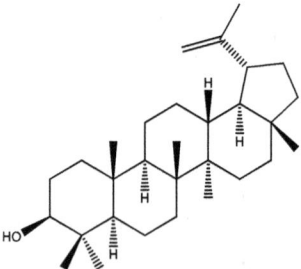

R = H; (IV) α-Amyrin
R = Ac (IVa)

R = H; (V) β-Amyrin
R = Ac; (Va)
R = Me(CH₂)₁₄CO; (Vb)

R = H; (VI) Lupeol
R = Ac; (VIa)
R=Me(CH₂)₂₆CO; (VIb)

(Fig.) contd.....

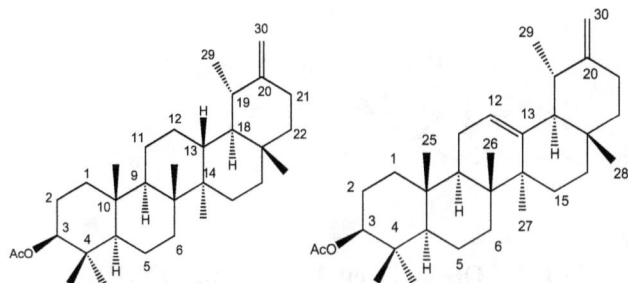

Taraxasteryl   acetate   (VII)   Hemidesterpene-$\Delta^{12,13}$-dehydro-taraxesteryl acetate (VIII)

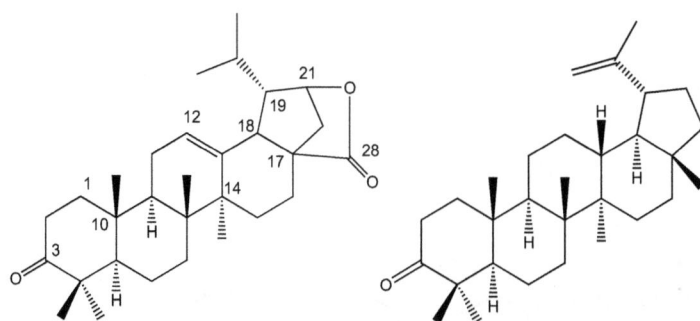

(IX)   **Lupanone   (X)**

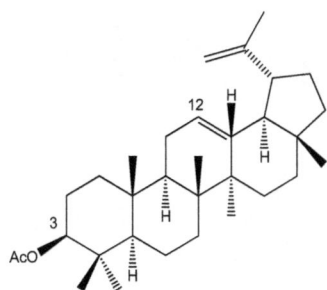

Δ^{12}-Dehydrolupeol acetate (XI)

(Fig.) contd.....

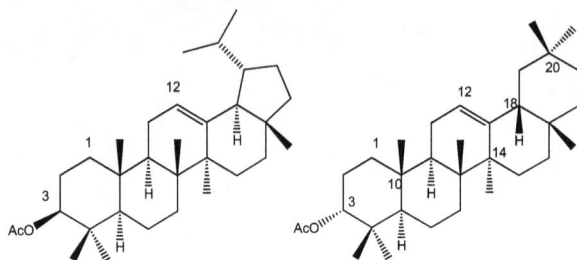

Δ¹²-Dehydrolupanyl-3β -acetate (XII)   **Olean-12-en-3α-yl acetate (XIII)**

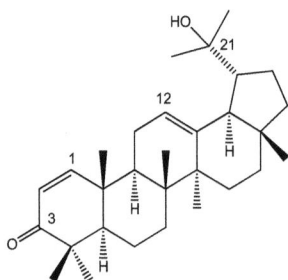

Lup-1,12-diene-3-on-21-ol (XIV)

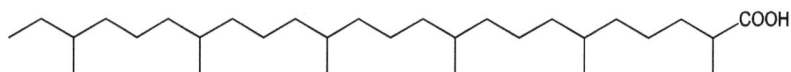

Hemidesmusoic acid: 2, 6, 10, 14, 18, 22–hexamethyltetracosoi-1-oic acid (XV)

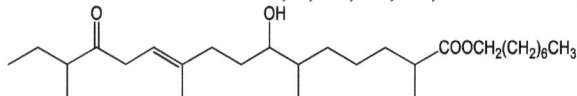

Octyl hemidesdisterpenoate (XVI)

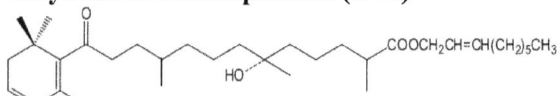

(XVII)

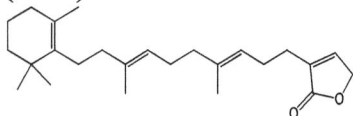

3-((3E,7E)-4,8-dimethyl-10-(2,6,6-trimethylcyclohex-1-enyl)deca-3,7-dienyl)-furan-2(5H)-one (XVIII)

(Fig.) contd.....

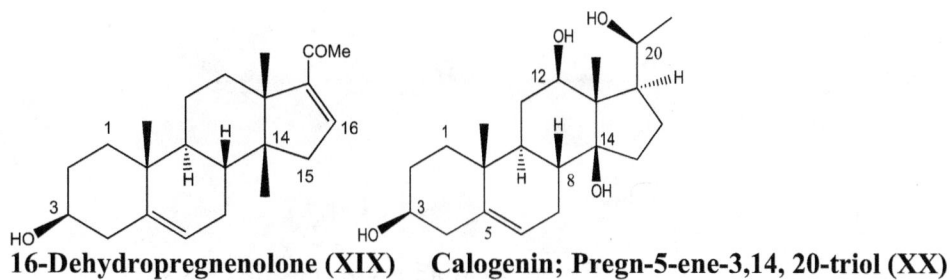

16-Dehydropregnenolone (XIX)   **Calogenin; Pregn-5-ene-3,14, 20-triol (XX)**

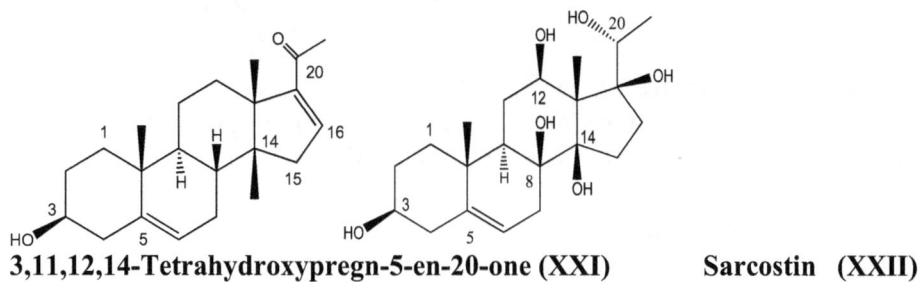

3,11,12,14-Tetrahydroxypregn-5-en-20-one (XXI)   **Sarcostin (XXII)**

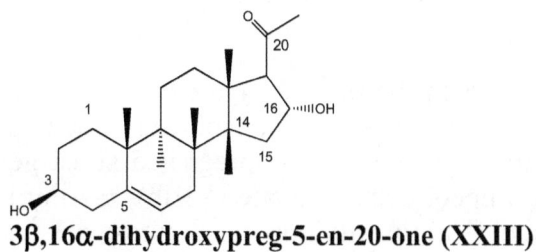

3β,16α-dihydroxypreg-5-en-20-one (XXIII)

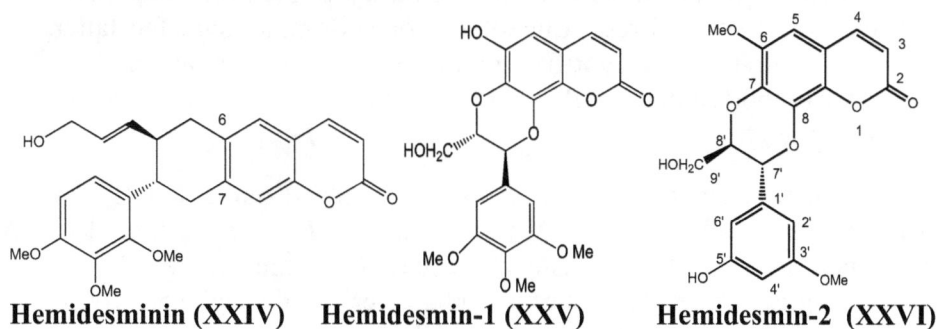

Hemidesminin (XXIV)   Hemidesmin-1 (XXV)   Hemidesmin-2 (XXVI)

(Fig.) contd.....

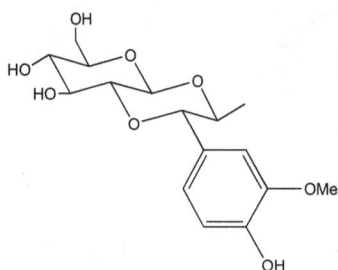

Phenylpropanoid glucoside (XXVII)

α-Amyrin (IV); α-Amyrin acetate (IVa); β-Amyrin (V); β-Amyrin acetate (Va); β-Amyrin palmitate (octadecanoate) (Vb); Lupeol (VI); Lupeol acetate (VIa); Lupeol octacosanoate (VIb); Taraxasteryl acetate (VII); Hemidesterpene - $\Delta^{12,13}$-dehydro-taraxesteryl acetate (VIII); 3-Keto-lup-12-ene-21→28-olide (IX); Lupanone (X); Δ^{12}-Dehydrolupeol acetate (XI); Δ^{12}-Dehydrolupanyl-3β -acetate; Olean-12-en-21β-yl acetate; Olean-12-en-3α-yl acetate (XIII);16(17)-*seco*-Ur--12,20(30)-dien-18α H-3β-yl acetate; 16(17)-*seco*-Urs-12,20(30)-dien-18αH-3β-ol; Urs-20(30)-en-18β H-3β -yl acetate; Lup-1,12-diene-3-on-21-ol (XIV).

One of the earliest studies which investigated the plant *H. indicus* reported the presence of many compounds [50]. Separation technologies included chromatography over previous innovative silver nitrate impregnated silica gel. Lupeol (VIII), Lupeol acetate (VIIIa), Lupeol octacosanoate (VIIIb), α-Amyrin (IV), β-Amyrin (V), β-Amyrin acetate (Va) in addition to β-Sitosterol and hexatriacontane were obtained from the petrol extract of the roots. Saponification of Lupeol octacosanoate afforded Lupeol and octacosanoic acid, the latter was converted to its methyl ester. Quantification of Lupeol octacosanoate in *H. indicus* root powder was reported using HPTLC [37]. Lupeol octacosanoate was used as the marker compound.

Further investigations related to *H. indicus* roots carried out at CARI, Kolkata showed the presence of the known triterpenoids - α-Amyrin acetate (IVa), β-Amyrin acetate (Va) and Taraxasteryl acetate (VI) and a new triterpene, designated Hemidesterpene. The latter was characterized through spectroscopical studies as $\Delta^{12,13}$-Dehydro-taraxesteryl acetate (VIII) [51].

Isolation of an active anti-diabetic compound β-amyrin palmitate (Vb), also has been reported from *H. indicus* roots [52] (see Section 2 on anti-diabetic activities). A CIMAP, Lucknow, based research group isolated several compounds from the ethanol extract of the stems of H. indicus [53] - the new triterpene lactone 3-Keto-lup-12-ene-21→ 28-olide (IX), Lupanone (X), Δ^{12}-Dehydrolupeol ?acetate

(XI), Δ^{12}-dehydrolupanyl-3β-acetate (XII), hexadecanoic acid, 4-hydroxy-3-methoxy-benzaldehyde and 3-hydroxy-4-methoxy-benzaldehyde.

A group of scientists at Hamdard University, New Delhi, reported the isolation and characterisation of several terpenoid constituents from the roots of *H. indicus* [54] - six new pentacyclic triterpenoids – Olean-12-en-21 β-yl acetate, Olean-1--en-3 α-yl acetate (XIII); 16(17)-*seco*-Urs-12,20(30)-dien-18 αH-3 β-yl acetate, 16(17)-*seco*-Urs- 12,20(30)-dien-18 αH-3 β-ol, Urs-20(30)-en-18 βH-3 β -yl acetate; Lup-1,12-diene-3-on-21-ol(XIV). They also obtained another three new terpenoids and two known steroids, from the ethanolic extract of the powdered roots of *H. indicus* [55] - Hemidesmusoic acid (2,6,10, 14,18,22-hexamethyltetracosoi-1-oic acid ; XV), the acyclic diterpenoid octyl hemidesdisterpenoate (n-octyl 2,6,10,14-tetramethyl- hexadec-7-ol-10-en-13-on-1-octanoate ; XVI), and the sesterpenoid ester *n*-non-2'- en-1'-yl-13(15, 19, 19-trimethyl-cyclohex-14,16-dienyl)- 2,6,10-trimethyl-tetradec-6-ol- 13-on-1-oate (XVII),

A new sesterterpenoid (XVIII), biogenetically derived by head to tail linkages of five isoprene units has been reported [20] - its structure was proposed as (XVIII) from detailed NMR and MS studies.

Steroids

Presence of *β*−sitosterol, a ubiquitous component of a few plants, has been reported in the roots of *H. indicus* [56]. The known phytosteroids *β*−sitosterol and *β*−sitosterol glucuronate have been isolated from the roots [50, 55]. Several studies have been carried out on the steroids present in cultured plant tissues and mature plants. Cultures made from stem, shoot, and roots of the plant through tissue culture techniques. Stem tissue cultures possessed organo-genetic potential, while shoot tip and root cultures grew as un-organized callus under different hormonal stimuli. All the cultures - leaves, stems and roots - contained phytosterols, *viz.* Cholesterol, Campesterol, *β*-sitosterol, and 16-Dehydropregnenolone (XIX). Concentration of 16-dehydropregnenolone (XIX) were - roots (0.04%) stem (0.006%), leaves (trace amounts) [57].

Glycosides

Several pregnane glycosides have been reported from *H. indicus* from research groups working at contributions from Lucknow University, as well as elsewhere. The Lucknow group has studied eleven new pregnane glycosides from the dried stems and twigs of this plant. In general, the extraction procedure involved extraction by chloroform-ethanol followed by column chromatography over silica gel. Structure elucidation was done on the basis of 15 detailed spectroscopic investigations (EI-MS, FABMS, 1H NMR, 13C NMR) and chemical transformations. Eight of these new pregnane glycosides were derived from calogenin, *i.e.* Pregn-5-ene-3,14,20-triol (XX). These are Hemidescine [59], Emidine [59], Indicine [60], Hemidine [60], Hemisine [61, 62], Desmisine [61, 62], Denicunine [64], and Heminine [64]. The structure of Desinine [58], was based on 3,11,12,14-Tetrahydroxypregn-5-en-20-one (XXI). The structure of Medidesmine [59] was based on Sarcostin, *i.e.* Pregn-5-ene-3,8, 12,14, 17,20-hexol (XXII).

The structure of new pregnane oligoglycoside indicusin [63] was isolated from the chloroform-ethanol extract of the stems of *H. indicus* defined as 11α, 12β-di-O-acetyl-orgogenin-3-O-β-D-cymaropyranosyl-(1→4)-*O*-β-D-cymaropyranosyl -(1→4)-*O*-β-D-cymaropyranoside. The new pregnane glycoside Hindicusine was isolated from the chloroform-ethanol extract of the stems of *H. indicus* [65]. Its structure has been established as 20-*O*-Benzoyl calogenin-3-*O*-β--digitoxopyranosideon the basis of spectroscopic investigations. Hindicusine and di- O-acetylhindicusine showed anti-hyperlipidemic activity comparable to gemfibrozil. Hindicusine and di- O-acetylhindicusine (200μg/ml) exhibited strong antioxidant activity and by preventing the formation of superoxide anion and hydroxyl radical.

A new condensed poly-propanoid glucoside and pregnane saponins were obtained from the *n*-butanol soluble fraction of a methanol extract of the roots of *H. indicus* [66]. The new compounds Hemidesmoside A-C in addition to the known Plocoside A. Separation involved droplet counter-current chromatography. Structure elucidation was achieved by spectroscopical investigations - IR, HR-ESI- MS, 1H- and 13C-NMR, including detailed two-dimensional (COSY, NOESY, HSQC, HMBC) analysis. The structures of the Hemidesimosides were based on 3?,16?-Dihydroxypreg-5-en-20-one (XXIII) [66].

Polyphenolics - Coumarino-lignoids, Flavonoids

Coumarino-lignoids

Three new Coumarino-lignoids were characterised after isolation from the roots of *H. indicus* at Calcutta University [67, 68]. The common structural feature of these compounds is that they have a coumarin unit linked to a lignoid C6-C3 unit through an *ortho*-dihydroxyl bridge. Hemidesmin (XXIV) [67] was a linearly fused coumarino-lignoid, whereas Hemidesmin-1 (XXV) [68] and Hemidesmin-2 (XXVI) [68] were non-linearly fused coumarino-lignoids.

Phenylpropanoid Glucoside

The new phenylpropanoid (XXVII) [66], belonging to a very rare class of compounds derived from a combination of a lignoid C6-C3 unit is also reported to be isolated through an *ortho*-dihydroxyl bridge with a hexose unit.

Flavonoids

Very few flavonoids have been isolated and identified. Methanolic extracts of the flowers and leaves of the plant yielded flavone glycosides - hyperoxide, isoquercetin, rutin from the flowers, hyperoxide, rutin from the leaves [69]. Secondary metabolites like vanillin, lupeol and rutin derived from *in-vivo* and *in-vitro* grown shoot and root culture of *H. indicus* have been estimated by a validated HPTLC method by Turrini [38].

ANTI-DIABETIC ACTIVITY OF *H. INDICUS*

Diabetes mellitus is one of the most investigated global health problems. India, which is becoming the diabetic capital of India has more than 40 million diabetic people who account for nearly 20% of the global diabetes population. The World Health Organization has also recommended the efficacy evaluation of traditional plant treatments for diabetes. In several countries, medicinal plants are traditionally used for controlling diabetes [70 - 73]. Among the medicinal plants which have been investigated for anti-diabetic activity is *H. indicus*. Ethno-botanical evidence suggests that *H. indicus* is popularly used in India as a potent anti-diabetic medicinal plant. Reported ethnomedical uses of *H. indicus* roots in diabetes reported from different places in India are compiled and presented in Table **4**.

Table 4. Ethnomedical uses of *H.indicus* in diabetes.

Part Used/Dosage Form	Route of Administration	Place of Use	Reference
Root paste with rhizome of *Zingiber officinale* and coconut fruit pulp	Oral	Shimoga district, Karnataka	[74]
Root decoction	Oral	Wayanad district, Kerala	[75]
Root decoction	Oral	Unakoti district, Tripura	[76]
Root infusion	Oral	Sirumalai hills, Dindigul district, Tamil Nadu	[77]

In view of the ethnobotanical evidence available, much work has been carried out to explore the anti-diabetic properties of extracts of *Hemidesmus indicus*. The first comprehensive report [18] was made by the research group of one of the co-authors of this review working at Calcutta University and collaborating with Dhaka University and BIRDEM, Dhaka. Following this report, several research groups, in India and Bangladesh have investigated the antidiabetic properties of *H.indicus* roots.

In the first report [18], shade-dried ground roots of *H. indicus* (Anantamul) were extracted thrice in the cold with 95% ethanol, and similarly with methanol. Removal of the solvent under reduced pressure, followed by freeze-drying, gave the ethanolic (HiRE) and methanolic (HirM) extracts [18]. Studies were conducted with male Long-Evans rats. The following investigations were carried out: HirE on diabetic (Type I and Type II) model rats for acute hypoglycaemic effects; HirM on Type II diabetic model rats for both acute and chronic effects. Both HirE and HirM had significant hypoglycaemic effects on Type II diabetic model rats [18]. Additionally, HirM had a beneficial effect on dyslipidaemia.

Extensive work has been done by K. Kannabiran and M. Gayathri of Vellore on roots collected from Tamilnadu and also on the active principle 2-hydroxy-4-methoxy benzoic acid [78, 79, 89 - 93].

The significant results of research done by the several research groups are summarised below:

i. Aqueous extract (HirW) roots of *H. indicus* exhibited significant antidiabetic and anti-oxidant activity on STZ-induced diabetic albino Wistar rats, and also restored metabolic parameters to near normal levels [78, 79]. The anti-hyperglycaemic activity was comparable to the standard drug Tolbutamide. Possible mechanisms of action were stimulation of the b-cells of Langerhans to produce insulin and due to increased peripheral glucose utilization.

ii. In vitro investigations were made the mechanism of anti-diabetic activity of aqueous extracts from *H.indicus* root, *Ficus benghalensis* bark, *Pterocarpus marsupium* bark. These extracts showed potent inhibition of glucose diffusion across bio-membrane, the *H. indicus* extract being the most effective. The authors opined that the hypoglycaemic activity was due to this inhibitory action [80].

iii. Sowmia and Kokilavani [81] carried out their experiments with lyophilized ethanolic extracts of the roots (HirE) on alloxan-induced diabetic male Wistar rats. Treatment with HirE (40mg/kg b.w./day) for four weeks showed hypoglycaemic effects comparable to the drug Glibenclamide. Sowmia et al. have also observed modulation of gluconeogenic and glycolytic enzymes in alloxan-induced diabetic rats [82, 83].

iv. Similar results have been reported by Zarei [84] with ethanol extracts (HirE) of Anatamool collected in Karnataka. Results of decrease in glucose levels in alloxan-induced diabetic rats were comparable for HirE (250 mg/kg b.w.) and Glibenclamide (3mg/kg, p.o.). The authors ascribed the effect to the free radical scavenging activity of HirE.

v. Subramanian [85] used a modified procedure for preparing the extract - the roots were sohxletted with petrol and then with ethanol. The concentrated ethanolic extract taken in water was orally administered to alloxan-induced diabetic rats. The results were comparable with orally administered gliclazide regarding anti-hyperglycemic, anti-dyslipidemic, and anti-oxidant activity.

vi. Siraj *et al.* have assayed the antidiabetic effect of HirE extracts by gut perfusion and six-segment methods on Long Evans rats [86]. In this study, the glucose absorption in control rats *vs.* rats fed with 250 mg/kg b.w. at intervals varying from 5 to 30 minutes. They observed a significant decrease in intestinal glucose absorption throughout the experimental time.

Treatment of Diabetes-induced Cataract and Wounds with *Hemidesmus indicus* Extracts

Diabetic cataract is a secondary complication due to Chronic hyperglycemia. Methanolic root extracts of *H.indicus* delays the progression of cataract in streptozotocin induced diabetic rats by inhibiting the rat lens aldose reductase enzyme activity by reducing the osmotic stress [87].

Reports suggest that diabetes slows down wound healing in affected humans and animals. Moideen *et al.* [21] and Vijaya Kumari*et al.* [88] observed that respectively ethanolic extract (5% ointment) of *H. indicus* leaves [21] and methanolic extract (5% w/w) of the roots [88] possessed marked wound healing activity on diabetic Wistar strain rats.

Isolation of Active Anti-diabetic Compounds and their Activity

In most of these studies, no attempts were made to isolate and study the components responsible for the anti-diabetic property in *H. indicus*. A limited number of investigations have endeavored to isolate the active principles responsible for antidiabetic activity in *H. indicus*.

β-Amyrin Palmitate

β-Amyrin palmitate (II) was identified as an anti-hyperglycemic active principle by anti- hyperglycaemic activity guided separation techniques, (II) exhibited significant antidiabetic activity in both alloxan and STZ- diabetic rats even at low concentrations. The optimum dose was (50 µg/kg b.w.) administered daily for 15 days; the non-fasted levels of blood glucose were reduced without affecting body and organ weight. Even activities detected in the glucose tolerance test were higher in oral administration in comparison to intraperitoneal applications. An elevated level of serum enzymes (SGOT, SGPT and ALP), cholesterol and urea in both STZ and alloxan-induced diabetic rats were reduced significantly. It was suggested that β-Amyrin palmitate blocks the entry of glucose molecules from the intestine [52].

2-Hydroxy 4-methoxy Benzoic Acid (HMBA)

Extensive studies [89 - 93] on HMBA, another active principle for antidiabetic activity, have been carried out. Oral HMBA administration (500 μg/kg b. w.) was done to *ad libitum* fed, fasted, and glucose-loaded diabetic and non-diabetic rats [89, 90]. A significant reduction in blood glucose levels was observed (F>0.05 and P< 0.05) in rats. Activities of glucose-6-phosphatase, fructose-1, 6-bisphosphatase, hexokinase, and phosphor-glucoisomerase in the liver and kidney in rats were restored to near normal levels of HMBA treated (7 weeks) diabetic rats. The significant reduction in glucose, glucose-6-phosphatase, and fructose-1,6-bisphosphatase activities in diabetic rats indicated the role of HMBA in suppressing gluco-neogenesis in diabetic rats [89 - 92].

The effect of HMBA on erythrocyte membrane-bound enzymes and antioxidant status in STZ induced diabetic rats has been reported [93]. Treatment with HMBA (dosage 500 μg/kg/day) for 7 weeks by oral intubation was comparable with the standard hypoglycemic agent glibenclamide (dosage 100 mg/kg).

These studies showed HMBA supports the restoration of antioxidant defense, reduces reactive oxygen species production, lipid peroxidation, and glycosylation of hemoglobin and elevates free radical quenching in tissues of diabetic rats.

In another *in vivo* study in rats, HMBA has shown anti-hyperlipidemic potential. Administration of HMBA at 200ug/kg/day for 30 days after oral administration of ethanol for decreased total cholesterol, triglycerides, low-density lipoproteins, phospholipids, free fatty acids, and increased high-density lipoprotein and plasma lipoprotein lipase concentration [94].

Aldose Reductase Inhibitors from H. indicus

A molecular docking study approach based on theoretical calculations on *H. indicus* phytoconstituents as Aldose reductase inhibitors were also reported [95]. As the role played by Aldose reductase primarily in type II Diabetes is widely documented; protein-ligand interaction studies were carried out on phyto-components of *H. indicus* with Aldose reductase as the target protein. Molecular docking studies of these into the 3D structure of 1H4G of Homo sapiens using FlexX were performed; top-scoring compounds were vanillin, hyperoside, isoquercetin, HMBA, and phenylpropanoid. These were evaluated as promising inhibitors showing a high binding affinity for the Aldose reductase enzyme.

CONCLUDING REMARKS

In the majority of pharmacological studies, the activity, anti-diabetic as well as other biological activities, were investigated with crude extracts. Future research must focus on Bioactivity-guided isolation and characterization of active principles, the establishment of modes of action as well as structure-activity relationship of the bioactive components.

What is remarkably surprising is that efforts to analyze aqueous and aqueous ethanolic extracts on which most of the work on anti-diabetic and other activities have been carried out have received very little attention as regards the isolation and characterization of components. Small organic molecules, glycosides, free amino- acids, and smaller peptide molecules which may be present in these extracts may contribute significantly to the various recorded activities of *Hemidesmus indicus*.

Toxicological investigations on *H. indicus* are virtually non-existent. Hence it is necessary to determine toxicity profiles of extracts as well as major active compounds on patients of different age groups and sex. Detailed phytopharmacognostic studies and HPTLC and HPLC analysis of extractives are necessary to differentiate *Anantamul* (*Hemidesmus indicus* roots) from the roots of four substitutes and adulterants, *viz.Ichnocarpus frutescens*, *Cryptolepis buchanani*, *Decalepis hamiltonii* and *Utleria salicifolia*.

CONSENT FOR PUBLICATION

Not applicable.

CONFLICT OF INTEREST

The authors declare no conflict of interest, financial or otherwise.

ACKNOWLEDGEMENTS

The authors thank the Indian Science Congress Association, Department of Science and Technology for the award of Sir Asutosh Mookerjee Fellowship and the Director General, CCRAS, New Delhi and Director, Central Ayurveda Research Institute, Kolkata for extending the facilities for working.

REFERENCES

[1]   Kirtikar KR, Basu BD. Blatter E, Caius JF, Mhaskar KS (Eds.),Indian Medicinal Plants, 1984, vol. I. Lalit Mohan Basu, Allahabad, India.

[2]   Chatterjee A, Pakrashi SC,1995. In: Prof (Mrs) Asima Chatterjee and Dr. SC Pakrashi (Eds.), The Treatise on Indian Medicinal Plants, vol. 3, Publications and Information Directorate, CSIR, New Delhi, India.

[3]   Chatterjee A, Pakrashi SC,2003. In: Prof (Mrs) Asima Chatterjee and Dr. SC Pakrashi (Eds.), The Treatise on Indian Medicinal Plants, vol. 6. Publications and Information Directorate, CSIR, New Delhi, India.

[4]   Anonymous, The Wealth of Indi, 1958. National Institute of Science Communications and Information Resources. CSIR,New Delhi, India.

[5]   Anonymous, The Wealth of Indi, 2002. National Institute of Science Communications and Information Resources. CSIR,New Delhi, India.

[6]   K V Tushar; K P Unnikrishnan; K M Hashim; I Balachandran. *Hemidesmus indicus*(L.) R. Br. A review. J Plant Sci 2008; 3: 146-56.

[7]   Austin A. A review on Indian sarsaparilla. J Biol Sci 2008; 8: 1-12.

[8]   Panchal GA, Panchal SJ, Patel JA. *Hemidesmus indicus*: a review. Pharmacologyonline 2009; 2: 758-71.

[9]   Chatterjee S. Aparna Banerjee; I Chandra. *Hemidesmusindicus*: A Rich Source of Herbal Medicine. Med Aromat Plants 2014; 3e: 155.

[10]   Iyer SR. Ayurvedic Yoga Samgraham, PS Varier's Arya Vaidya Sala. Kottakal 1983.

[11]   Anonymous . The Ayurvedic Pharmacopeia of India. 1st ed. New Delhi: Ministry of Health and Family Welfare, Department of Health, Government of India 1989; pp. 107-8.

[12]   Anonymous . Quality Standards of Indian Medicinal Plants. New Delhi: Indian Council for Medical Research 2005; Vol. 2: pp. 119-28.

[13]   Lakshmi T, Rajendran R. *Hemidesmus indicus* commonly known as Indian Sarasaparilla- An Update. Int J Pharm Bio. Sci 2013; 4(4): 397 – 340.

[14]   Sharma P C, Yelne M B, Dennis T J. Database on Medicinal Plants Used in Ayurveda. 3rd ed. New Delhi. India: Central Council for Research in Ayurveda and Siddha;2005. p. 282-4.

[15]   Das M, Banerji A, Dutta S, Saha S, Hazra J. Phyto-pharmacognostical evaluation and HPTLC study on Anantamul. Pharmacy (Basel) 2017; 8(3): 68-72.
        [http://dx.doi.org/10.7897/2277-4343.083146]

[16]   Churchill J, Churchill A. An Introduction to the Study of Materia Medica. London: Kessinger Publishing 2009; p. 348.

[17]   Weissner W. Anantamul (*Hemidesmus indicus*) A Review of Biomedical Studies and U.S. Products. Ayurveda Journal of Health 2014, Vol. XII, (4); 52.

[18]   Murshed S, Rokeya B, Nahar N, *et al.* Hypoglycemic and Hypolipidaemic effect of *Hemidesmus indicus* root on diabetic model rats. Diabetes Res 2005; 39(1): 15-23.

[19]   Subramaniam S, Abarna A, Thamizhiniyan T. Antihyperglycemic, antioxidant and antidyslipidemic properties of *Hemidesmus indicus* root extract studied in alloxan-induced experimental diabetes in rats. Int J Pharm Sci Res 2012; 3(1): 227-34.

[20]   Sowmiya C, Divya Priya S. Int Res J Pharm 2014; 5(4): 343-7.

[21]   Mohammed Moideen M, Verghese R, Krishna Kumar E, Dhanapal CK. Wound healing activity of ethanolic extract of *Hemidesmus indicus* (Linn) R.Br. leaves in rats. Res J Pharm Biol Chem Sci 2011; 2(3): 643-51.

[22] Vijayalakshmi K, Shyamala R, Thirumurugan V, *et al.* Physico-Phytochemical investigation and anti-inflammatory. Anc Sci Life 2010; 29(4): 35-40.
[PMID: 22557366]

[23] Sayeed M, Khan M, Devanna N, Syed YH, Ansari JA. J Pharm Biosci 2013; 4: 141-5.

[24] Saryam R, Seriya C, Khan S. Physico-chemical and preliminary phytochemical screening of *Hemidesmusindicus*. J Chem Pharm Res 2012; 4(11): 4695-7.

[25] Ravishankara MN, Shrivastava N, Padh H, Rajani M. Evaluation of antioxidant properties of root bark of *Hemidesmus indicus* R. Br. (Anantmul). Phytomedicine 2002; 9(2): 153-60.
[http://dx.doi.org/10.1078/0944-7113-00104] [PMID: 11995949]

[26] Nagarajan S, Jagan M R, Gurudatt K N. Chemical composition of the volatiles of *Hemidesmus indicus* R Br Flavour Fragr J 2001; 16: 212-4.

[27] Nagarajan S, Jagan Mohan Rao L. Determination of 2-hydroxy-4-methoxybenzaldehyde in roots of *Decalepis hamiltonii* (Wight & Arn.) and *Hemidesmus indicus* R.Br. J AOAC Int 2003; 86(3): 564-7.
[http://dx.doi.org/10.1093/jaoac/86.3.564] [PMID: 12852577]

[28] Sreekumar S, Seeni S, Pushpangadan P. Production of 2-hydroxy 4-methoxy benzaldehyde using root cultures of *Hemidesmus indicus*. Biotechnol Lett 1998; 20(7): 631-5.
[http://dx.doi.org/10.1023/A:1005354003727]

[29] Sreekumar S, Seeni S, Pushpangadan P. Micropropagation of *Hemidesmus indicus*for cultivation and production of 2-hydroxy 4-methoxy benzaldehyde. Plant Cell Tissue Organ Cult 2000; 62(3): 211-8.
[http://dx.doi.org/10.1023/A:1006486817203]

[30] Darekar R, Khetre A, Singh S, Damle M. HPTLC quantitation of 2-hydroxy-4-methoxybenzaldehyde in *Hemidesmus indicus* R.Br. root powder and extract. J Planar Chromatogr Mod TLC 2009; 22(6): 453-6.
[http://dx.doi.org/10.1556/JPC.22.2009.6.13]

[31] Sircar D, Dey G, Mitra A. A validated HPLC method for simultaneous determination of 2-hydroxy-4-methoxybenzaldehyde and 2-hydroxy-4-methoxybenzoic acid in root organs of *Hemidesmus indicus*. Chromatographia 2007; 65(5-6): 349-53.
[http://dx.doi.org/10.1365/s10337-006-0146-x]

[32] Alam MI, Gomes A. Viper venom-induced inflammation and inhibition of free radical formation by pure compound (2-hydroxy-4-methoxy benzoic acid) isolated and purified from anantamul (*Hemidesmus indicus* R.Br) root extract. Toxicon 1998; 36(1): 207-15.
[http://dx.doi.org/10.1016/S0041-0101(97)00070-6] [PMID: 9604294]

[33] Jirovetz L, Buchbauer G, Höferi M, Shafi MP, Sagaran PG. Essential oil analysis of *Hemidesmus indicus* R. Br. roots from southern India. J Essent Oil Res 2002; 14(6): 437-8.
[http://dx.doi.org/10.1080/10412905.2002.9699914]

[34] Sreelekha M, Jirovetz L, Shafi MP. Comparative study of the essential oils from *Hemidesmus indicus*and *Decalepis hamiltonii*. Asian J Chem 2007; 19(6): 4942-4.

[35] Kavitha D, Sudhakar P, Reddy PR. Phytochemical studies on the roots of *Hemidesmusindicus* (L.) R. Br. ecotypes. Ann Phytomed 2017; VI(I): 83-7.
[http://dx.doi.org/10.21276/ap.2017.6.1.12]

[36] Kundu A, Jawali N, Mitra A. Shikimate pathway modulates the elicitor-stimulated accumulation of fragrant 2-hydroxy-4-methoxybenzaldehyde in *Hemidesmus indicus* roots. Plant Physiol Biochem 2012; 56: 104-8.
[http://dx.doi.org/10.1016/j.plaphy.2012.04.005] [PMID: 22609460]

[37] Darekar RS, Khetre AB, Sinha PK, Jaswani RM, Damle M. Quantification of lupeol Rasayan J Chem 2008; 1(3): 526-31.

[38] Turrini E, Calcabrini C, Tacchini M, *et al.* 2018a. In vitro study of the cytotoxic, cytostatic, and

antigenotoxic profile of *Hemidesmus indicus* (L.) R.Br. (Apocynaceae) crude drug extract on T lymphoblastic cells. Toxins (Basel) 2018; 10(2): 70.
[http://dx.doi.org/10.3390/toxins10020070] [PMID: 29415441]

[39]   Fimognari C, Lenzi M, Ferruzzi L, *et al.* Mitochondrial pathway mediates the antileukemic effects of *Hemidesmus indicus*, a promising botanical drug. PLoS One 2011; 6(6): e21544.
[http://dx.doi.org/10.1371/journal.pone.0021544] [PMID: 21738701]

[40]   Ferruzzi L, Turrini E, Burattini S, *et al.* *Hemidesmus indicus* induces apoptosis. J Ethnopharmacol 2013; 147: 84-91.
[http://dx.doi.org/10.1016/j.jep.2013.02.009] [PMID: 23500881]

[41]   Dharmesh SM, Jayaram S. Assessment of antioxidant potentials of free and bound phenolics of *Hemidesmus indicus* (L) R.Br against oxidative damage. Pharmacognosy Res 2011; 3(4): 225-31.
[http://dx.doi.org/10.4103/0974-8490.89741] [PMID: 22224044]

[42]   Misra N, Misra P, Datta SK, Mehrotra S. *In vitro* biosynthesis of antioxidants from *Hemidesmus indicus* R. Br. cultures. In Vitro Cell Dev Biol Plant 2005; 41(3): 285-90.
[http://dx.doi.org/10.1079/IVP2004627]

[43]   Nandy S, Dey A, De A, Bhattacharyya R, Ray P, Mukherjee S. Enhanced Bioactivity exhibited by In vitro grown Hemidesmus indicus(L.) R. Br. extracts in terms of antioxidation and anti human pathogenic bacterial activity.Medicinal Plants: Phytochemistry, Pharmacology and Therapeutics 4. New Delhi: Daya Publisher 2015; pp. 255-64.

[44]   Verma SC, Rani R, Nigam S, *et al.* Development and validation of precise and rapid HPTLC method for determination of ferulic acid in *Hemidesmus indicus* roots. Asian J Res Chem 2011; 4(11): 1747-51.

[45]   Murti PB, Seshadri TR. A study of the chemical components of the roots of *Decalepis hamiltonii* (Makaliveru), Part III- comparison with *Hemidesmus indicus* (Indian sarsparilla). Proc Indiana Acad Sci 1941; 13: 399-403.
[http://dx.doi.org/10.1007/BF03049299]

[46]   Murti PB, Seshadri TR. A study of the chemical components of the roots of *Decalepis hamiltonii* (Makaliveru), Part IV- Resinol of *Decalepis hamiltonii* and *Hemidesmus indicus*. Proc Indiana Acad Sci 1941; 14: 93-9.
[http://dx.doi.org/10.1007/BF03046552]

[47]   Nair GA, Ramiah N. Physiochemical methods of identification and estimation of genuine and substitute/adulterant in single drug mixtures. Part 1. *Hemidesmus indicus*and *Ichnocarpus frutescens*. J Sci Res Plants Med 1982; 3: 57-60.

[48]   Fiori J, Leoni A, Fimognari C, *et al.* Determination of phytomarkers in pharmaceutical. Anal Lett 2014; 47(16): 2629-42.
[http://dx.doi.org/10.1080/00032719.2014.917423]

[49]   Das S, Devaraj SN. Antienterobacterial activity of *Hemidesmus indicus* R. Br. root extract. Phytother Res 2006; 20(5): 416-21.
[http://dx.doi.org/10.1002/ptr.1879] [PMID: 16619372]

[50]   Padhy SN, Mahato SB, Dutta NL. Asclepiadaceous terpenoids. Phytochemistry 1973; 12(1): 217-8.
[http://dx.doi.org/10.1016/S0031-9422(00)84656-7]

[51]   Banerji A, Banerji J, Das M, Hazra J. Hemidesterpene, a new Triterpenoid J Indian Chem Soc 2016; 93(12): 1401-4.

[52]   Nair SA, Sabulal B, Radhika J, Arunkumar R, Subramoniam A. Promising anti-diabetes mellitus activity in rats of *β*-amyrin palmitate isolated from *Hemidesmus indicus* roots. Eur J Pharmacol 2014; 734: 77-82.
[http://dx.doi.org/10.1016/j.ejphar.2014.03.050] [PMID: 24726843]

[53]   Gupta MM, Verma RK, Misra LN. Terpenoids from *Hemidesmus indicus*. Phytochemistry 1992;

31(11): 4036-7.
[http://dx.doi.org/10.1016/S0031-9422(00)97582-4]

[54] Roy SK, Ali M, Sharma MP, Ramachandram R. New pentacyclic triterpenes from the roots of *Hemidesmus indicus*. Pharmazie 2001; 56(3): 244-6.
[PMID: 11265594]

[55] Roy SK, Ali M, Sharma MP, Ramachandran R. Phytochemical investigation of *Hemidesmus indicus* R. Br. Roots. Indian J Chem 2002; 41B(11): 2390-4.

[56] Chatterjee RC, Bhattacharya BK. A note on the isolation of β-sitosterol from *Hemidesmus indicus*. J Indian Chem Soc 1955; 32: 485-96.

[57] Heble MR, Chadha MS. Steroids in cultured tissues and mature plant of *Hemidesmus indicus*R. Br. (Asclepiadiaceae). ZeitschriftfürPflanzenphysiologie 1978; 89(5): 401-6.

[58] Oberoi K, Khare MP, Khare A. A pregnane ester diglycoside from *Hemidesmus indicus*. Phytochemistry 1985; 24(10): 2395-7.
[http://dx.doi.org/10.1016/S0031-9422(00)83049-6]

[59] Chandra R, Deepak D, Khare A. Pregnane glycosides from *Hemidesmus indicus*. Phytochemistry 1994; 35(6): 1545-8.
[http://dx.doi.org/10.1016/S0031-9422(00)86891-0]

[60] Prakash K, Sethi A, Deepak D, Khare A, Khare MP. Two pregnane glycosides from *Hemidesmus indicus*. Phytochemistry 1991; 30(1): 297-9.
[http://dx.doi.org/10.1016/0031-9422(91)84141-E]

[61] Deepak D, Srivastava S, Khare A. Pregnane glycosides from *Hemidesmus indicus*. Phytochemistry 1997; 44(1): 145-51.
[http://dx.doi.org/10.1016/S0031-9422(96)00393-7] [PMID: 8983217]

[62] Deepak D, Srivastava S, Khare A. Deepak, D., Srivastav, S., Khare, A. Pregnane Glycosides. In: Fortschritte der Chemie organischer Naturstoffe / Progress in the Chemistry of Organic Natural Products, Springer, Vienna. 1997;71.

[63] Deepak D, Srivastav S, Khare A. Indicusin-A pregnane diester Triglycoside from *Hemidesmus indicus* R. Br. Nat Prod Lett 1995; 6(2): 81-6.
[http://dx.doi.org/10.1080/10575639508044094]

[64] Sigler P, Saksena R, Deepak D, Khare A. C_{21} steroidal glycosides from *Hemidesmus indicus*. Phytochemistry 2000; 54(8): 983-7.
[http://dx.doi.org/10.1016/S0031-9422(99)00611-1] [PMID: 11014302]

[65] Sethi A, Bhatia A, Srivastava S, *et al.* Pregnane glycoside from *Hemidesmus indicus* as a potential anti-oxidant and anti-dyslipidemic agent. Nat Prod Res 2010; 24(15): 1371-8.
[http://dx.doi.org/10.1080/14786410802265084] [PMID: 20169502]

[66] Zhao Z, Matsunami K, Otsuka H, Negi N, Kumar A, Negi DS. A condensed phenylpropanoid glucoside and pregnane saponins from the roots of *Hemidesmus indicus*. J Nat Med 2013; 67(1): 137-42.
[http://dx.doi.org/10.1007/s11418-012-0659-6] [PMID: 22456894]

[67] Mandal S, Das PC, Joshi PC, Das A, Chatterjee A. Hemidesminin - A New Coumarino-Lignoid from *Hemidesmus indicus* Indian J Chem 1991; 30B(7): 712-3.

[68] Das PC, Joshi PC, Mandal S, Das A, Chatterjee A, Banerji A. New coumarinolignoids from *Hemidesmus indicus*R. Br. Indian J Chem 1992; 31B(3): 342-5.

[69] Subramanian S, Nair AGR. Flavonoids of some Asclepiadaceous plants. Phytochemistry 1968; 7: 1703-4.

[70] Bailey CJ, Day C. Traditional plant medicines as treatments for diabetes. Diabetes Care 1989; 12(8): 553-64.

[http://dx.doi.org/10.2337/diacare.12.8.553] [PMID: 2673695]

[71] Grover J K, Yadav S, Vats V. Medicinal Plants of India with Antidiabetic Potential. J Ethnopharmacol 2002; 81: 81-100.

[72] Marles R, Farnsworth N. Economic and Medicinal Plant Research. UK: Academic Press 1994; Vol. 6: p. 149.

[73] Modak M, Dixit P, Londhe J, Ghaskadbi S, Devasagayam TPA, Devasagyam T. Indian herbs and herbal drugs used for the treatment of diabetes. J Clin Biochem Nutr 2007; 40(3): 163-73. [http://dx.doi.org/10.3164/jcbn.40.163] [PMID: 18398493]

[74] Rajakumar N, Shivanna MB. Ethno-medicinal application of plants in the eastern region of Shimoga district, Karnataka, India. J Ethnopharmacol 2009; 126(1): 64-73. [http://dx.doi.org/10.1016/j.jep.2009.08.010] [PMID: 19686831]

[75] Silja VP, Varma KS, Mohanan KV. Ethnomedicinal plant knowledge of the Mullukuruma tribe of Wayanad district, Kerala. Indian J Tradit Knowl 2008; 7: 604-12.

[76] Ghosh Tarafdar R, Nath S, Das Talukdar A, Dutta Choudhury M. Antidiabetic plants used among the ethnic communities of Unakoti district of Tripura, India. J Ethnopharmacol 2015; 160: 219-26. [http://dx.doi.org/10.1016/j.jep.2014.11.019] [PMID: 25457986]

[77] Maruthupandian A, Mohan VR, Kottaimuthu R. Ethnomedicinal plants used for the treatment of diabetics and jaundice by palliyartribals in Sirumalai hills, Western Ghats, Tamil Nadu, India. Indian J Nat Prod Resour 2011; 2: 493-7.

[78] Krishnan Kannabiran. Hypoglycemic activity of *Hemidesmus indicus*R. Br. on streptozotocin-induced diabetic rats. Int J Diabetes Dev Ctries 2008; 28(1): 6-10. [http://dx.doi.org/10.4103/0973-3930.41979] [PMID: 19902032]

[79] Kannabiran K, Mahalingam G. *Hemidesmus indicus* root extract ameliorates diabetes-mediated metabolic changes in rats. Int J Green Pharm 2009; 3(4): 314-8. [http://dx.doi.org/10.4103/0973-8258.59739]

[80] Archit R, Gayathri M, Punnagai M. An *in vitro* investigation into the Mechanism of Anti-Diabetic activity of selected Medicinal Plants. International Journal of Drug Development and Research 2013; 5(3): 221-6.

[81] Sowmia C, Kokilavani R. Antidiabetic and antihypercholesterolemic effect of *Hemidesmus indicus* Linn.R. root in Alloxan induced diabetic rats. Anc Sci Life 2007; 26(4): 4-10. [PMID: 22557243]

[82] Sowmia C, Gurusamy K, Kokilavani R, *et al.* Assesment of glycemic potential and activity of marker enzymes on *Hemidesmus indicus* ethanolic root extract in alloxan induced diabetic rats. Drugline 2008; 10(1-2): 14-20.

[83] Sowmia C, Kokilavani R, Gurusamy K. Modulation of Glycolytic and Gluconeogenic Enzymes by Treatment with *Hemidesmus indicus* R. Br. Ethanolic Root Extract in Alloxan Induced Diabetic Rats. Res J Biotechnol 2009; 4(1): 15-9.

[84] Zarei M, Baker S, Zarei M. Effect of *Hemidesmus indicus* root extract on the blood glucose level in alloxan induced diabetic rats. J Microbiol Biotechnol Res 2013; 3(2): 64-7.

[85] Subramanian S, Abarna A, Thamizhiniyan V. Antihyperglycemic, antioxidant Int J Pharm Sci Res 2012; 3(1): 227-34.

[86] Siraj MA, Shams MR, Hossain E, Salahuddin M, Tahsin F. A AKhalid; S P Paul.Assay of antidiabetic activity of *Hemidesmus indicus* by gut perfusion and six segment methods on Long Evans rats. Pharmacologyonline 2013; 3: 81-7.

[87] Tirumani P, Venu S, Sridhar G, Praveen kumar M, Rajashekhar AV, Naga Raju T. Delaying of cataract through intervention of *Hemidesmus indicus* in STZ induced diabetic rats. Nat Prod Res 2018; 32(11): 1295-8.

[http://dx.doi.org/10.1080/14786419.2017.1333991] [PMID: 28580798]

[88]   Vijaya Kumari K, Niteswar K. Phytochemical and clinical evaluation of Sariba (*Hemidesmus indicus*) on wound healing. International Research Journal of Pharmacy 2012; 3: 277-81.

[89]   Kannabiran K, Gayathri M. Effect of 2-hydroxy-4-methoxy benzoic acid from the roots of *Hemidesmus indicus* on streptozotocin-induced diabetic rats. Indian J Pharm Sci 2009; 71(5): 581-5. [http://dx.doi.org/10.4103/0250-474X.58180] [PMID: 20502585]

[90]   Gayathri M, Kannabiran K. Hypoglycemic effect of 2-hydroxy 4-methoxy benzoic acid isolated from the roots of *Hemidesmus indicus* on streptozotocin-induced diabetic rats. Pharmacologyonline 2010; 1: 144-54.

[91]   Gayathri M, Kannabiran K. Antidiabetic activity of 2-hydroxy 4-methoxy benzoic acid isolated from the roots of *Hemidesmus indicus*on streptozotocin-induced diabetic rats. Int J Diabetes Metab 2009; 17(1): 53-7.

[92]   Gayathri M, Kannabiran K. 2-hydroxy 4-methoxy benzoic acid isolated from roots of *Hemidesmus indicus* ameliorates liver, kidney and pancreas injury due to streptozotocin-induced diabetes in rats. Indian J Exp Biol 2010; 48(2): 159-64.
[PMID: 20455325]

[93]   Gayathri M, Kannabiran K. Effect of 2-hydroxy-4-methoxy benzoic acid isolated from *Hemidesmus indicus* on erythrocyte membrane bound enzymes and antioxidant status in streptozotocin-induced diabetic rats. Indian J Pharm Sci 2012; 74(5): 474-8.
[http://dx.doi.org/10.4103/0250-474X.108438] [PMID: 23716880]

[94]   Anoop A, Jegadeesan M. Biochemical studies on the anti-ulcerogenic potential of *Hemidesmus indicus* R.Br. var. *indicus*. J Ethnopharmacol 2003; 84(2-3): 149-56.
[http://dx.doi.org/10.1016/S0378-8741(02)00291-X] [PMID: 12648808]

[95]   Gunda SK, Bandi S, Sahithi P. *Hemidesmus indicus* Plant Derived Compounds as Aldose Reductase Inhibitors – A Molecular Docking Study Int J Pharm Sci Rev Res 2015; 34(1): 114-7.

Utilization of Tea Polyphenols Against Pesticide Induced Toxicity: International and National Scenario

Devojit K. Sarma[1], Manoj Kumar[1], Swasti Shubham[1], Meenakshi Samartha[3], Pritom Chowdhury[4] and Ravindra M. Samarth[1,2,*]

[1] *ICMR-National Institute for Research in Environmental Health, Bhopal, India*

[2] *ICMR-Bhopal Memorial Hospital & Research Centre, Bhopal, India*

[3] *Department of Zoology, RKDF University, Bhopal, India*

[4] *Department of Biotechnology, Tea Research Association, Tocklai Tea Research Institute, Jorhat, Assam, India*

Abstract: Exposure to pesticides has become a major toxic threat to human and non-target species in India due to the extensive use of chemical-based pesticides in agriculture and for public health purposes. Pesticide induced DNA damage is caused by exposure to certain carcinogenic pesticides through DNA adduct formation and generating altered cells, and subsequently leading to health hazards including cancer. Bio-pesticides are available to prevent the menace of pesticides on human health, such as integrated pest management, use of personal protective measures, or use of non-chemical. Being an agrarian country and its sole dependency on agriculture sectors for most rural employment, India continues to expect its dependency on chemical pesticides, as evident from the high annual demand for pesticides. Therefore, there is an urgent need for an effective approach to reduce the harmful impacts of unavoidable human encounters with toxic pesticides. In this endeavor, preventive measures in the form of functional foods and dietary antioxidants could be employed as one of the complementary and alternative therapeutic approaches to counteract against the ill effects of pesticides in humans. In the past, tea polyphenols have demonstrated an excellent ability to reduce toxicant-induced cellular damage, and DNA damage through mutations, apoptosis, and cancer. In the present review, we have summarized the research carried out on the use of tea polyphenols to counter pesticide toxicity so far and discussed it further from the viewpoint of International and national importance.

Keywords: Bioavailability, DNA damage, Genotoxicity, Nano-formulations, Pesticides, Polyphenols.

---

* **Corresponding author Ravindra M. Samarth:** Department of Research, ICMR-Bhopal Memorial Hospital & Research Centre, Bhopal, India; Tel: +91-755-2749987; E-mail: rmsamarth@gmail.com

Mukesh Kumar Sharma and Pallavi Kaushik (Eds.)

INTRODUCTION

Pollution from environmental mutagens, such as chemical pesticides, is an increasing concern. Many times, adverse impacts on the environment as well as on non-target species dominate the favourable consequences of pesticide use. Agricultural workers and their family members are at high risk of pesticide-induced DNA damage, which prolongs many disease conditions or even death in countries like India. An effective and sustainable method to reduce the adverse impact of pesticide use on health is highly demanded.

There is a high demand for pesticides in India. Most of these pesticides have a residual effect on the environment and human body, leading to many complications. DNA damage in the human body is a molecular marker indicative of pesticide exposure and can be informative in pesticide management through biomonitoring. The biomonitoring DNA damage in pesticide-exposed people is necessary for managing the health issues caused.

Being an agrarian country, there is a high demand for chemical pesticides in India. Out of 234 registered pesticides in India, includes WHO classified Class Ia (4), Class Ib (15), and Class II (76) represent about 40 percent of the registered pesticides in India.

Several of these pesticides have a residual effect on the environment and human body, leading to many short-term and long-term complications. Effective therapeutic agents are required in this endeavor to protect against pesticide-induced DNA damage and for biomonitoring purposes in farmers, thereby preventing further development of complications such as cancers. Tea polyphenols have been studied for their excellent ability as a protective antioxidant agent against many cancers and other diseases in laboratory conditions indicating their potential use as an alternative therapy. The use of tea polyphenols can be an effective and sustainable method to reduce the effect of pesticides on human health. Here, in the present review, we emphasized the role of tea polyphenols against pesticide-induced toxicity at both the national and international levels.

International Scenario

Pesticides are the substances or mixtures of substances having agricultural utility to protect crops from pests, weeds, and diseases as well as in public health for use against diseases like malaria, dengue, and schistosomiasis, mostly vector-borne diseases. Several pesticides that adversely affect human and environmental health are banned for their use in agriculture [1]. In a rural area, the agricultural workers and residents are often exposed to toxic pesticides and thus are at high risk of pesticide toxicity. The type, duration, route, and health condition of the exposed individual are the main factors in imparting toxicity of the pesticide. After encountering a pesticide, it may be metabolized in the body, excreted, stored, or bioaccumulated [2].

Various adverse effects were found to be linked to the toxic nature of pesticides. Several health effects such as diseases of the skin, GI, respiratory, endocrine, reproductive, neurological as well as carcinogenic effects were seen as health hazards of pesticides in the exposed population [3 - 5]. Pesticide exposure in any form accidental, occupational, or intentional, may lead to severe health hazards, including death [6]. World Health Organization has estimated about 500,000-1,000,000 people as victims of pesticide poisoning every year around the world; of these two third belong to developing countries [7].

One of the main mechanisms of chronic and severe pesticide toxicity is oxidative stress induced by several pathways such as free radical overproduction, modification of antioxidant defense system, or detoxification and scavenging enzymes [8]. Various pesticides, such as organochlorines, organophosphates, carbamates, and pyrethroids, are known to induce toxicity mainly through oxidative stress [9 - 11].

Free radical production through increased oxidative stress damages cellular structures and molecules like DNA, RNA, and proteins disrupting the normal cellular process. When the capacity of the body to neutralize or repair such damage is overwhelmed, damaged molecules accumulate and disrupt normal cellular processes. In the long run, as seen with chronic exposure to pesticides, these disruptions lead to several diseases, including neurodegenerative diseases, congenital anomalies, and cancers [12]. Pesticides or their metabolites-induced toxicity involves various processes which can cause direct damage to DNA or induce single-strand DNA breaks employing DNA excision, replication, and recombination or apoptosis [13]. Damages to DNA can be considered markers for the onset of cancer risk; therefore, reducing DNA damage as an initial event of the carcinogenesis process must have significance in reducing the risk of cancer [14].

Therefore, many studies, are focused on pesticide-induced DNA strand breaks, chromosomal aberrations (CA), micronuclei (MN), sister chromatid exchange (SCE), as well as epigenetic modifications [15 - 20]. Due to chronic exposure to pesticides, epigenetic alterations occur, which are known to interfere with gene expression that took place without any modification of DNA sequence [21]. In South Brazil, soybean farmers showed increased values of DNA damage due to chronic exposure to multiple pesticides; this persistent genetic instability due to hypermethylation of DNA may be held responsible for the critical events in the development of ill health effects, including cancer [22]. Therefore, it is necessary and important to determine the toxicity of several genotoxic agents of pesticides affecting human health [18].

There are several standardized tests and assays which are developed for the extensive assessment of genotoxicity of a wide variety of substances and chemical agents of interest. Among these tests, the comet assay and MN test became popular in comparison to other tests and have been found useful in environmental monitoring and screening studies for assessing the mutagenic properties of new chemicals and drugs on a routine basis [23]. The formation of micronuclei takes place during the telophase, where the nuclear envelope is reconstituted in daughter cells [24]. Micronuclei are formed due to either clastogenic *i.e.*, acentric chromosome fragments, or aneugenic effect *i.e.*, partial migration of the whole chromosome that escaped from the main core. The formation of micronuclei are considered as chromatin loss due to damaged or lost chromosomes or loss of the mitotic apparatus. The early modifications in cellular metabolism are recognized by the formation of bilobed nuclei [25].

The comet assay is also known as single-cell gel electrophoresis, in this technique, the property of migration of DNA when the electric field is applied has been exploited [26]. This has been utilized for the assessment of the DNA damage and alkaline labile sites of eukaryotic cells at alkaline pH [27]. This technique has been successfully used for genotoxicity testing of several mutagenic substances and biomonitoring of human exposure to potential mutagens [28], evaluating the efficacy of DNA repair systems can also be tested using comet assay [29, 30]. Oxidative damage to DNA can be studied by combining standard comet assay with enzymes (that distinguish the oxidized nucleotides) that cut the DNA backbone [31].

Though the use of pesticides is harmful to both environment and humans, there is no other way to control its menace other than judicious use based on scientific judgment and use of bio-pesticides. Particularly because of the rising population and increasing demand for food and agricultural products, it is expected that the use of pesticides will continue to rise shortly unless a viable alternative is discovered. Another approach to mitigate the harmful effects of pesticides is through protective measures. Such measures can be either in the form of protective devices that reduce the exposure or therapies or bioactive substances that mitigate the biological effects of pesticides on cells of the body. There has been a concerted effort to identify such complementary and alternative therapies. Oxidative stress plays an important role in pesticide toxicity; therefore, it is identified as the obvious target for preventive therapies. Naturally occurring antioxidants have drawn attention in recent years and have been used by human beings in protecting against oxidative stress induced by pesticides [32]. However, these natural antioxidants have an advantage over synthetic antioxidants in terms of toxicity issues [33]. Therefore, natural antioxidants from the tea plant are considered safe and non-toxic in their extract form.

Tea is consumed as a popular beverage all over the world and is considered to have health-promoting effects and a pleasant aroma. Commercial beverage-grade tea is primarily manufactured from the leaves of *Camellia sinensis* and is available in three forms, *i.e.*, green tea, black tea, and oolong tea [34]. Green tea is manufactured from the unfermented leaves of *Camellia sinensis*, it contains mainly polyphenols called catechins. The green tea catechins are mainly comprised of (-)-epicatechin, (-)-epicatechin-3-gallate, (-)-epigallocatechin, and (-)- epigallocatechin-3-gallate (EGCG). Black tea is manufactured through extensive enzymatic oxidation of polyphenols that give rise to theaflavins. The black tea contains the main theaflavin are TF-3-gallate, TF-3'-gallate, and TF--3'-digallate [35]. Various studies on the animal model system have shown that tea and its polyphenols have chemopreventive action in various organs and animals [36]. Other studies on black and green tea in the mammalian model have reported the significant role of polyphenols in inhibiting skin carcinogenesis [37, 38]. Several polyphenolic compounds obtained from the green tea leaves extract had significant antioxidant activity against lipid peroxidation [39] and against DNA damage [40 - 42], most of which are due to radiation exposures. Green tea extracts were also found to be effective against UVB-induced DNA damage [43]. Similarly, black tea extracts were also found protective against radioactive DNA damage in humans [44].

However, an inverse association between various cancers or chronic diseases and tea consumption was observed in certain epidemiological studies [45]. A prospective cohort study has shown a positive association between tea consumption and a lower risk of cancers in postmenopausal women [46]. Another prospective cohort study showed tea consumption was associated with a low risk of digestive system cancers in women [47]. A similar trend was reported in prostate cancer risk and green tea consumption in older men in Japan in another prospective study [48]. The protective effects result from the interaction of several activities *via* antioxidant, anti-inflammatory, antimutagenic, hepatoprotective, neuroprotective, and anticarcinogenic mechanisms (Fig. **1**).

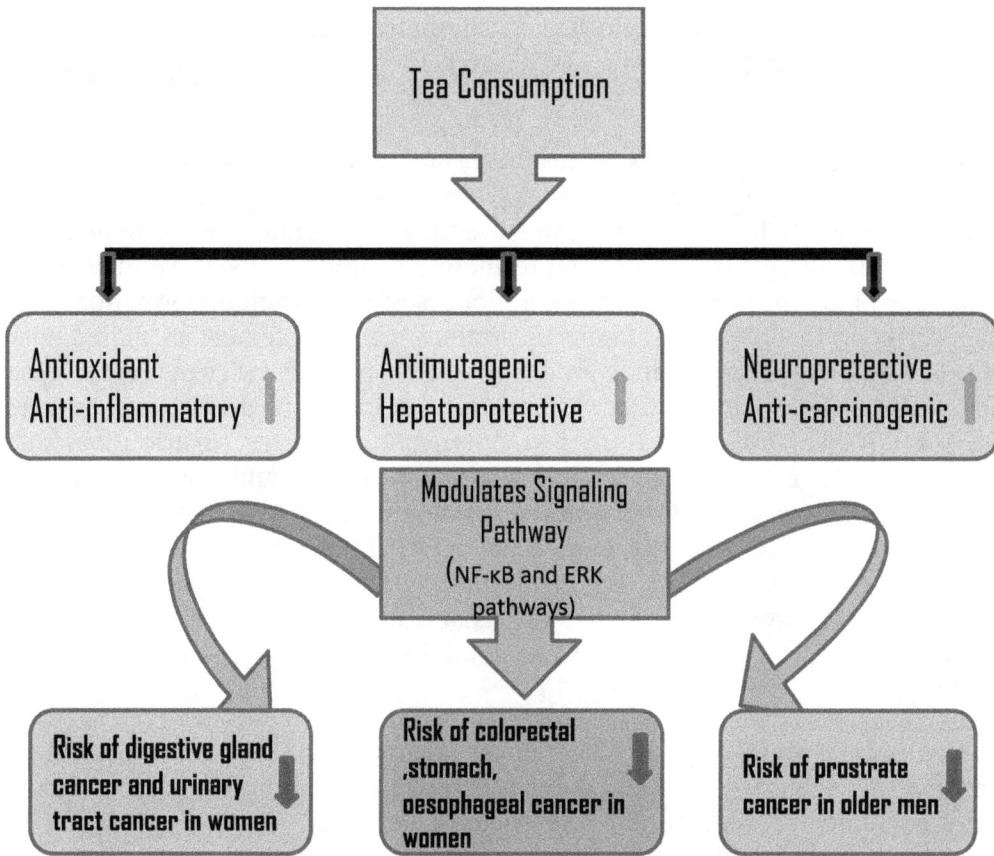

Fig. (1). Association of various cancers and chronic diseases with tea consumption.

Green tea is known to act through modulation of NF-kB and ERK signalling pathways, mitochondrial membrane potential, caspase-3 activity, proapoptotic proteins, and phase II detoxification system [49]. Although protective effects of other phytochemicals such as mate tea, *Allium sativum*, or honey, and vitamin c and E have been demonstrated against pesticide-induced DNA damage [50 - 53], however, despite its potential, very limited numbers of reports available on the protective role of tea polyphenols against pesticide-induced toxicity. Heikal et al. [54] described the protective role of synthetic antioxidants against organophosphate pesticide-induced DNA damage in rats.

Despite sizable evidence regarding the protective properties of tea polyphenols against oxidative damage, its therapeutic use has been fraught with challenges. Poor bioavailability is the main hindrance to oral formulations because several intrinsic and extrinsic factors, as well as chemical structure, molecular weight, solubility, metabolism, and eliminations from the system, are considered responsible [55, 56]. Thus, exploring an alternative delivery mechanism of tea polyphenols, especially for both EGCG and Theaflavin, is highly required to assign the therapeutic role.

The important aspects such as permeability and chemical stability need to be increased by means of many modifications to these active agents. The chemical additives mainly reducing agents can be added to maintain the structure and certain dissolving agents can be used to increase solubility [57]. Another is the use of phase I and/or phase II enzyme inhibitors to mask biotransformation [58]. Other strategies include adding lipids or proteins, *i.e.* complementary ingredients, and conjugation with promoiety groups [59, 60]. In recent development, nano vectors like cyclodextrins, matrix systems, solid dispersions, and liposomes were used for encapsulation to ensure fast polyphenol delivery, distribution, and bioactivity [61, 62]. However, these systems differ and depend on the encapsulated active ingredients' internal structure and physical state. In drug delivery systems, the effective use of nanoparticles needs at least 60 percent encapsulation efficiency [62]. For nano-particle-mediated polyphenol delivery studies, various biocompatible and biodegradable polymers were recruited such as cyclodextrins, nanospheres, nanocapsule, solid lipid nanoparticles, liposomes, and micelles [62].

In the intestinal tract, EGCG gets rapidly degraded *via* oxidative processes; therefore, to enhance its intake, stability, and bioavailability, incorporation in nano-sized delivery vectors is being tried successfully. The encapsulation of EGCG in poly (l-lactide)-poly (ethylene glycol) nanoparticles was done for assessment of its efficacy against human prostate cancer PC3 cells [63]. The encouraging results were obtained and showed that encapsulated EGCG retained biological effectiveness in the inhibition of PC3 proliferation with 10 fold dose advantage, was biocompatible and permitted the control of time and rate of polymer degradation. EGCG was incorporated in bovine serum albumin (BSA) nanoparticles in another study to study the effect on PC3 cell's lethality [64]. Synthesized PLGA based nanovectors were also used with 70% loading efficiency and increased antioxidant efficiency *in vivo*, oral administration was more effective than parenteral administration [65]. A strong (30 fold dose advantage) *in vivo* protective effect of PGLA based nanoparticles of tea polyphenols as compared to bulk EGCG or Theaflavin was observed [66]. The carbohydrate matrix (maltodextrin 60% and gum arabic 40%) was constituted for encapsulating EGCG with 85% of encapsulation efficiency, resulting in inhibition of the tumorigenesis process [67]. The nanolipidic EGCG particles improved the neuronal alpha-secretase enhancing ability (91%) *in vitro* and its oral bioavailability (more than 2 fold) *in vivo* [68]. The MBA-MD-231 cells showed that EGCG within the membrane helped protect antioxidant properties and prevent the production of hepatocyte growth factors. A gelatin nanoparticle loaded with EGCG showed a significant inhibitory effect on HGF-induced cell scattering [69].

EGCG was also encapsulated in chitosan nanoparticles to assess the ability to enhance EGCG stability and bioavailability. It was noted that it resulted in 2-fold enhancement in bioavailability and a 1.8-fold increase in absorption [70]. These nanoparticles also increased oral bioavailability 1.5 fold in mice [71]. A great property of chitosan nanoparticles noticed was an increase in retention time, ultrafine size with the potential to release bioactive molecules for a longer time, this property merits it as the ideal oral delivery vehicle [72]. It is also known for additional properties of low toxicity and biocompatibility [73]. A variety of factors affect the stability of chitosan nanoparticles therefore, it is necessary to take care of these factors like pH, and digestive enzymes (GI tract and mucus layer) thereby impacting the nanoparticle delivery system. Thus, studies must focus on the development of chitosan-based nanoparticles of tea polyphenols appropriately designed for oral administration and should have better GI stability, better mucus penetrating activity, and better intestinal epithelial cell targeting action.

National Scenario

Agriculture is the backbone of the Indian economy, has as much as 17% contribution in total GDP, and has a stronghold of about 70% for direct or indirect employment in rural India [74]. By overcoming the high dependency on monsoon and irrigation facilities and losses due to pests, weeds, and diseases. An extraordinary growth has been registered by Indian agriculture during the last few decades, with an increase in food grain production from 51 million tons in 1950-51to 250 million tons in 2011-12, the maximum since Indian independence. In this enhanced productivity, the usage of pesticides plays a vital role in countries like India. Presently, 234 pesticides are registered in India with yearly consumption of 57000 MT in 2016-17, covering approximately 17.25 million hectares of agricultural land useful for cultivation [75]. However, this paves the way for the rigorous use of pesticides reflected on severe hazards to the food chain and ecological environment and showed a significant increase of pesticide residue in food and body tissues [76]. It is implied that agricultural workers and farmers form the largest occupational group at the highest risk of undesirable health effects. Public health workers, manufacturing, and formulating industry workers are also at risk of exposure [77].

There are a handful of studies from different parts of India that looks into the effect of pesticides on DNA damage of agricultural workers, tea garden workers, and public health workers such as sprayers [77 - 82], which mostly detects a strong correlation of DNA damage and exposure to pesticides in the population group studied (Fig. **2**). The interaction between the pesticide and tea polyphenols has been depicted in Fig. (**3**).

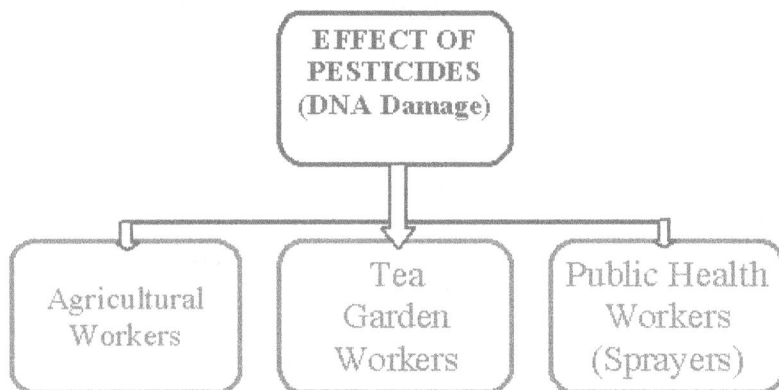

Fig. (2). Association between different pesticide exposed groups and DNA damage.

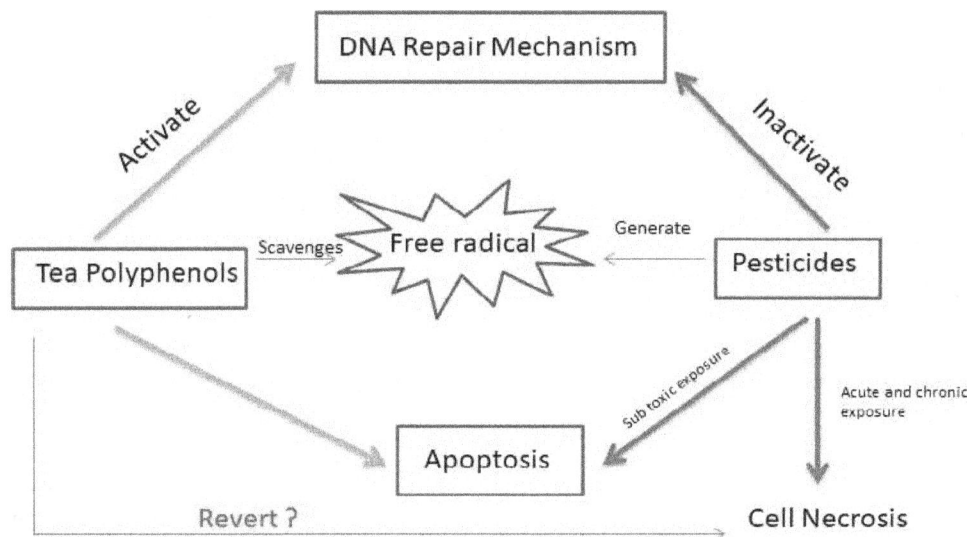

Fig. (3). Interaction between polyphenols and Pesticides.

Looking into the potential genetic hazard caused by pesticides in the human body, its preventive measures are very important in India. Presently, personal protective measures are the only way to reduce the effect of pesticide exposure. However, shortfalls such as inadequate clothing, leakage or defects in spray equipment, handling of pesticides without proper hand gloves, improper use of mask while spraying pesticides in the field, as well as environmental factors such as temperature, wind direction, *etc.* are also contributing factors for enhanced or uncontrolled toxicity due to pesticide exposure. Therefore, alternative preventive measures are urgently required to reduce the pesticide burden on human health in India.

Although tea is a very common beverage in India, and the Assam variety of tea was found to contain the highest level of catechin, its potential role in therapeutics remains unexplored. Tea polyphenols have already proved to be a potential therapeutic against many human diseases, including cancer, diabetes, and cardiovascular diseases [83 - 86]. The limited studies cover the protective effects of tea polyphenols or studies against pesticide-induced DNA damage in India. Similarly, there is a very limited study [66] from India on the nano-formulation of tea polyphenols to increase its bioavailability and its potential use as a therapeutic agent against pesticide-induced illness. Therefore, it is necessary as well as important to study in detail the effects of both natural and nano-formulated tea polyphenols such as EGCG and theaflavins on pesticide-induced DNA damage so that a cost-effective and sustainable preventive measure can be developed to protect the population group who often get exposed to pesticides in India.

Identified Research Gaps

From the review of the literature, the following research gaps have been identified:

- It has been found that there is very limited study on the use of tea polyphenols against pesticide-induced toxicity in India.
- Moreover, it has also been observed that scanty available information regarding the evaluation of effective doses of tea polyphenols that can be used as defensive agents for DNA damage caused by various classes of pesticides (like class Ia, Ib, or II) and chemical types (such as organophosphate, pyrethroid or carbamate, *etc.*) of pesticides.
- Finally, the considerable scope has been observed to increase the bioavailability of tea polyphenols to develop it as a potent functional food or therapeutic agent that can be used to safeguard human health from the undesirable effects of pesticide exposure.

In recent exploratory research, the polyphenols from black tea (theaflavin) have been evaluated for their anti-viral capacity against the hepatitis C virus (HCV). It was observed that all theaflavins (theaflavin (TF1)), theaflavin-3'-monogallate (TF2), and the theaflavin-3-3'-digallate (TF3) extracted from black tea possess inhibitory properties against infection [87]. The ability of black tea polyphenols like TF1, TF2, TF3, and procyanidin B2 has been recently evaluated *in silico* [88] against manifold targets of SARS-Cov2 (RdRp, 3CLpro, and PLpro) using molecular dynamic approaches and found very promising. Because of the limitations of *in vitro* cell models, that only they express part of the metabolic capabilities voiced in the tissues of their origin and exhibit variations in sensitivity to toxic compounds; therefore the cytotoxic and genotoxic actions demand a wide array of testing using various cell lines [89].

It has been observed from many preclinical studies that several polyphenols have displayed the ability to be considered an effective candidates, but the main hindrance remains the poor bioavailability of active ingredients, which costs unsuitability as a therapeutic agent. Nanotechnology-based oral formulations have shown the way forward to overcome this shortcoming by encapsulating suitable bioactive tea polyphenols for regulated release [90].

Since higher doses of polyphenols may exert cytotoxic and genotoxic effects [91], it is wise to conduct dose-response studies at a wide range of doses of polyphenols [14]. Although it has been observed from earlier studies that EGCG (10μmol/L) has shown *in vitro* toxicity in primary rat hepatocytes, however, such information for theaflavin is warranted. Similarly, the toxicity of a novel nanoparticulate system needs to be subjected for verification before use in *in vivo* system [73]. The clonogenic efficacy assay [92], methyl thiazolyl tetrazolium (MTT) assay [93] and γ-H2AX assay [94] can be used to determine the cytotoxicity of different doses of the purified polyphenols in the cell lines. Similarly, CBMN and comet assays must be carried out to determine the dose-sensitive genotoxicity effects of the purified polyphenols. Additionally, as mentioned, molecular assays about mRNA expression of DNA damage responsive genes along with DNA repair genes may be determined using qRT-PCR [66, 95].

The research should be intended to develop new or modified method/protocol for a nanotechnology-derived delivery system for tea polyphenols with high bioavailability, which can act more efficiently against pesticide-induced DNA damage in human populations.

CONCLUSION

Looking into the potential preventive effects of green tea polyphenols against pesticide-induced DNA damage, more research is needed to assess the dose-dependent effect of tea polyphenols, understand its pharmacodynamics and pharmacokinetics, and generate clinical evidence in the coming time. Also, biomarkers need to be identified for the beneficial effects of green tea polyphenols with potential use as biomonitoring tools for human populations. These biomarkers need to explain the sound understanding of interactions of polyphenols with internal and external factors The effective doses for human consumption of tea polyphenols need to be established for effective and sustainable use to manage pesticide-related morbidity and mortality.

CONSENT FOR PUBLICATION

All authors approved the final version and consented to publication.

CONFLICT OF INTEREST

The authors declare no conflict of interest, financial or otherwise.

AUTHOR CONTRIBUTION

DKS, MK, and RMS conceptualized, reviewed, and wrote the manuscript. SS, MS, and PC contributed to gathering literature and helped in writing the manuscript.

ACKNOWLEDGEMENTS

The authors made excellent efforts to integrate and cite all relevant recent literature, however, any unintended oversight is genuinely regretted.

REFERENCES

[1]   Alewu B, Nosiri C. Pesticides and human health. In: Stoytcheva M, Ed. Pesticides in the Modern World – Effects of Pesticides Exposure. InTech 2011; pp. 231-50.

[2]   Pirsaheb M, Limoee M, Namdari F, Khamutian R. Organochlorine pesticides residue in breast milk: a systematic review. Med J Islam Repub Iran 2015; 29: 228.
[PMID: 26478886]

[3]   Sanborn M, Kerr KJ, Sanin LH, Cole DC, Bassil KL, Vakil C. Non-cancer health effects of pesticides: systematic review and implications for family doctors. Can Fam Physician 2007; 53(10): 1712-20.
[PMID: 17934035]

[4]   Semchuk KM, Love EJ, Lee RG. Parkinson's disease and exposure to agricultural work and pesticide chemicals. Neurology 1992; 42(7): 1328-35.
[http://dx.doi.org/10.1212/WNL.42.7.1328] [PMID: 1620342]

[5]   Khot R, Joshi PP, Pandharipande M, Nagpure K, Thakur DS. Glyphosate poisoning with acute pulmonary edema. Toxicol Int 2014; 21(3): 328-30.
[http://dx.doi.org/10.4103/0971-6580.155389] [PMID: 25948977]

[6]   Gunnell D, Eddleston M, Phillips MR, Konradsen F. The global distribution of fatal pesticide self-poisoning: Systematic review. BMC Public Health 2007; 7(1): 357.
[http://dx.doi.org/10.1186/1471-2458-7-357] [PMID: 18154668]

[7]   World Health Organization. Public health impact of pesticides used in agriculture 1990.

[8]   Abdollahi M, Ranjbar A, Shadnia S, Nikfar S, Rezaie A. Pesticides and oxidative stress: a review. Med Sci Monit 2004; 10(6): RA141-7.

[PMID: 15173684]

[9]   Ranjbar A, Pasalar P, Abdollahi M. Induction of oxidative stress and acetylcholinesterase inhibition in organophosphorous pesticide manufacturing workers. Hum Exp Toxicol 2002; 21(4): 179-82.
[http://dx.doi.org/10.1191/0960327102ht238oa] [PMID: 12099619]

[10]   Lee CH, Kamijima M, Kim H, *et al.* 8-Hydroxydeoxyguanosine levels in human leukocyte and urine according to exposure to organophosphorus pesticides and paraoxonase 1 genotype. Int Arch Occup Environ Health 2007; 80(3): 217-27.
[http://dx.doi.org/10.1007/s00420-006-0128-1] [PMID: 16915393]

[11]   Kale M, Rathore N, John S, Bhatnagar D. Lipid peroxidative damage on pyrethroid exposure and alterations in antioxidant status in rat erythrocytes: a possible involvement of reactive oxygen species. Toxicol Lett 1999; 105(3): 197-205.
[http://dx.doi.org/10.1016/S0378-4274(98)00399-3] [PMID: 10355540]

[12]   Kaur R, Kaur K. Occupational pesticide exposure, impaired DNA repair, and diseases. Indian J Occup Environ Med 2018; 22(2): 74-81.
[http://dx.doi.org/10.4103/ijoem.IJOEM_45_18] [PMID: 30319227]

[13]   Møller P, Wallin H. Adduct formation, mutagenesis and nucleotide excision repair of DNA damage produced by reactive oxygen species and lipid peroxidation product. Mutat Res Rev Mutat Res 1998; 410(3): 271-90.
[http://dx.doi.org/10.1016/S1383-5742(97)00041-0] [PMID: 9630671]

[14]   Azqueta A, Collins A. Polyphenols and DNA Damage: A Mixed Blessing. Nutrients 2016; 8(12): 785.
[http://dx.doi.org/10.3390/nu8120785] [PMID: 27918471]

[15]   Zeljezic D, Garaj-Vrhovac V. Chromosomal aberration and single cell gel electrophoresis (Comet) assay in the longitudinal risk assessment of occupational exposure to pesticides. Mutagenesis 2001; 16(4): 359-63.
[http://dx.doi.org/10.1093/mutage/16.4.359] [PMID: 11420406]

[16]   Zeljezic D, Garaj-Vrhovac V. Sister chromatid exchange and proliferative rate index in the longitudinal risk assessment of occupational exposure to pesticides. Chemosphere 2002; 46(2): 295-303.
[http://dx.doi.org/10.1016/S0045-6535(01)00073-X] [PMID: 11827288]

[17]   Alves JS, Silva FRD, Silva GFD, *et al.* Investigation of potential biomarkers for the early diagnosis of cellular stability after the exposure of agricultural workers to pesticides. An Acad Bras Cienc 2016; 88(1): 349-60.
[http://dx.doi.org/10.1590/0001-3765201520150181] [PMID: 26839999]

[18]   Bolognesi C, Holland N. The use of the lymphocyte cytokinesis-block micronucleus assay for monitoring pesticide-exposed populations 2016.
[http://dx.doi.org/10.1016/j.mrrev.2016.04.006]

[19]   Varona-Uribe ME, Torres-Rey CH, Díaz-Criollo S, *et al.* Exposure to pesticide mixtures and DNA damage among rice field workers. Arch Environ Occup Health 2016; 71(1): 3-9.
[http://dx.doi.org/10.1080/19338244.2014.910489] [PMID: 24972111]

[20]   Zhang X, Wallace AD, Du P, *et al.* DNA methylation alterations in response to pesticide exposure *in vitro.* Environ Mol Mutagen 2012; 53(7): 542-9.
[http://dx.doi.org/10.1002/em.21718] [PMID: 22847954]

[21]   Das R, Thakur K, Shrivastava A, Puri A, Mutsuddi M. Identifying epigenetic endpoints of pesticide exposure can curtail risk to develop cancer: a review. Int J Adv Res (Indore) 2017; 5(1): 1093-107.
[http://dx.doi.org/10.21474/IJAR01/2857]

[22]   Benedetti D, Lopes Alderete B, de Souza CT, *et al.* DNA damage and epigenetic alteration in soybean farmers exposed to complex mixture of pesticides. Mutagenesis 2018; 33(1): 87-95.
[http://dx.doi.org/10.1093/mutage/gex035] [PMID: 29244183]

[23]   Bücker A, Carvalho W, Alves-Gomes JA. Avaliation of mutagenicity and gentotoxicity in Eigenmanniavirescens (Teleostei: Gymnotiformes) exposed to benzene. Acta Amazon 2006; 36(3): 357-64.

[24]   Udroiu I. The micronucleus test in piscine erythrocytes. Aquat Toxicol 2006; 79(2): 201-4.
[http://dx.doi.org/10.1016/j.aquatox.2006.06.013] [PMID: 16846653]

[25]   Fenech M. The *in vitro* micronucleus technique. Mutat Res 2000; 455(1-2): 81-95.
[http://dx.doi.org/10.1016/S0027-5107(00)00065-8] [PMID: 11113469]

[26]   Lindahl T, Andersson A. Rate of chain breakage at apurinic sites in double-stranded deoxyribonucleic acid. Biochemistry 1972; 11(19): 3618-23.
[http://dx.doi.org/10.1021/bi00769a019] [PMID: 4559796]

[27]   Azqueta A, Slyskova J, Langie SA, O'Neill Gaivão I, Collins A. Comet assay to measure DNA repair: approach and applications. Front Genet 2014; 5: 288.
[http://dx.doi.org/10.3389/fgene.2014.00288] [PMID: 25202323]

[28]   Anderson D, Dhawan A, Laubenthal J. The comet assay in human biomonitoring. Methods Mol Biol 2013; 1044: 347-62.
[http://dx.doi.org/10.1007/978-1-62703-529-3_18] [PMID: 23896886]

[29]   Rojas E, Lopez MC, Valverde M. Single cell gel electrophoresis assay: methodology and applications. J Chromatogr, Biomed Appl 1999; 722(1-2): 225-54.
[http://dx.doi.org/10.1016/S0378-4347(98)00313-2] [PMID: 10068143]

[30]   Collins AR. The comet assay for DNA damage and repair: principles, applications, and limitations. Mol Biotechnol 2004; 26(3): 249-61.
[http://dx.doi.org/10.1385/MB:26:3:249] [PMID: 15004294]

[31]   Collins AR. Measuring oxidative damage to DNA and its repair with the comet assay. Biochim Biophys Acta, Gen Subj 2014; 1840(2): 794-800.
[http://dx.doi.org/10.1016/j.bbagen.2013.04.022] [PMID: 23618695]

[32]   Scalbert A, Johnson IT, Saltmarsh M. Polyphenols: antioxidants and beyond. Am J Clin Nutr 2005; 81(1) (Suppl.): 215S-7S.
[http://dx.doi.org/10.1093/ajcn/81.1.215S] [PMID: 15640483]

[33]   Frei B. Reactive oxygen species and antioxidant vitamins: Mechanisms of action. Am J Med 1994; 97(3): S5-S13.
[http://dx.doi.org/10.1016/0002-9343(94)90292-5] [PMID: 8085584]

[34]   Weisburger JH. Tea and health: a historical perspective. Cancer Lett 1997; 114(1-2): 315-7.
[http://dx.doi.org/10.1016/S0304-3835(97)04691-0] [PMID: 9103320]

[35]   McKay DL, Blumberg JB. The role of tea in human health: an update. J Am Coll Nutr 2002; 21(1): 1-13.
[http://dx.doi.org/10.1080/07315724.2002.10719187] [PMID: 11838881]

[36]   Leone M, Zhai D, Sareth S, Kitada S, Reed JC, Pellecchia M. Cancer prevention by tea polyphenols is linked to their direct inhibition of antiapoptotic Bcl-2-family proteins. Cancer Res 2003; 63(23): 8118-21.
[PMID: 14678963]

[37]   Yang CS, Maliakal P, Meng X. Inhibition of carcinogenesis by tea. Annu Rev Pharmacol Toxicol 2002; 42(1): 25-54.
[http://dx.doi.org/10.1146/annurev.pharmtox.42.082101.154309] [PMID: 11807163]

[38]   Choudhury SR, Balasubramanian S, Chew YC, Han B, Marquez VE, Eckert RL. (-)-Epigallocatech-n-3-gallate and DZNep reduce polycomb protein level *via* a proteasome-dependent mechanism in skin cancer cells. Carcinogenesis 2011; 32(10): 1525-32.
[http://dx.doi.org/10.1093/carcin/bgr171] [PMID: 21798853]

[39]   Kondo K, Kurihara M, Miyata N, Suzuki T, Toyoda M. Mechanistic studies of catechins as antioxidants against radical oxidation. Arch Biochem Biophys 1999; 362(1): 79-86.
[http://dx.doi.org/10.1006/abbi.1998.1015] [PMID: 9917331]

[40]   Anderson RF, Fisher LJ, Hara Y, *et al.* Green tea catechins partially protect DNA from middle dotOH radical-induced strand breaks and base damage through fast chemical repair of DNA radicals. Carcinogenesis 2001; 22(8): 1189-93.
[http://dx.doi.org/10.1093/carcin/22.8.1189] [PMID: 11470748]

[41]   Hakim IA, Chow HHS, Harris RB. Green tea consumption is associated with decreased DNA damage among GSTM1-positive smokers regardless of their hOGG1 genotype. J Nutr 2008; 138(8): 1567S-71S.
[http://dx.doi.org/10.1093/jn/138.8.1567S] [PMID: 18641208]

[42]   Ho CK, Choi S, Siu PM, Benzie IFF. Effects of single dose and regular intake of green tea (*Camellia sinensis*) on DNA damage, DNA repair, and heme oxygenase-1 expression in a randomized controlled human supplementation study. Mol Nutr Food Res 2014; 58(6): 1379-83.
[http://dx.doi.org/10.1002/mnfr.201300751] [PMID: 24585444]

[43]   Schwarz A, Maeda A, Gan D, Mammone T, Matsui MS, Schwarz T. Green tea phenol extracts reduce UVB-induced DNA damage in human cells *via* interleukin-12. Photochem Photobiol 2008; 84(2): 350-5.
[http://dx.doi.org/10.1111/j.1751-1097.2007.00265.x] [PMID: 18179621]

[44]   Ježovičová M, Koňariková K, Ďuračková Z, Keresteš J, Králik G, Žitňanová I. Protective effects of black tea extract against oxidative DNA damage in human lymphocytes. Mol Med Rep 2016; 13(2): 1839-44.
[http://dx.doi.org/10.3892/mmr.2015.4747] [PMID: 26718244]

[45]   Tang J, Zheng JS, Fang L, Jin Y, Cai W, Li D. Tea consumption and mortality of all cancers, CVD and all causes: a meta-analysis of eighteen prospective cohort studies. Br J Nutr 2015; 114(5): 673-83.
[http://dx.doi.org/10.1017/S0007114515002329] [PMID: 26202661]

[46]   Zheng W, Doyle TJ, Kushi LH, Sellers TA, Hong CP, Folsom AR. Tea consumption and cancer incidence in a prospective cohort study of postmenopausal women. Am J Epidemiol 1996; 144(2): 175-82.
[http://dx.doi.org/10.1093/oxfordjournals.aje.a008905] [PMID: 8678049]

[47]   Nechuta S, Shu XO, Li HL, *et al.* Prospective cohort study of tea consumption and risk of digestive system cancers: results from the Shanghai Women's Health Study. Am J Clin Nutr 2012; 96(5): 1056-63.
[http://dx.doi.org/10.3945/ajcn.111.031419] [PMID: 23053557]

[48]   Kurahashi N, Sasazuki S, Iwasaki M, Inoue M, Tsugane S. Green tea consumption and prostate cancer risk in Japanese men: a prospective study. Am J Epidemiol 2007; 167(1): 71-7.
[http://dx.doi.org/10.1093/aje/kwm249] [PMID: 17906295]

[49]   Chen L, Mo H, Zhao L, *et al.* Therapeutic properties of green tea against environmental insults. J Nutr Biochem 2017; 40: 1-13.
[http://dx.doi.org/10.1016/j.jnutbio.2016.05.005] [PMID: 27723473]

[50]   Miranda DDC, Arçari DP, Pedrazzoli J Jr, *et al.* Protective effects of mate tea (Ilex paraguariensis) on H2O2-induced DNA damage and DNA repair in mice. Mutagenesis 2008; 23(4): 261-5.
[http://dx.doi.org/10.1093/mutage/gen011] [PMID: 18308716]

[51]   Ahmad W, Shaikh S, Nazam N, Lone MI. Protective Effects of Quercetin against Dimethoate-Induced Cytotoxicity and Genotoxicity in *Allium sativum* Test. Int Sch Res Notices 2014; 2014: 1-6.
[http://dx.doi.org/10.1155/2014/632672] [PMID: 27379342]

[52]   Zalata A, Elhanbly S, Abdalla H, *et al.* *In vitro* study of cypermethrin on human spermatozoa and the possible protective role of vitamins C and E. Andrologia 2014; 46(10): 1141-7.

[http://dx.doi.org/10.1111/and.12206] [PMID: 24329529]

[53]   Alleva R, Manzella N, Gaetani S, *et al.* Organic honey supplementation reverses pesticide-induced genotoxicity by modulating DNA damage response. Mol Nutr Food Res 2016; 60(10): 2243-55.
[http://dx.doi.org/10.1002/mnfr.201600005] [PMID: 27129605]

[54]   Heikal TM, Mossa ATH, Nawwar GA. El-SherbinyM, Ghanem HZ. Protective effect of a synthetic antioxidant "Acetyl Gallate Derivative" against dimethoate induced DNA damage and oxidant/antioxidant status in male rats. J Environ Anal Toxicol 2012; 2(155): 2161-0525.

[55]   Scalbert A, Williamson G. Dietary intake and bioavailability of polyphenols. J Nutr 2000; 130(8S Suppl): 2073S-85S.

[56]   D'Archivio M, Filesi C, Varì R, Scazzocchio B, Masella R. Bioavailability of the polyphenols: status and controversies. Int J Mol Sci 2010; 11(4): 1321-42.
[http://dx.doi.org/10.3390/ijms11041321] [PMID: 20480022]

[57]   Ader P, Wessmann A, Wolffram S. Bioavailability and metabolism of the flavonol quercetin in the pig. Free Radic Biol Med 2000; 28(7): 1056-67.
[http://dx.doi.org/10.1016/S0891-5849(00)00195-7] [PMID: 10832067]

[58]   Brand W, Padilla B, van Bladeren PJ, Williamson G, Rietjens IMCM. The effect of co-administered flavonoids on the metabolism of hesperetin and the disposition of its metabolites in Caco-2 cell monolayers. Mol Nutr Food Res 2010; 54(6): 851-60.
[http://dx.doi.org/10.1002/mnfr.200900183] [PMID: 20112299]

[59]   Lesser S, Cermak R, Wolffram S. Bioavailability of quercetin in pigs is influenced by the dietary fat content. J Nutr 2004; 134(6): 1508-11.
[http://dx.doi.org/10.1093/jn/134.6.1508] [PMID: 15173420]

[60]   Lam WH, Kazi A, Kuhn DJ, *et al.* A potential prodrug for a green tea polyphenol proteasome inhibitor: evaluation of the peracetate ester of (−)-epigallocatechin gallate [(−)-EGCG]. Bioorg Med Chem 2004; 12(21): 5587-93.
[http://dx.doi.org/10.1016/j.bmc.2004.08.002] [PMID: 15465336]

[61]   Musthaba SM, Baboota S, Ahmed S, Ahuja A, Ali J. Status of novel drug delivery technology for phytotherapeutics. Expert Opin Drug Deliv 2009; 6(6): 625-37.
[http://dx.doi.org/10.1517/17425240902980154] [PMID: 19505192]

[62]   Conte R, Calarco A, Napoletano A, Valentino A, Margarucci S, *et al.* Polyphenols Nanoencapsulation for Therapeutic Applications. J Biomol Res Ther 2016; 5: 139.

[63]   Siddiqui IA, Adhami VM, Bharali DJ, *et al.* Introducing nanochemoprevention as a novel approach for cancer control: proof of principle with green tea polyphenol epigallocatechin-3-gallate. Cancer Res 2009; 69(5): 1712-6.
[http://dx.doi.org/10.1158/0008-5472.CAN-08-3978] [PMID: 19223530]

[64]   Zu YG, Yuan S, Zhao XH, Zhang Y, Zhang XN, Jiang R. Preparation, activity and targeting ability evaluation *in vitro* on folate mediated epigallocatechin-3-gallate albumin nanoparticles. Yao Xue Xue Bao 2009; 44(5): 525-31.
[PMID: 19618731]

[65]   Italia JL, Datta P, Ankola DD, Kumar MNVR. Nanoparticles enhance per oral bioavailability of poorly available molecules: epigallocatechin gallate nanoparticles ameliorates cyclosporine induced nephrotoxicity in rats at three times lower dose than oral solution. J Biomed Nanotechnol 2008; 4(3): 304-12.
[http://dx.doi.org/10.1166/jbn.2008.341]

[66]   Srivastava AK, Bhatnagar P, Singh M, *et al.* Synthesis of PLGA nanoparticles of tea polyphenols and their strong *in vivo* protective effect against chemically induced DNA damage. Int J Nanomedicine 2013; 8: 1451-62.
[PMID: 23717041]

[67]   Rocha S, Generalov R, Pereira MC, Peres I, Juzenas P, Coelho MAN. Epigallocatechin gallate-loaded polysaccharide nanoparticles for prostate cancer chemoprevention. Nanomedicine (Lond) 2011; 6(1): 79-87.
        [http://dx.doi.org/10.2217/nnm.10.101] [PMID: 21182420]

[68]   Smith A, Giunta B, Bickford PC, Fountain M, Tan J, Shytle RD. Nanolipidic particles improve the bioavailability and α-secretase inducing ability of epigallocatechin-3-gallate (EGCG) for the treatment of Alzheimer's disease. Int J Pharm 2010; 389(1-2): 207-12.
        [http://dx.doi.org/10.1016/j.ijpharm.2010.01.012] [PMID: 20083179]

[69]   Shutava TG, Balkundi SS, Vangala P, *et al.* Layer-by-layer-coated gelatin nanoparticles as a vehicle for delivery of natural polyphenols. ACS Nano 2009; 3(7): 1877-85.
        [http://dx.doi.org/10.1021/nn900451a] [PMID: 19534472]

[70]   Dube A, Ng K, Nicolazzo JA, Larson I. Effective use of reducing agents and nanoparticle encapsulation in stabilizing catechins in alkaline solution. Food Chem 2010; 122(3): 662-7.
        [http://dx.doi.org/10.1016/j.foodchem.2010.03.027]

[71]   Dube A, Nicolazzo JA, Larson I. Chitosan nanoparticles enhance the intestinal absorption of the green tea catechins (+)-catechin and (−)-epigallocatechin gallate. Eur J Pharm Sci 2010; 41(2): 219-25.
        [http://dx.doi.org/10.1016/j.ejps.2010.06.010] [PMID: 20600878]

[72]   Siddiqui IA, Bharali DJ, Nihal M, *et al.* Excellent anti-proliferative and pro-apoptotic effects of (−)-epigallocatechin-3-gallate encapsulated in chitosan nanoparticles on human melanoma cell growth both *in vitro* and *in vivo*. Nanomedicine 2014; 10(8): 1619-26.
        [http://dx.doi.org/10.1016/j.nano.2014.05.007] [PMID: 24965756]

[73]   Liang J, Yan H, Puligundla P, Gao X, Zhou Y, Wan X. Applications of chitosan nanoparticles to enhance absorption and bioavailability of tea polyphenols: A review. Food Hydrocoll 2017; 69: 286-92.
        [http://dx.doi.org/10.1016/j.foodhyd.2017.01.041]

[74]   Arjun KM. Indian agriculture-status, importance and role in Indian Economy. Int J Agric Food Sci Technology 2013; 4(4): 343-6.

[75]   Devi PI, Thomas J, Raju RK. Pesticide consumption in India: A spatiotemporal analysis. Agric Econ Res Rev 2017; 30(1): 163-72.
        [http://dx.doi.org/10.5958/0974-0279.2017.00015.5]

[76]   Kori RK, Jain AK, Yadav RS. Biomarkers: an essential gizmo in pesticide toxicity. Biom J 2016; 2: 1-5.

[77]   Yadav RS, Kori RK, Thakur RS, Kumar R. Assessment of Adverse Health Effects Among Chronic Pesticide-Exposed Farm Workers in Sagar District of Madhya Pradesh, India. Int J Nutr Pharmacol Neurol Dis 2018; 8(4): 153-61.
        [http://dx.doi.org/10.4103/ijnpnd.ijnpnd_48_18]

[78]   Yadav AS, Sehrawat G. Evaluation of genetic damage in farmers exposed to pesticide mixtures. Int J Hum Genet 2011; 11(2): 105-9.
        [http://dx.doi.org/10.1080/09723757.2011.11886131]

[79]   Kaur R, Lata M, Kaur S. Evaluation of DNA damage in agricultural workers exposed to pesticides using single cell gel electrophoresis (comet) assay. Indian J Hum Genet 2011; 17(3): 179-87.
        [http://dx.doi.org/10.4103/0971-6866.92100] [PMID: 22345990]

[80]   Hazarika R, Deka P. Assessment of DNA damage in agricultural workers exposed to mixture of pesticides in Assam (India). Nature Environment and Pollution Technology 2017; 16(4): 1081-6.

[81]   Dhananjayan V, Ravichandran B, Panjakumar K, *et al.* Assessment of genotoxicity and cholinesterase activity among women workers occupationally exposed to pesticides in tea garden. Mutat Res Genet Toxicol Environ Mutagen 2019; 841: 1-7.
        [http://dx.doi.org/10.1016/j.mrgentox.2019.03.002] [PMID: 31138404]

[82] Dutta S, Bahadur M. Comet assay genotoxicity evaluation of occupationally exposed tea-garden workers in northern West Bengal, India. Mutat Res Genet Toxicol Environ Mutagen 2019; 844: 1-9.
[http://dx.doi.org/10.1016/j.mrgentox.2019.06.005] [PMID: 31326030]

[83] Prasad S, Kaur J, Roy P, Kalra N, Shukla Y. RETRACTED: Theaflavins induce G2/M arrest by modulating expression of p21waf1/cip1, cdc25C and cyclin B in human prostate carcinoma PC-3 cells. Life Sci 2007; 81(17-18): 1323-31.
[http://dx.doi.org/10.1016/j.lfs.2007.07.033] [PMID: 17936851]

[84] Gupta J, Siddique YH, Beg T, Ara G, Afzal M. A review on the beneficial effects of tea polyphenols on human health. Int J Pharmacol 2008; 4(5): 314-38.
[http://dx.doi.org/10.3923/ijp.2008.314.338]

[85] Patel R, Krishnan R, Ramchandani A, Maru G. Polymeric black tea polyphenols inhibit mouse skin chemical carcinogenesis by decreasing cell proliferation. Cell Prolif 2008; 41(3): 532-53.
[http://dx.doi.org/10.1111/j.1365-2184.2008.00528.x] [PMID: 18400024]

[86] Roy P, George J, Srivastava S, Tyagi S, Shukla Y. Inhibitory effects of tea polyphenols by targeting cyclooxygenase-2 through regulation of nuclear factor kappa B, Akt and p53 in rat mammary tumors. Invest New Drugs 2011; 29(2): 225-31.
[http://dx.doi.org/10.1007/s10637-009-9349-y] [PMID: 19936622]

[87] Chowdhury P, Sahuc ME, Rouillé Y, et al. Theaflavins, polyphenols of black tea, inhibit entry of hepatitis C virus in cell culture. PLoS One 2018; 28;13(11): e0198226.

[88] Gogoi M, Borkotoky M, Borchetia S, Chowdhury P, Mahanta S, Barooah AK. Black tea bioactives as inhibitors of multiple targets of SARS-CoV-2 (3CLpro, PLpro and RdRp): a virtual screening and molecular dynamic simulation study. J Biomol Struct Dyn 2021; 1-24.
[http://dx.doi.org/10.1080/07391102.2021.1897679] [PMID: 33715595]

[89] Huang R, Southall N, Cho MH, Xia M, Inglese J, Austin CP. Characterization of diversity in toxicity mechanism using in vitro cytotoxicity assays in quantitative high throughput screening. Chem Res Toxicol 2008; 21(3): 659-67.
[http://dx.doi.org/10.1021/tx700365e] [PMID: 18281954]

[90] Khan N, Bharali DJ, Adhami VM, et al. Oral administration of naturally occurring chitosan-based nanoformulated green tea polyphenol EGCG effectively inhibits prostate cancer cell growth in a xenograft model. Carcinogenesis 2014; 35(2): 415-23.
[http://dx.doi.org/10.1093/carcin/bgt321] [PMID: 24072771]

[91] Mennen LI, Walker R, Bennetau-Pelissero C, Scalbert A. Risks and safety of polyphenol consumption. Am J Clin Nutr 2005; 81(1) (Suppl.): 326S-9S.
[http://dx.doi.org/10.1093/ajcn/81.1.326S] [PMID: 15640498]

[92] Franken NAP, Rodermond HM, Stap J, Haveman J, van Bree C. Clonogenic assay of cells in vitro. Nat Protoc 2006; 1(5): 2315-9.
[http://dx.doi.org/10.1038/nprot.2006.339] [PMID: 17406473]

[93] Takenouchi T, Munekata E. Amyloid beta-peptide-induced inhibition of MTT reduction in PC12h and C1300 neuroblastoma cells: effect of nitroprusside. Peptides 1998; 19(2): 365-72.
[http://dx.doi.org/10.1016/S0196-9781(97)00377-X] [PMID: 9493870]

[94] Graillot V, Takakura N, Hegarat LL, Fessard V, Audebert M, Cravedi JP. Genotoxicity of pesticide mixtures present in the diet of the French population. Environ Mol Mutagen 2012; 53(3): 173-84.
[http://dx.doi.org/10.1002/em.21676] [PMID: 22389207]

[95] Hreljac I, Zajc I, Lah T, Filipič M. Effects of model organophosphorous pesticides on DNA damage and proliferation of HepG2 cells. Environ Mol Mutagen 2008; 49(5): 360-7.
[http://dx.doi.org/10.1002/em.20392] [PMID: 18418871]

CHAPTER 11

Therapeutically Important Bioactive Compounds Derived from Fungal Origin

Neha Jain[1], Mukesh Kumar Sharma[2,*] and Pallavi Kaushik[1]

[1] *Department of Zoology, University of Rajasthan, Jaipur-302004, India*

[2] *Department of Zoology, SPC Government College, Ajmer-305001, India*

Abstract: The rising of chronic ailments impinged on humans worldwide has paved the urgent need for newer therapeutic vital compounds that are biologically active and have the capacity to endeavour without exerting any adverse or cytotoxic effects. This necessitates extensive research to investigate unexplored natural sources for such promising sources. A diverse array of fungi species has garnered considerable attention over the past century due to the assortment of their opportunities to generate novel active ingredients with multifunction mechanisms towards recuperative applications. Some of the fungal bioactive compounds possess exclusive therapeutic potential and pharmaceutical importance. These efficacious bioactive compounds including Paclitaxel, Podophyllotoxin, Enniatins, Camptothecin, Ascophytatin with their properties like anti-bacterial, antiviral, anti-parasitic, anti-diabetic, anti-cancerous, immunomodulatory are discussed in this chapter.

Keywords: Endophytes, Topoisomerase, Karyokinetics, Anti malignant, Paclitaxel , Podophyllotoxin, Enniatins, Camptothecin, Ascophytatin.

INTRODUCTION

From the dawn of time, nature has played a significant role in pharmaceutical research for humankind by offering therapeutic medications. The exploration of natural products has a lot of untapped potential, and several pieces of research have emphasized the considerable benefits of the same in the development process. The use of natural compounds is also considered a revolutionary development in the study and application of chemical complexes from biological origins with new curative capacities to achieve complex objectives of disease control [1, 2].

* **Corresponding author Mukesh Kumar Sharma:** Department of Zoology, SPC Government College, Ajmer-305001; Rajasthan, India; Tel: +91-98291 99444; E-mail: mkshrma@hotmail.com

Additionally, there has been a substantial shift in the current scenario to a more sustainable, environmental, and green lifestyle due to the emergence of contemporary diseases as well as the encroachment of drug-resistant pathogens escalating tremendously and rendering the existing antimicrobial medicines ineffectual [3, 4].

However, an extensive investigation for better and more effective agents to cope with these health issues is indeed ongoing and microorganisms offer a unique source of impending compliant chemicals. These are endowed with an excellent opportunity to get a constant supply of biologically active metabolites in order to serve the needs of development with safety research and/or industrial output [5, 6].

The research on bioactive compounds of fungal origin has found importance since the discovery of penicillin in the 1930s. Fungi have become a dominant contributor to pharmaceutical drugs that helps in generating life-saving medications such as antibiotics, antiparasitic, antibacterial, antifungal, antioxidant, immunosuppressant, antiviral, anti-inflammatory, anticancer, and cholesterol-lowering compounds. This has raised scientists' awareness of bioactive compounds produced by fungus in the rhizosphere or floral endosphere that might be utilized for a spectrum of activities versus human infections [4, 7 - 9].

Moreover, fungi are one of the greatest resources among living organisms from land and marine sources that have been exploited by humans since prehistoric times as these tend to play a critical role in economic and environmental balances. These have a unique metabolism that encourages and promotes a plethora of functional metabolites with a variety of chemical configurations of diverse classes allied with phenylpropanoids, terpenes, polyketides, alkaloids, *etc* [10].

Furthermore, medicinal herbs are the abode of a wide range of microbial domains. Their reliance on the biosynthesis of bioactive metabolites as a remedy to combat the rise of new drug-resistant infections has heightened the search for a non-chemosynthetic substitute to treat human illnesses. According to studies, just 7% of the 1.5 million fungal species have been discovered; despite new results utilizing next-generation sequencing reveal that there are between 3.5 and 5.1 million fungal species on the planet. As a result, fungal endophytes have taken over the environment and might be a viable source of many bioactive compounds [8].

As per studies, about 18 percent of plant-derived molecules can also be generated by their related fungus. Taxol, for example, is a bioactive chemical produced from the medicinal plant Taxus and the endophytic fungus *Taxomyces andreanae*. As a result, the Taxol from *T. andreanae* has a distinct advantage over its host plant in terms of fermentation and biosynthesis [8].

The present chapter deals with major bioactive compounds derived from various endophytic or non-endophytic fungal strains with established therapeutic potential. These varieties can be used for the mass production of bioactives for pharmacological uses.

Important Fungal Bioactive Constituents with their Therapeutic Uses

Podophyllotoxin [C22H22O8]

A non alkaloid, lignan metabolite (Fig. **6**) with chemopreventive capacity, extracted from endophytes *Aspergillus fumigatus, Fusarium oxysporum, Trametes hirsute, Phialocephala fortinii* as well as some genera belonging to *Trichoderma, Phomopsis Penicillium* [1], and *Alternaria sp* [11]. The chemical tends to adhere to tubulin and limits its action in a reversible manner, causing the karyokinetic spindle structure to be disrupted. Moreover, Podophyllotoxin promotes cell cycle arrest in the G2 phase by eliciting single and double stranded DNA breaks due to their interactions with DNA topoisomerase II [12]. Major derivatives of Podophyllotoxin are Teniposide and Etoposide, which bear diverse therapeutic properties like antiviral, anti-helminthic, antibacterial and chiefly antitumor as mentioned in Fig. (**1**). Additionally, these have been exploited as purgative and cathartic agents in the world of medical science [1, 3, 4, 8, 11, 13].

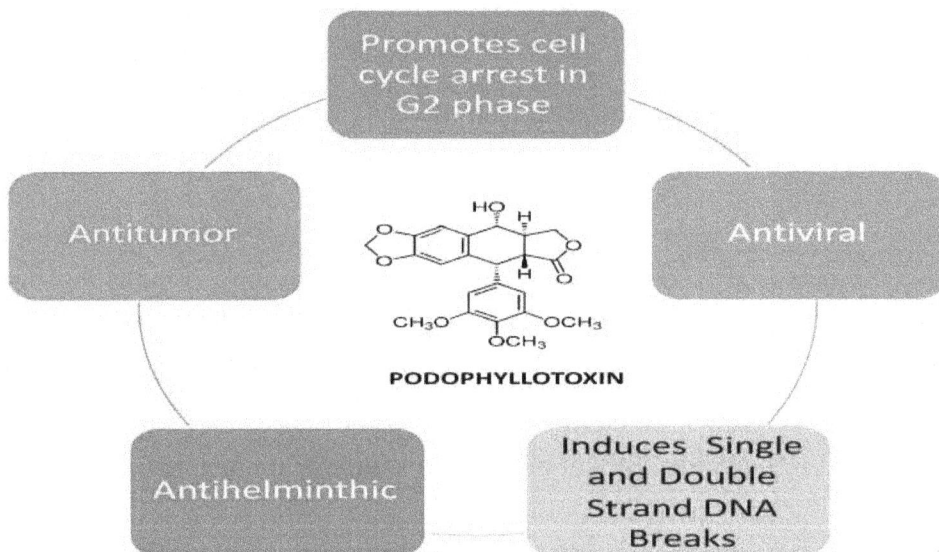

Fig. (1). Major therapeutic properties of Podophyllotoxin.

Paclitaxel [TAXOL]

Paclitaxel, a tetra cyclic, diterpenoid bioactive compound, is traded under the name, Taxol (Fig. **6**). It has anticancer [1, 4, 8] and antiviral (anti HIV) [1] properties and is derived from various endophytic fungi such as *Taxomyces andreanae, Grammothele lineate, Metarhizium, Ozonium, Pestalotiopsis guepini, Aspergillus aculeatinus* and *Periconia* sps., *Fusarium solani, Fusarium oxysporum, Alternaria brassicicola, Pestalotia, Monochaetia, Botryodiplodia, Tubercularia, Botrytis, Colletotrichum, Taxomyces, Cladosporium, Mucor, Ectostroma, Phyllosticta, Papulaspora, Acremonium, Pithomyces sp* [1, 3, 4, 10, 11]. The metabolite has been approved by FDA to treat advanced breast, refractory ovarian [4, 11], lung cancer [4], and Kaposi's sarcoma [11]. Molecularly, the taxol's gene influences non-mevalonate (MEP) and mevalonate (MVA) pathways to get itself articulated [4]. It exhibits the antineoplastic capacity by inhibiting microtubule depolymerization thereby, interfering in the segregation of chromosomes and assemblage of mitotic spindles eventually leading to mitotic arrest and cell death [11]. Additionally, its efficacy has also been investigated in preventing viral replication by restraining HIV-1 integrase and viral protease displaying valuable antiviral properties as specified in Fig. (**2**) [1].

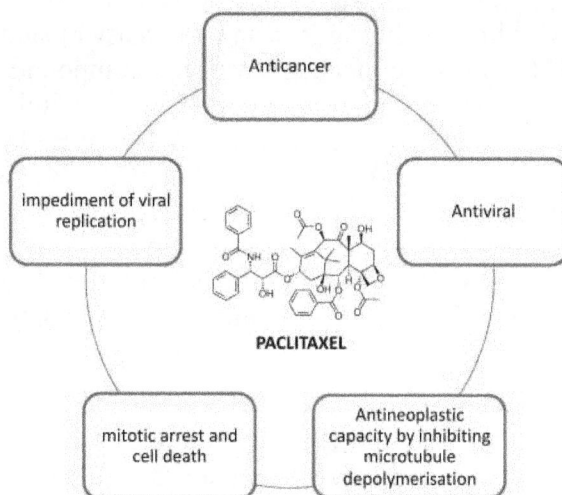

Fig. (2). Major therapeutic properties of Paclitaxel.

Enniatins

A cyclohexapeptide compound (Fig. **6**) extracted from mangrove fungus *Fusarium* sp. (*F. proliferatum, F. subglutinans, F. avenaceum, F. tricinctum, F. poae, F. oxysporum, F. sambucinum, F. sporotrichioides, and F. acuminatum*), *Halosarpheia, Verticillium, Alternaria* [3, 14, 15] has been investigated for their beneficial features including insecticidal, anti-fungal, anti-cancer, anti-parasitic, anti-viral and anti-microbial activities [16 - 23]. Anti-bacterial competence has been successfully reported against *B. subtilis, C. perfringen, E. faecalis, S. aureus, A. baumannii, E. coli, H. pylori,* and *P. aeruginosa* whereas and anti-mycobacterium consequence against *M. smegmatis*. The compound's antifungal attribute has been explored in *A. flavus, A. niger, A. ochraceus, C. albicans, F. graminearum, F. oxysporum, F. verticillioides, P. verrucosum,* and *S. chartarum.* The major mode of action represents interaction, depolarization, and permeabilization of the membrane of bacteria as well as getting itself inserted in the lipid portion of the same, leading to the integrity reduction of the membrane [15]. An alternate prospective pathway against microbes of the remedial compound is associated with its ionophoric properties [3, 15].

Moreover, the metabolite has also been recognized for its anti-malignant activity in tumour cells [3] comprising Caco-2 (human intestine), BEAS-2B (human normal lung epithelial cells), HEPG2 (human liver cells), HEK (human normal keratinocytes), N87 (human gastric cells) and HUVEC (human normal vascular endothelial cells) cell lines enduring it as an exemplary bioactive compound in the restorative use [15]. Cytotoxic mechanism of the compound includes membrane insertion by forging cation-selective pores to persuade cellular ionic homeostasis, triggering calcium rise and cytochrome C release that precedes elevated caspase-3 activity ensuing in apoptosis as shown in Fig. (**3**) [24]. There are about 29 enniatins identified and classified so far, either as a single metabolite or as mixes of separate homologs. Furthermore, Fusafungine, a drug synthesized from a combination of enniatins, is now productively exploited as a topical therapy for upper respiratory tract infections *via* oral and/or nasal inhalation [14].

Camptothecin

A pentacyclic, quinoline alkaloid (Fig. **6**) is known for its potential as an anti-tumour agent. The compound and its derivatives are isolated from endophytic fungus *Entrophospora infrequens* [10], *Neurospora sp., Fusarium solani,* and fungal strain XK001 [3]. Mechanistically, Camptothecin inhibits topoisomerase-1 (intranuclear enzyme), causing DNA cleavage and cytotoxicity during the molecular processes of replication and transcription as shown in Fig. (**4**). Furthermore, the compound's semi-synthetic derivatives *i.e.* Camtostar (irinotecan) and Hycamtin (topotecan), have been identified and accredited by FDA for clinical purposes against small cell lung and refractory ovarian cancers, cervical cancer, and rectum and large intestine cancers with a reduced amount of toxicity than the parent compound [3, 4, 8, 9, 11, 12, 25, 26].

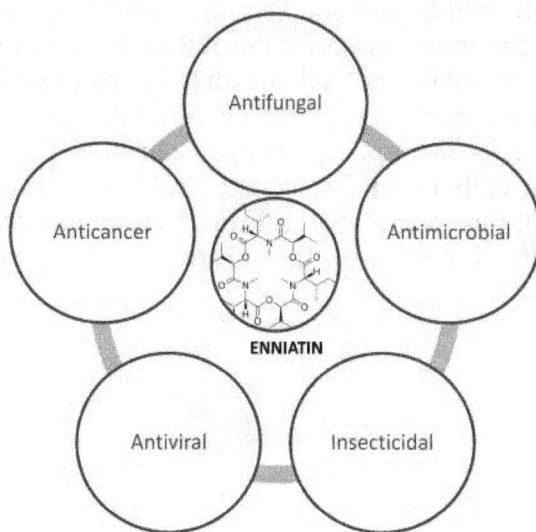

Fig. (3). Major therapeutic properties of Enniatin.

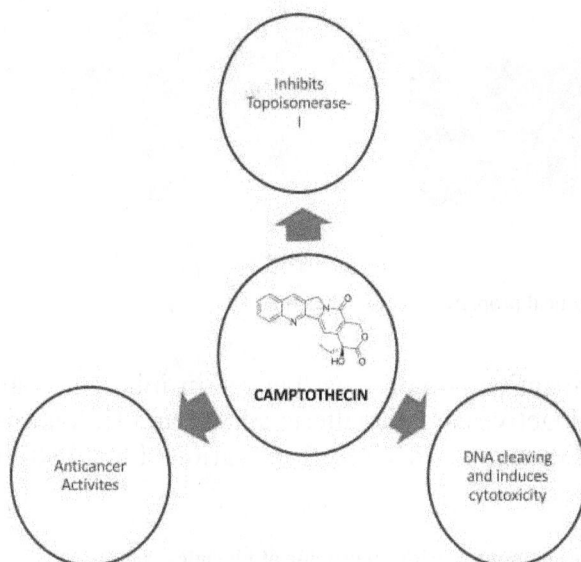

Fig. (4). Major pharmaceutical properties of Camptothecin.

Ascochytatin

Ascochytatin is a spirodioxynaphthalene metabolite (Fig. **6**) which is primarily isolated from *Ascochyta* sp. NGB4 (marine-derived Japanese fungus). The compound is known for its excellent antimicrobial activity against *B. subtilis* CNM2000 and 168 (wild) bacterial strains, gram-positive bacteria, and *C. albicans* yeast. The foremost reason for this tremendous attribute of Ascochytatin resides in its ability to inhibit crucial encoding genes (YycG/YycF) responsible for the two-component regulatory system (TCS) of the bacteria. Additionally, the compound also exhibits cytotoxic potential against several mammalian cancer cells such as Jurkat cells (human leukaemia cell line) and A549 (human lung carcinoma cell line), thus exerting therapeutic effects in clinical use [2, 27, 28]. Some important properties of the compound are shown in Fig. (**5**).

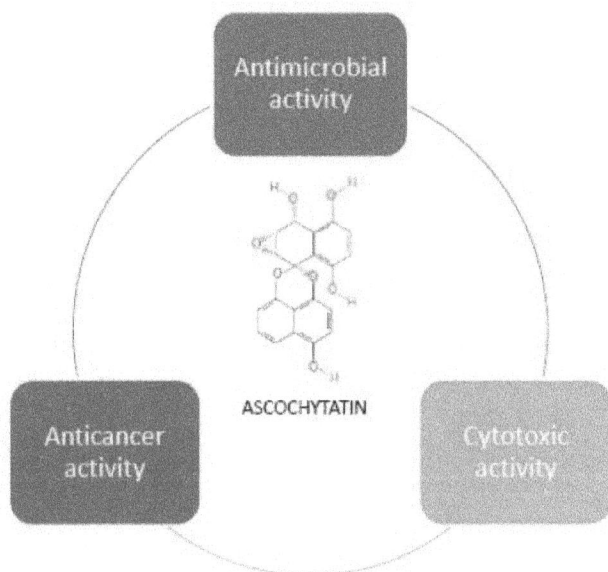

Fig. (5). Major pharmaceutical properties of Ascochytatin.

Other important bioactive compounds that retain inherent characteristics to act towards assorted bioactives are Xanalteric acids I and II, Vincristine, Ergoflavin, Fusidilactones, Aflatoxin, *etc.* derived from various fungal strains are mentioned in Table **1**.

Table 1. Major bioactive compounds with their mode of biological action.

S.No.	Bioactive Compound	Fungal Source	Bioactivity	Refs.
1	Xanalteric acids I and II	*Alternaria* sp	Antibacterial, anticancer	[2, 10, 29]

(Table 1) cont.....

2	Vincristine	*Fusarium oxysparum*	Anticancer	[8, 10, 13]
3	Ergoflavin	*Pyrenochaeta terrestris, Penicillium oxalicum, Phoma terrestris* and *Aspergillus* sp.	Anticancer	[8, 11]
4	Fusidilactones	*Fusidium* sp	Antifungal	[13, 29]
5	Aflatoxin	*Aspergillus flavus*	Antibacterial	[1, 30]
6	Capsaicin	*Alternaria alternata*	Anticancer, Cardiovascular diseases	[11, 31-33]
7	Diorcinol K, D, I	*Aspergillus* sp. CUGB-F046 strain	Antibacterial	[34]
8	Tyrosol	*Penicillium chrysogenum DXY-1*	Antibacterial	[6, 35]
9	Coccoquinone A	*Aspergillus versicolor*	Anti-HSV-, Antifouling, Antioxidant	[34, 36]
10	Cyclosporin	*Sabina recurve*	Antiviral	[8]

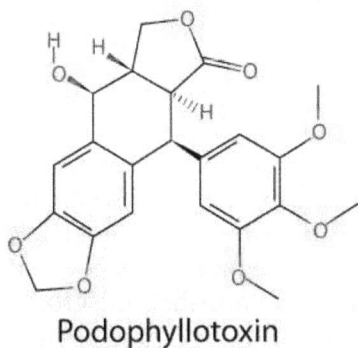

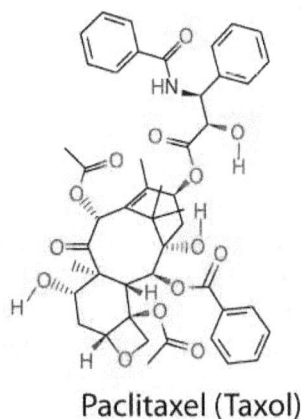

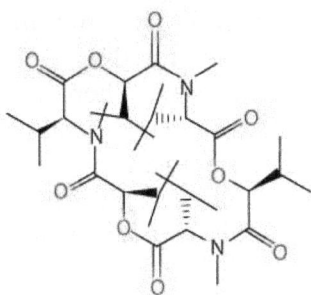

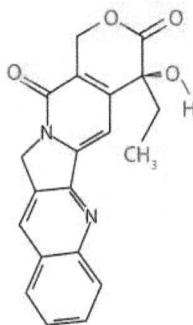

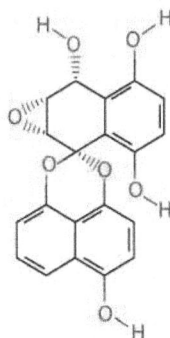

Podophyllotoxin

Paclitaxel (Taxol)

Enniatin   Camptothecin   Ascochytatin

Fig. (6). Chemical structures of important bioactive compounds obtained by various fungus.

CONCLUSION

Microbial [fungal] research is currently intriguing, with enormous potential in agriculture, pharmacology, and medicine. Screening fungal organisms for probable beneficial metabolite production can aid in the identification of their pharmacological functions as well as research into the bioprospecting of fungal species as biological entities that will assure long-term public welfare.

Myriad studies have successfully isolated novel, beneficial bioactive compounds from fungi that have biological properties such as anti-diabetic, anti-bacterial, immunomodulatory, insecticidal, anti-fungal, anti-protozoan, anti-inflammatory, anti-tuberculosis, anti-viral, anti-helminthic, anti-cancer activities, *etc.* Despite this, only a limited number of fungal species have been thoroughly characterized for secondary metabolite production. Thus, the great genetic diversity of fungi which needs to be explored and documented. Priorities in research must switch to biotechnological advancements in order to speed up the screening of novel biomolecules for the treatment of a wide range of life-threatening illnesses for protecting human health.

FUTURE CHALLENGES

Fungal sources provide fresh hope and prospects for the synthesis of bioactive chemicals, which has been hampered by poor yields, a lack of understanding of biochemical interactions, scaling-up difficulties, and axenic expansion. There is a continual need to express these natural active compounds *in vitro,* which has limited success in commercialization albeit being accomplished in certain cases. The interplay of fungal organisms with other related microorganisms is poorly understood. Plant tissue culture approaches have failed to provide larger yields owing to genetic instability in the culture, limited fungal development, cell aggregation formation, and sensitivity to shearing. Furthermore, tissue culture upkeep is both expensive and more time-consuming than fermentation methods. Although, fungal fermentation establishes a methodology for the synthesis of bioactive molecules that is both powerful and long-lasting. There are some advantages of fungal fermentation processes, such as a basic fungal cell medium, low cost, faster fungi growth with minimal risk of contamination, and *in vitro* enhanced fermentation conditions that facilitate the growth of naturally occurring substances, but generally, it falls short of the requirements for long-term production.

Another significant roadblock is the difficulty of generating complex metabolites of bioactive chemicals utilizing a combinatorial chemical synthesis method. These flaws can be addressed by using inducers/elicitors of a certain metabolic pathway, which can eventually enhance yield.

Nevertheless, the constraints might be solved by using signalling molecules and cheap precursor loading in the culture media to trigger the optimal biochemical pathway in order to obtain a higher yield. Furthermore, the presence of numerous superfluous compounds in the growth media might impair the overall production.

The negative feedback loop is a crucial component of the fungal fermentation strategy that must be thoroughly explored in order to obtain increased productivity. Fungal research using genetic engineering approaches, transformation studies, mutagenesis, gene cluster amplification, culture condition optimization, medium manipulation, and elicitor addition should all assist to boost secondary metabolite yields.

CONSENT FOR PUBLICATION

Not applicable.

CONFLICT OF INTEREST

The authors declare no conflict of interest, financial or otherwise.

ACKNOWLEDGEMENTS

The authors extend their gratitude to the CSIR New Delhi, for providing financial assistance in the form of CSIR-JRF to Neha Jain (File no. 09/149(0753)/2019-EMR-1).

REFERENCES

[1]   Cadamuro RD, da Silveira Bastos IMA, Silva IT, *et al.* Bioactive Compounds from Mangrove Endophytic Fungus and Their Uses for Microorganism Control. J Fungi (Basel) 2021; 7(6): 455.
[http://dx.doi.org/10.3390/jof7060455] [PMID: 34200444]

[2]   Debbab A, Aly AH, Lin WH, Proksch P. Bioactive compounds from marine bacteria and fungi. Microb Biotechnol 2010; 3(5): 544-63.
[http://dx.doi.org/10.1111/j.1751-7915.2010.00179.x] [PMID: 21255352]

[3]   Selvakumar V, Panneerselvam A. Fungi and their role in sustainable development: Current perspectives. Fungi their Role Sustain Dev Curr Perspect 2018; 1-779.

[4]   Manganyi MC, Ateba CN. Untapped potentials of endophytic fungi: A review of novel bioactive compounds with biological applications. Microorganisms 2020; 8(12): 1934.
[http://dx.doi.org/10.3390/microorganisms8121934] [PMID: 33291214]

[5]   Vacchelli E, Ma Y, Baracco EE, *et al.* Chemotherapy-induced antitumor immunity requires formyl peptide receptor 1. Science (80-) 2015; 350(6263): 972-8.

[6]   Sharma D, Pramanik A, Agrawal PK. Evaluation of bioactive secondary metabolites from endophytic fungus Pestalotiopsis neglecta BAB-5510 isolated from leaves of Cupressus torulosa D.Don. 3 Biotech 2016; 6(2): 1-14.

[7]   Lin L, Xu J. Fungal Pigments and Their Roles Associated with Human Health. J Fungi (Basel) 2020; 6(4): 280.

[http://dx.doi.org/10.3390/jof6040280] [PMID: 33198121]

[8]   Adeleke B, Babalola O. Pharmacological potential of fungal endophytes associated with medicinal plants: A review. J Fungi (Basel) 2021; 7(2): 147.
[http://dx.doi.org/10.3390/jof7020147] [PMID: 33671354]

[9]   Deshmukh S, Gupta M, Prakash V, Reddy MS. Mangrove-Associated Fungi: A Novel Source of Potential Anticancer Compounds. J Fungi (Basel) 2018; 4(3): 101.
[http://dx.doi.org/10.3390/jof4030101] [PMID: 30149584]

[10]   Srivastava AK. The role of fungus in bioactive compound production and nanotechnology Role of Plant Growth Promoting Microorganisms in Sustainable Agriculture and Nanotechnology. INC 2019; pp. 145-62.

[11]   Uzma F, Mohan CD, Hashem A, *et al.* Endophytic fungi-alternative sources of cytotoxic compounds: A review. Front Pharmacol 2018; 9(APR): 309.
[http://dx.doi.org/10.3389/fphar.2018.00309] [PMID: 29755344]

[12]   Lichota A, Gwozdzinski K. Anticancer Activity of Natural Compounds from Plant and Marine Environment 2018.
[http://dx.doi.org/10.3390/ijms19113533]

[13]   Gunatilaka AAL. Natural products from plant-associated microorganisms: distribution, structural diversity, bioactivity, and implications of their occurrence. J Nat Prod 2006; 69(3): 509-26.
[http://dx.doi.org/10.1021/np058128n] [PMID: 16562864]

[14]   Sy-Cordero AA, Pearce CJ, Oberlies NH. Revisiting the enniatins: a review of their isolation, biosynthesis, structure determination, and biological activities. J Antibiot (Tokyo) 2014; 23(1): 1-7.
[PMID: 24463294]

[15]   Olleik H, Nicoletti C, Lafond M, *et al.* Comparative Structure–Activity Analysis of the Antimicrobial Activity, Cytotoxicity, and Mechanism of Action of the Fungal Cyclohexadepsipeptides Enniatins and Beauvericin. Toxins (Basel) 2019; 11(9): 514.
[http://dx.doi.org/10.3390/toxins11090514] [PMID: 31484420]

[16]   Firáková S, Proksa B, Sturdíková M. Biosynthesis and biological activity of enniatins. Pharmazie 2007; 62(8): 563-8.
[PMID: 17867547]

[17]   Jayasinghe L, Abbas HK, Jacob MR, Herath WHMW, Nanayakkara NPD. *N*-Methyl-4-hydro-y-2-pyridinone Analogues from *Fusarium oxysporum*. J Nat Prod 2006; 69(3): 439-42.
[http://dx.doi.org/10.1021/np050487v] [PMID: 16562855]

[18]   Jeschke P, Benet-Buchholz J, Harder A, Etzel W, Schindler M, Thielking G. Synthesis and anthelmintic activity of cyclohexadepsipeptides with (S,S,S,R,S,R)-configuration. Bioorg Med Chem Lett 2003; 13(19): 3285-8.
[http://dx.doi.org/10.1016/S0960-894X(03)00688-7] [PMID: 12951110]

[19]   Fukuda T, Arai M, Tomoda H, Omura S. New beauvericins, potentiators of antifungal miconazole activity, Produced by Beauveria sp. FKI-1366. II. Structure elucidation. J Antibiot (Tokyo) 2004; 57(2): 117-24.
[http://dx.doi.org/10.7164/antibiotics.57.117] [PMID: 15112960]

[20]   Sharom FJ, Lu P, Liu R, Yu X. Linear and cyclic peptides as substrates and modulators of P-glycoprotein: peptide binding and effects on drug transport and accumulation. Biochem J 1998; 333(3): 621-30.
[http://dx.doi.org/10.1042/bj3330621] [PMID: 9677321]

[21]   Dornetshuber R, Heffeter P, Kamyar MR, *et al.* Enniatin Exerts p53-Dependent Cytostatic and p53 Independent Cytotoxic Activities against Human Cancer Cells. Chem Res Toxicol 1945; 2007(III): 202-3.
[PMID: 17326668]

[22]   Zhang H, Ruan C, Bai X, Zhang M, Zhu S, Jiang Y. Isolation and identification of the antimicrobial. BioMed Res Int 2016; 2016: 1084670.
[PMID: 27413733]

[23]   Tong Y, Liu M, Zhang Y, *et al.* Beauvericin counteracted multi-drug resistant *Candida albicans* by blocking ABC transporters. Synth Syst Biotechnol 2016; 1(3): 158-68.
[http://dx.doi.org/10.1016/j.synbio.2016.10.001] [PMID: 29062940]

[24]   Fraeyman S, Croubels S, Devreese M, Antonissen G. Emerging fusarium and alternaria mycotoxins: Occurrence, toxicity and toxicokinetics. Toxins (Basel) 2017; 9(7): 228.
[http://dx.doi.org/10.3390/toxins9070228] [PMID: 28718805]

[25]   Choudhari AS, Mandave PC, Deshpande M, Ranjekar P, Prakash O. Phytochemicals in Cancer Treatment: From Preclinical Studies to Clinical Practice. Front Pharmacol 2020; 10(January): 1614.
[http://dx.doi.org/10.3389/fphar.2019.01614] [PMID: 32116665]

[26]   Prakash O, Kumar A, Kumar P, Ajeet A. Anticancer Potential of Plants and Natural Products: A Review. Am J Pharmacol Sci 2013; 1(6): 104-15.
[http://dx.doi.org/10.12691/ajps-1-6-1]

[27]   Kanoh K, Okada A, Adachi K, *et al.* Ascochytatin, a novel bioactive spirodioxynaphthalene metabolite produced by the marine-derived fungus, Ascochyta sp. NGB4. J Antibiot (Tokyo) 2008; 61(3): 142-8.
[http://dx.doi.org/10.1038/ja.2008.123] [PMID: 18503192]

[28]   Mayer AMS, Rodríguez AD, Berlinck RGS, Fusetani N. Marine pharmacology in 2007–8: Marine compounds with antibacterial, anticoagulant, antifungal, anti-inflammatory, antimalarial, antiprotozoal, antituberculosis, and antiviral activities; affecting the immune and nervous system, and other miscellaneous mechanisms of action. Comp Biochem Physiol C Toxicol Pharmacol 2011; 153(2): 191-222.
[http://dx.doi.org/10.1016/j.cbpc.2010.08.008] [PMID: 20826228]

[29]   Deshmukh SK, Verekar SA, Bhave SV. Endophytic fungi: a reservoir of antibacterials. Front Microbiol 2015; 5(DEC): 715.
[PMID: 25620957]

[30]   Frisvad JC, Hubka V, Ezekiel CN, *et al.* Taxonomy of *Aspergillus* section *Flavi* and their production of aflatoxins, ochratoxins and other mycotoxins. Stud Mycol 2019; 93(1): 1-63.
[http://dx.doi.org/10.1016/j.simyco.2018.06.001] [PMID: 30108412]

[31]   Popescu GDA, Scheau C, Badarau IA, *et al.* The Effects of Capsaicin on Gastrointestinal Cancers. Molecules 2020; 26(1): 94.
[http://dx.doi.org/10.3390/molecules26010094] [PMID: 33379302]

[32]   Bao Z, Dai X, Wang P, Tao Y, Chai D. Capsaicin induces cytotoxicity in human osteosarcoma MG63 cells through TRPV1-dependent and -independent pathways. Cell Cycle 2019; 18(12): 1379-92.
[http://dx.doi.org/10.1080/15384101.2019.1618119] [PMID: 31095448]

[33]   Fattori V, Hohmann M, Rossaneis A, Pinho-Ribeiro F, Verri W. Capsaicin: Current understanding of its mechanisms and therapy of pain and other pre-clinical and clinical uses. Molecules 2016; 21(7): 844.
[http://dx.doi.org/10.3390/molecules21070844] [PMID: 27367653]

[34]   Zain ul Arifeen M, Ma YN, Xue YR, Liu CH. Deep-sea fungi could be the new arsenal for bioactive molecules. Mar Drugs 2019; 18(1): 9.
[http://dx.doi.org/10.3390/md18010009] [PMID: 31861953]

[35] Yurchenko AN, Girich EV, Yurchenko EA. Metabolites of Marine Sediment-Derived Fungi: Actual Trends of Biological Activity Studies. Mar Drugs 2021; 19(2): 88.
[http://dx.doi.org/10.3390/md19020088] [PMID: 33557071]

[36] Vitale GA, Coppola D, Palma Esposito F, *et al.* Antioxidant molecules from marine fungi: Methodologies and perspectives. Antioxidants 2020; 9(12): 1183.
[http://dx.doi.org/10.3390/antiox9121183] [PMID: 33256101]

CHAPTER 12

Immunomodulatory Potential of Bioactives from Selected Ayurvedic Plants

Parvathy G. Nair[1]**, Amit Kumar Dixit**[2,*] **and Deepti Dixit**[3]

[1] *National Ayurveda Research Institute for Panchakarma, Central Council for Research in Ayurvedic Sciences, Ministry of AYUSH, Government of India, Cheruthuruthy, Thrissur, Kerala, India*

[2] *Central Ayurveda Research Institute, Central Council for Research in Ayurvedic Sciences, Ministry of AYUSH, Government of India, Kolkata, India*

[3] *School of Biochemistry, Devi Ahilya University, Khandwa Road, Indore, Madhya Pradesh, India*

Abstract: The history of usage of herbal medicine is as old as human civilization. Plant-based drugs have been an invaluable and incredible source for several medical treatments in the traditional system of medicine. With technological advances, it has become possible to get a clear understanding of active compounds behind the therapeutic effectiveness of these drugs. Plant-derived immunomodulators are one such class of compounds, considered safe alternatives than synthetic immunomodulators which cause serious side effects. These agents can increase the body's immune responsiveness against pathogens by activating both the innate and adaptive immune systems. Phyto drugs have gained more interest due to their multi-pharmacological potential of being antioxidant, adaptogen, *etc.* along with immunomodulator. The current book chapter focuses on a few extensively scrutinized immunomodulatory phytocompounds from medicinal plants such as *Tinospora cordifolia*, *Andrographis paniculata*, Curcuma longa, *Zingiber officinale, Allium sativum, Terminalia chebula,* and *Piper longum*. Phytomedicines from these plants have displayed significant immunomodulatory potential in a variety of experimental (*in vitro* and *in vivo*) models, few compounds have exhibited good therapeutic potential in clinical trials also.

Keywords: Herbal medicine, Immunomodulators, Medicinal plants, Ayurveda, Traditional medicine, Immune system, Phytocompounds.

INTRODUCTION

Human immune system is quite capable to maintain immunity required for protecting the body against diseases or other potentially damaging foreign bodies. Still, certain chemical, biological, physical, physiological factors and adverse en-

---

* **Corresponding author Amit Kumar Dixit:** Central Ayurveda Research Institute, Central Council for Research in Ayurvedic Sciences, Ministry of AYUSH, Government of India, Kolkata, India; Tel: +91-89205 74307; E-mail: deepdixit20@gmail.com

Mukesh Kumar Sharma and Pallavi Kaushik (Eds.)

vironmental conditions can alter its normal functioning. In such conditions, immunomodulatory drugs can modify the immune system by either selective inhibition or intensification of immune responsive cells and facilitate the healing in a disease. These drugs can sometimes directly influence a specific immune function or modify components of the immunoregulatory network to achieve an indirect effect on a specific immune function [1].

Discovery of drugs which can selectively stimulate or suppress the immune system paved a new pathway in the management of many diseases where immune dysfunction plays a major role, like autoimmune and infection-associated immunopathologic diseases. Modulators can either be immunostimulatory (developed for their potential applicability to infection, immunodeficiency, and cancer) or immunosuppressive (employed to inhibit the immune response in many immune-mediated diseases *i.e.*, in organ transplantation and autoimmune diseases). Another category is immunoadjuvants, which are usually administered in combination with a main drug to facilitate the immune system by increasing magnitude, duration and induction of antigen specific immune response. Natural, synthetic, recombinant immunomodulatory compounds are widely used as adjuvant/supportive supplementary therapy for prophylaxis and treatment of such clinical conditions. Most of these drugs stimulate the natural and adaptive defence mechanisms enabling the body to heal itself. Monoclonal antibodies, fusion proteins, cytokines and other chemically synthesised compounds are extensively used as immunomodulatory drugs. But major limitations of the use of these agents are their detrimental side effects on general usage. Immunostimulant cytokines like interleukins are also found not fit for prolonged use because of its cost-effectiveness and adverse effects. Therefore, for additional safety and effectiveness, the focus shifted on to herbs and polyherbal preparations which are used traditionally in ethnomedical practices for effective management of wide range of inflammatory and infectious diseases. Exploring the pharmacological action of herbal drugs and its combinations, which bring forth particular therapeutic effect, is an impossible job due to its complex nature. But, from the reverse pharmacological leads, biomolecules isolated from these plants are being widely studied for their immunomodulatory and biological response modifying action. Further research and development are done on these compounds, synthetic modifications are also done at times to optimize the bioavailability and pharmacokinetics [2 - 5]. This chapter presents a review on plant derived biomolecules which have exhibited potent immunomodulatory effects in pre-clinical investigations with wide potential to be used as clinical immunomodulatory agents.

Components of Immune System and Role of Immunomodulators

Immune system is a unique defence arrangement for maintaining homeostasis and providing protection from invading foreign agents by generating interdependent cells. Immune responses are maintained by various organs and cells. Main organs are Bone marrow, Thymus, Spleen and lymph nodes. Bone marrow, the main lymphoid organ, is responsible for production of all blood cells through a process known as Haematopoiesis. From here, the immature thymocytes (prothymocytes) migrate to the thymus and undergo the maturation process (Thymic education) and finally are released in blood stream. These cells with specialized functions work in collaboration to protect the body from infectious microorganisms and also from the growth of tumor cells on account of their capacity to recognize and eliminate the invading pathogens. This capability of resistance against diseases in multi-cellular organisms is described as immunity. Leukocytes developed from bone marrow precursors are the major immune response mediators. Cells like lymphocytes, neutrophils and monocytes/ macrophages, being the fundamental units, act collectively for immune system of the body. The front-line host defence in case of a pathogenic attack is handled by macrophages and mast cells. Macrophages become actively involved in phagocytosis and mast cells recruit eosinophils and basophils to trigger exocytosis. Thymus cells (T cells), bone marrow cells (B cells) and natural killer (NK) cells are the major lymphocytes involved in initiating immune responses. T cells generally differentiate into antigen specific effector cells and B cells into antibody secreting cells. Dendritic cells (DC) are the classical antigen presenting cells with unique ability to capture and present antigens to T cells which are critical for initiating adaptive immune response against infectious agents. Spleen is a blood filter that captures the foreign materials (antigens) mainly by macrophages or dendritic cells and initiates the immune response after presenting the antigen to B and T cells to produce antibodies. Another important organ, lymph nodes, are present throughout the body to act as an immunologic filter for lymph. Here also macrophages or dendritic cells capture the antigen from the site of infection to initiate the immune response. Other than these, there are mucosal-associated lymphoid tissues (MALT), which collect antigens from the epithelial surfaces of the body [6, 7].

Immunity has two components innate and adaptive immunity. In both types of immunity, cells and molecules play a significant role in engulfing bacteria and killing parasites, viruses or tumor cells by secreting activation signals in the form of cytokines, lymphokines or interleukins mediated by T-helper cells. A non-specific (antigen independent) first line barrier for defence against an invading pathogen and injury is innate immunity which leaves no memory. It works efficiently to keep the organism healthy but its deterioration can result in secondary infections leading to serious illness and death. Cytokines, NK cells and gamma delta T cells are involved in activation by means of receptors. Two main receptors DAMP (damage associated molecular pattern) or PAMP (Pathogen – associated molecular pattern) is associated for the generation of pro-inflammatory responses following a cascade of signal initiated by PRR (Pathogen recognition receptors) after recognizing a pathogen. Whereas, adaptive immunity is unique to vertebrates, being a more complicated, specific and diversified defence mechanism that leaves memory of an infection. It acts by two mechanisms humoral and cellular. Humoral immunity is an antibody-mediated immunity which involves antibody secreting plasma cells following proliferation of antigen-stimulated B- lymphocytes. While, the cellular component is mediated by cells, mainly T lymphocytes, macrophages and natural killer cells. In response to antigen presentation process, T cells differentiate primarily into either cytotoxic T cells (CD8+ cells) or T-helper (Th) cells (CD4+ cells). By expressing appropriate antigens cytotoxic cells kill foreign agents such as viruses and tumor cells. Th cells "mediate" the immune response by directing other cells to perform cytotoxic and phagocytic activity, thereby these establish and maximise immune responses. Th1, Th2 and Th17 are several types of Th cells which are induced by antigen presenting cells. Regulatory T cells, a subset of Th cells also limit and suppress immune responses and develop "immune tolerance" to certain foreign antigens [8, 9].

Nowadays, to cure various diseases, not only a proper immune system but modulation of immune response is also required. Immunomodulators are such compounds which can change the immune response by involving induction, expression, amplification or inhibition of any part or phase of the immune response. Plants based immunomodulators act on diverse components of immune system to regulate the immune responses in the body (Fig. **1**) [10, 11].

Immunomodulatory Potential of Traditional Medicinal Plants

Indian traditional system of medicine like Ayurveda has a database of various medicinal plants which can strengthen the body's defence and contribute to general physical and mental well-being. The original Ayurvedic treatises like Charak Samhita and Sushrutha Samhita are written in Sanskrit and do not give any direct references to drugs which can be used as immunomodulators. But Ayurveda specifically describes a group of drugs called *rasayanas,* which help humans to attain longevity, regain youth, and get a sharp memory/intellect and freedom from diseases. Its properties like anti-ageing, increasing the life-span and resistance to disease has attracted the research attention to explore their immunomodulatory potential [12]. Some other non *rasayana* drugs which can trigger the metabolic functions, antipathogenic and anti-allergic properties can also act as immunomodulators. Apart from these some drugs have been mentioned as strengthening (*jeevaniya*), vitalising (*balya*) and life maintaining (*vayasthapana*) are also extensively explored for their influences on immune system. This is because it is hypothesised that immune system has a bidirectional link to several organ systems in the body in maintaining the homeostasis, which includes drugs which can strengthen and maintain the functioning of these organs can play a pivotal role in modulating immunity. It is also interesting to note that, few plants mentioned under these groups are found to be overlapping, suggesting immune system as their common target for therapeutic action (Table **1**) [13 - 16].

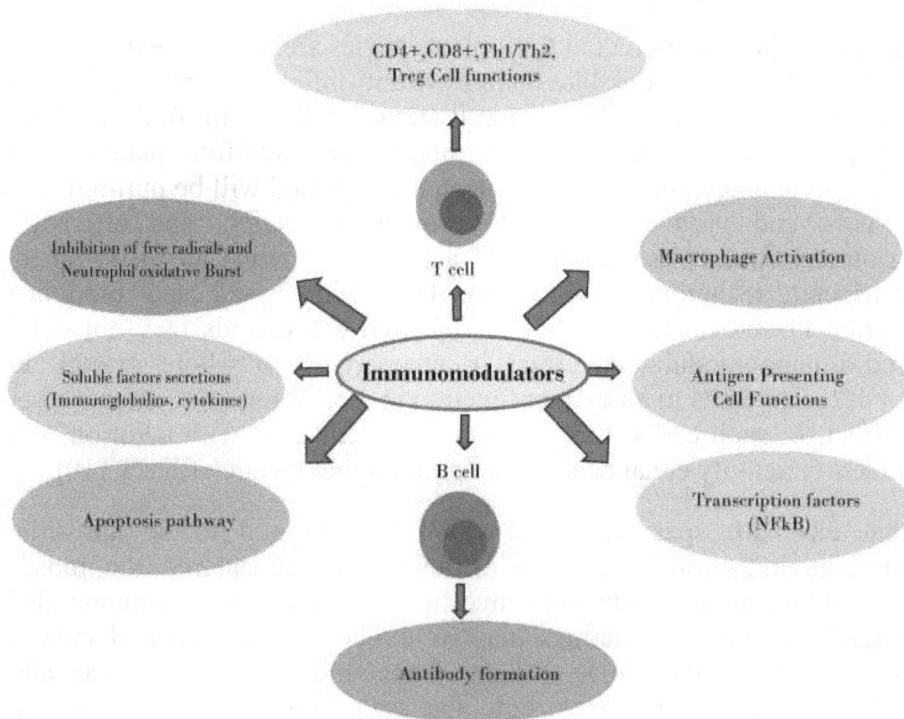

Fig. (1). Role of Immunomodulators in human immune system.

Table 1. Botanical sources of few plants listed as *rasayana, jeevaniya, balya* and *vayasthapana*in Ayurveda [17].

Rasayana	Jeevaniya	Balya	Vayasthapana
Allium sativum	Microstylis wallichi	Bacopa monnieri	Tinospora cordifolia
Centella asiatica	Microstylis mucifera	Mucuna pruriens	Terminalia chebula
Piper longum	Polygonatum verticillate	Asparagus racemosus	Emblica officinalis
Semecarpus anacardium	Polygonatum cirrhifolium	Teramnus labialis	Boerrhavia diffusa
Tinospora cordifolia	Fritillaria royeli	Ipomea digitata	Desmodium gangecticum
Curcuma longa	Roscoea purpurea	Withania somnifera	Centella asiatica

(Table 1) cont.....

Emblica officinalis	Phaseolus trilobus	Desmodium gangecticum	Asparagus racemosus
Terminalia chebula	Teramnus labialis	Sida cordifolia	Leptadenia reticulata
Terminalia bellerica	Leptadinia reticulata	Abutilon indicum	Pluchea lanceolata
Plumbago zeylanica	Glycyrrhiza glabra	Soymida febrifuga	Clitoria ternata

*Botanical identity of Ayurvedic drugs is compiled from different Medicinal plant compendia's, Ayurvedic Pharmacopeia of India

Immunomodulatory Phytocompounds

The phytocompounds extracted from plant species are found to exhibit wide range of pharmacological actions like analgesic, anti-inflammatory, *etc*. Based on the traditional claims, each plant drug is first screened to find leading active principles. The active compounds will then be separated from plant extract using chromatographic techniques. The separated compound will be purified and tested in *in-vitro* and *in-vivo* models to evaluate its safety and efficacy. After experimental studies the structure of active compounds are determined using spectroscopic techniques, which are later synthesised and modulated for evaluation in clinical trials. At times purified compounds may not exhibit the desired immunomodulatory effect in comparison to whole extract, because different components in an extract function in a combinatorial manner to produce that effect. In such cases, the compound is modulated with addition of natural stabilizers or activity enhancers to get optimum therapeutic efficacy [10].

Among all plant species, those which are claimed to be anti-infectious, antitumoral, anti-viral or anti- parasiticidal are considered the most suited candidates for immunomodulatory investigations. The leading compounds behind immunopharmacological actions may be either low or high molecular weight compounds. Low molecular weight compounds mainly include alkaloids, phenolic compounds, quinones, saponins, sesquiterpenes, di- and triterpenoids, tryptamine, phytoestrogens. Polysaccharides, glycoprotein like lectins, nucleotides are the major high molecular weight phytocompounds. These plant products are reported to affect the immune system by enhancement of macrophagic phagocytosis, induction of cytokines and release of inducible nitric oxides and reactive oxygen intermediates [18, 19].

Numerous studies have been conducted on bioactive compounds from *rasayana* and non *rasayana* medicinal plants and to study their effects on the immune system. Such reported preclinical and clinical immunomodulatory activities of phytocompounds in few traditional medicinal plants are compiled and presented below (Table **2**). Chemical structures of the compounds reported are also given in Fig. (**2**).

Table 2. Major plant based biomolecules with proven immunomodulatory potential.

Plant species	Phytocompound (class)	Isolated Compound	Reference
Tinospora cordifolia (Menispermacea)	Glycoside Polysaccharide	Cordifolioside A Syringin 1,4-α-D-glucan (RR1)	[21] [20]
	Alkaloid	Berberine	[26]
Andrographis paniculata (Acanthaceae)	Diterpene lactone	Andrographolide	[29]
Curcuma longa (Zingiberacea)	Polyphenol	Curcumin	[42]
Zingiber officinale (Zingiberacea)	Polyphenol	[6]-gingerol	[47]
Allium sativum (Alliaceae)	Organosulfur	Allicin	[52]
Terminalia chebula (Combretaceae)	Tannin	Chebulagic acid Gallic acid	[67] [69]
Piper longum (Piperaceae)	Alkaloid	Piperine	[74]

Tinospora cordifolia (Willd.) Miers ex Hook.f. & Thomas

Tinospora cordifolia is an important medicinal plant known for its immunomodulatory potential. This activity is due to the synergistic effects of multiple compounds present in various parts of the plant. These compounds include low molecular weight alkaloids, clerodane diterpenoids, sesquiterpenoids, and phenyl propanoids. High molecular weight arabinogalactan named G1- 4A, 1,4-α-D-glucan (RR1) are also found to stimulate the immune system. Glycosides like cordioside, cordiofolioside A, cordiofoliside B, cordial, syrigin are reported to stimulate the immune response by macrophage activation. Polysaccharide (1→4)-α-D-glucan (named RR1) isolated from *T.cordifolia* is reported to be non-cytotoxic which can uniquely activate the lymphocyte subsets like natural killer cells (NK) along with T and B cells. In normal lymphocytes, RR1 elicited immunomodulation by synthesis of IL-1β, IL-6, IL-12 p70, IL-12 p40, IL-18, IFN-γ, tumor necrosis factor (TNF-α) and monocyte chemoattractant protein (MCP)-1 without inducing the production of IL-2, IL-4, IL-10, interferon (IFN)- α and TNF-h. Immunomodulator protein (ImP), a single chain acidic protein without glycans, isolated from its stem has shown lymphocyte proliferation and macrophage activating properties *in vitro*. Mucosal (intranasal) administration of purified *T.cordifolia* ImP provided natural antibodies (serum IgG and IgA) in BALB/c mice indicating its intrinsic immunogenic potential. *T.cordifolia* ImP also acted as an adjuvant for a weak antigen like OVA by increasing the serum anti-OVA IgG and IgA, promising its usage as a mucosal adjuvant for experimental antigens in further studies on humans. N-formylannonain and 11-hydroxymustakone isolated from stem of *T. cordifolia* were found to have good immunomodulatory potential by means of its splenocyte proliferation activity [20 - 25]. Berberine, another isoquinoline alkaloid found in *T.cordifolia,* is already reported to play a role in ameliorating various autoimmune inflammatory diseases. Berberine administered intragastrical, and successfully alleviated experimental autoimmune neuritis (EAN- an established animal model of human Guillain–Barre syndrome) by suppressing both cellular and humoral immunity. It suppressed the proliferation of lymphocytes (CD4+ T cells), downregulated both Th1 (TNF-a) and Th2 (IL-10) cytokines and reduced anti-P0 peptide 180–199 IgG1 and IgG2a. Proapoptotic effect of berberine specific to certain dendritic cells (DC) are already reported. Chronic proliferative synovitis and joint destruction in autoimmune diseases like rheumatoid arthritis (RA) are always driven by DC. Hence they represent a novel and important target for immunosuppressive therapy for these diseases. Berberine showed strong apoptosis to murine bone marrow derived myeloid DCs, in a time and dose dependent manner in animal models. It could also limit the maturation of DCs, shorten their lifespan by selective induction of apoptosis in mature DCs only [26, 27].

Molecular docking simulation investigations confirmed that the cordifolioside exhibited high inhibitory activity on the binding pocket of main protease (M pro), one of the attractive drug targets of SARS-CoV-2, due to its immune modulatory activity on human TGF-β and TNF-α. It is proposed that after further investigations, cordifolioside can be used as a possible anti COVID drug which can reduce human cytokine storm [28].

Andrographis paniculata (Burm. F) Nees

Andrographis paniculata commonly known as the "King of bitters" is a traditionally used medicinal plant with broad range of biological activities. Three diterpene compounds, *i.e.,* andrographolide, 14-deoxyandrographolide and 14-deoxy-11,12-didehydroandrographolide isolated from *A.paniculata* had shown immunomodulatory activity by means of increasing human peripheral blood lymphocytes (HPBLs) proliferation at 1μm concentration. These compounds also enhanced IL-2 induction in HPBLs, although higher concentration of andrographolide showed cytotoxicity towards HPBLs. But hollow fiber assay done *in vivo* immunocompromised Swiss albino mice showed that andrographolide significantly inhibits the cancer cell proliferation without any signs of toxicity in mice even at high doses.Purified diterpenes, andrographolide and neo andrographolide extracted from crude extract of AP induced significant stimulation of antibody and delayed type hypersensitivity (DTH) response to sheep red blood cells (SRBC) in mice. Stimulation of innate immune response of the andrographolides was measured *in vitro* by phagocytosis of C-leucine labelled *Escherichia coli* and increased in peritoneal macrophage migration index (MMI)of the treated animals. Andrographolide was shown to interfere with the capacity of antigen-pulsed dendritic cells to activate T cells on a series of *in vitro* and *in vivo* assays. Dendritic cells (DCs) are ideal therapeutic targets for pharmacological modulation of immune responses especially in autoimmune diseases. Andrographolide inhibited the DC function and was in turn able to down-modulate T cell-mediated immunity to ameliorate experimental autoimmune encephalomyelitis (EAE- an ideal animal model for mimicking human multiple sclerosis). It was reported to prevent initial T cell priming by interfering with DC maturation and modulating the antigen presentation capacity. Excessive production of inflammatory mediators like Tumor necrosis factor (TNF- α) and IL-12 can induce conditions like tissue injury, septic shock and autoimmune diseases. Andrographolide was observed to inhibit the production of both TNF-α and IL-12 in LPS (lipopolysaccharide)-stimulated mouse peritoneal macrophages. Suppression of ERK1/2 signalling pathway by andrographolide was hypothesised to be the probable reason for inhibition of production of TNF-α [29 - 32].

A phase 1 clinical trial of Andrographolide conducted in 13 HIV-positive patients and 05 normal volunteers reported that oral administration of the drug in an escalating manner (5 mg/kg bodyweight for 3 weeks, escalating to 10 mg/kg bodyweight for 3 weeks, and to 20 mg/kg bodyweight for a final 3 weeks) didn't develop any serious adverse events in majority of patients. But one patient in positive group developed an anaphylactic reaction at 6th week. A significant rise in the mean CD4+ lymphocyte levels was observed in HIV-1 infected individuals with administration of 10 mg/kg andrographolide dose. No significant changes were seen in mean plasma HIV-1 RNA levels throughout the trial. It was reported that if the actions of andrographolide allow for the appropriate progress of HIV-1 infected lymphocytes through the cell cycle, this may play a role in inhibiting or reversing the decline of the CD4+ population in HIV infection. Andrographolide sulfonate, a sulfonation derivative of andrographolide, is widely used in Chinese traditional medicine for effective management of inflammatory/infectious diseases. Another clinical study which compared conventional therapy for hand foot mouth therapy with a combination of andrographolide sulfonate with conventional therapy have reported that the latter showed the latter group showed comparatively good clinical efficacy. *In vitro* analysis showed that andrographolide sulfonate inhibited LPS-stimulated neutrophil activation, inferred by a decrease in production of reactive oxygen species and cytokines. The clinical efficacy of andrographolide sulfonate against HFMD may be due to its ability to inhibit neutrophil activation, indicating its role as a clinical immune cell modulator. Multiple clinical trials on andrographolide in patients with multiple sclerosis, cancer, and bronchitis could be found in different clinical trial registries [33 - 37].

Curcuma longa L.

Curcuma longa, also known as "Indian saffron" is a spice plant cultivated mainly in southeast Asian countries. Traditional medicine uses its rhizome as a safe and active medicine in treatment of various chronic diseases. Curcumin is a potent phytocompound in *C.longa* explored much experimentally for its diverse biological actions. Curcumin is basically a polyphenolic compound with three molecules, together called curcuminoids. It is represented by curcumin (60-70%), followed by demethoxycurcumin (20-27%) and bisdemethoxycurcumin (10-15%). Immunomodulatory activity of curcumin is mostly immunosuppressive, but in certain studies, immunostimulant effects are also reported. It can impact a diverse range of molecular targets and selectively modulate multiple cell signaling pathways linked to different chronic diseases. Curcumins immunomodulatory activity is by means of its interaction with various immune mediators, including B and T lymphocytes, macrophages, DCs, cytokines, transcription factors with their downstream signalling pathways. Cytokines like B lymphocyte stimulator (BLYS) trigger the B cell proliferation and autoantibody secretion in autoimmune conditions. Curcumin has been suggested to serve as a good therapeutic agent in management of such diseases, as this can inhibit the BLYS expression. This inhibitory effect is indirectly due to the reduction in nuclear factor kappa B (NF-κB) activity, further resulted in the inhibition of DNA binding capacity of NF- κB and nuclear translocation of p65. Curcumin also exerts an inhibitory effect on DC maturation in a dose-dependant manner, comparable to the activity of immunomodulatory drugs like IL-10, TGF-β, corticosteroids, cyclosporine,1,25-dihydroxyvitamin D_3 and aspirin. This inhibitory effect on DC maturation is associated with suppressed activation of MAPKs (Mitogen-Activated Protein Kinase) and NF-κB. Imbalance in functions is commonly found in autoimmune conditions. In various experimental models (*in vitro/ in vivo*) curcumin has been found as an effective therapeutic agent for the management of autoimmune conditions like Systemic lupus erythematosus, as it can modulate and restore the functions of imbalanced T-helper cell subsets (Th1/Th17), regulatory T cells (Tregs) and DCs. DCs play a crucial role in the initiation of hypersensitivity and autoimmunity. Curcumin can inhibit the maturation and function of murine bone marrow-derived DCs (BMDCs) by reducing the expression of CD80, CD86, and MHC-II molecules. Under the influence of curcumin, phenotypic maturation and modulation of the cytokine production of BMDC happens, which results in the inhibition of Th1 development. Curcumin is reported to enhance the number and function of Treg cells through upregulation of Foxp3 and CD69 and suppress the differentiation of Treg cells into Th17 cells. Th17 cell responses are further reduced by inhibition of cell proliferation and functioning of relevant inflammatory cytokines and transcription factors. The immunomodulatory action of curcumin has exhibited a protective effect in large number of chronic inflammatory conditions including inflammatory bowel diseases and psoriasis [38 - 42].

Safety and efficacy of curcumin are well established in healthy volunteers. But in spite of this, poor pharmacological properties of curcumin in terms of its limited aqueous solubility and poor oral bioavailability have posed many hindrances to its therapeutic applicability. Coupling with bioenhancers like piperine, extracted from black pepper has been reported to increase the bioavailability of curcumin by 2000%. New research development in terms of nanotechnology based delivery systems of curcumin has also shown to induce higher humoral immune response compared with the free curcumin in animal models, by means of its higher bioavailability and controlled release [43, 44]. Large number of clinical trials are reported on the immunomodulatory potential of curcumin on diseases like cancer (colorectal cancer, pancreatic cancer, breast cancer, prostate cancer, multiple myeloma, lung cancer, oral cancer, and head and neck squamous cell carcinoma), rheumatoid arthritis and inflammatory bowel diseases (Ulcerative colitis and Crohn's disease) [4, 45].

Zingiber officinale Roscoe

Ginger (*Zingiber officinale* Roscoe) is a commonly consumed spice in the world and is also used as a medicinal plant in traditional medicine. The oleoresin from the rhizomes of ginger contains many bioactive components which exert a variety of remarkable pharmacological and physiological activities. Zingerone, gingerols, paradol and shogaols are the major constituents of ginger. Gingerols are the major constituents, found slightly higher in fresh forms of ginger than in dried one, but higher concentration of Shogaols is reported in dried ginger. Among all [6]-gingerol(6G) is the most abundant active constituent in ginger with diverse biological activities. Experimental studies have found 6G as an effective adjunct anti-mycobacterial and immunomodulatory drug for the treatment of drug-susceptible and drug-resistant strains of tuberculosis. Decreased survival of mycobacteria was found in mouse peritoneal macrophages and mouse model of TB infection after treatment with 6G as compared to untreated controls. 6G significantly induced the number of antigen-presenting cells like macrophages and dendritic cells, which are required for the activation of adaptive immunity. Enhanced Th1/Th17 immune response was also seen in the spleens of infected mice treated with 6G as compared to the untreated counterparts, resulting in reduction of bacillary load in the lungs and spleen of the mice. 6G treatment also exhibited *Mycobacterium tuberculosis* (Mtb) specific nature of immune responses, as confirmed by adoptive transfer experiments. 6G treatment induced Mtb specific host protective IFN–γ and IL-17, which thereby produced more CD4+ and CD8+ T cells by inhibiting the other T cell subsets which are associated with disease progression. Anti-bacterial and immunomodulatory effects of 6G are developed from its ability to influence intracellular signalling in host macrophages [46, 47].

6G shows good larvicidal activity against *Echinococcus granulosus* and is reported to be useful in the treatment of human hydatidosis due to its immunomodulatory potential. Protoscoleces (PSC) are targets which can easily be attacked by host immune mechanisms to kill the parasite. 6G significantly killed PSC *in vitro* both in culture and coculture, prepared from the hydatid cyst removed surgically from lungs and liver of patients. Pro-inflammatory cytokine (IFN-γ) and inducible nitric oxide (iNOS) pathways are involved in the protective mechanism against *E.granulosus*. 6G could reduce the production of inflammatory mediators like nitric oxide (NO) by host mononuclear cells in response to parasitic infection. Vitality and viability of PSC and NO production could be directly influenced by 6G, thereby protecting the vital functions of infected organs through its immunomodulatory. This active component in ginger has shown to selectively inhibit the lymphokine production in lipopolysaccharide stimulated macrophages in animal models. It was found useful to treat inflammation without interfering with the antigen presenting function of macrophages. 6G have been studied in various *in vitro, in vivo* models of carcinogenesis, also tested in early phase human clinical trials and is found to exhibit antiproliferative, antitumor, anti-invasive and anti-inflammatory effects in chronic diseases and carcinoma. It is also reported to induce apoptosis in prostate cancer cell lines. Another compound 6-shogaol has also shown anticancer activities against breast cancer *via* inhibition of cell invasion reduction of matrix metalloproteinase-9 expression [48 - 51].

Allium sativum L.

Garlic (*Allium sativum* L.) has long been used in traditional medicine worldwide for its wide spectrum of pharmacological activities. The bio active compounds in garlic bulb are mainly of two categories, the non-volatile sulfur containing precursors in intact garlic and the second group of organosulfur compounds, which are generated during the process of garlic product preparation. The major non-volatile sulfur containing compound is alliin, which is also the precursor of compounds like allicin, methiin, and cycloalliin. Allicin (diallyl thiosulfinate or diallyl disulfide) is found in garlic only when it is crushed, cut, chewed, dehydrated, pulverized, or exposed to water. These processes activate the enzyme alliinase in it to metabolize alliin to allicin. Several of these garlic compounds were reported to be efficient in producing modulation of immune responses in various experimental models [52].

Aged garlic extract has been reported to show more immunomodulatory response than fresh ones, mainly due to transformation of organosulfur compounds in it. Two major proteins, garlic agglutinins (ASA I and II), isolated from aged garlic extract, also displayed good immunomodulatory potential as confirmed by specific hemagglutination and mannose-binding activities. Fructan, a fructooligosaccharide found in aged garlic extract, has also been reported to promote its immunomodulatory response. Both high molecular weight and low molecular weight fructans isolated from aged garlic, showed significant immunomodulatory effects on responder cells like murine lymphocytes, and peritoneal exudates cells *in vitro*. It also displayed mitogenic activity and activation of macrophages including phagocytosis, comparable to known polysaccharide immunomodulators such as zymosan and mannan. Aged garlic fructans have also been reported to show immunoadjuvant activity for the humoral immune response of a weak antigen (OVA) in BALB/c mice [53, 54, 55, 56].

Diallyl sulphide (DAS), another flavor compound isolated from garlic, could diminish the *Porphyromonas gingivalis* lipopolysaccharide-stimulated proinflammatory cytokine expression and the NF-kB activation in human gingival fibroblasts. It was also found beneficial in inhibiting the TNF-α and histamine induced inflammation in rat smooth muscle thoracic aorta A7r5 cell lines. DAS could block the nuclear accumulation of phospho-p65 protein in TNF-α induced A7r5 cells by attenuating the TNF-α receptor complex by inducing the dissociation of TNF receptor-associated death domain and TNF receptor-associated factor 2. DAS also inhibited histamine-induced inflammation by decreasing the level of reactive oxygen species (ROS) formation by enhancing the nuclear factor-erythroid 2 -related antioxidative enzyme. Moreover, it suppressed the expression of IL-1 and TNF-α mRNAs by inhibiting the ROS-induced PI3K/Akt pathway and downstream NF-kB and AP-1 proteins [57, 58].

Alliin is reported to exert a significant effect on the immune response functions of certain peripheral blood cells. Increase in pokeweed mitogen induced cell proliferation, spontaneous production of IL-1b, as well as an increase in both a number of phagocytic cells and latex particles engulfed by each individual cell were the noticeable effects of alliin on these cells. Another *in vitro* study reported alliin could control the inflammatory state of adipocytes by decreasing IL-6 and monocyte chemoattractant protein 1(MCP-1) expressions (both at mRNA and protein levels), as well as diminish extracellular signal regulated kinase (ERK)1/2 phosphorylation in LPS-stimulated 3T3-L1 adipocytes by modifying their metabolic profile. It could also modify the mRNA expression of genes involved in phospholipid and organophosphate metabolic processes, in positive regulation of the related immune process (expressing immunoglobulin (Ig) and in T-cell receptor-related genes) [59, 60].

Allicin had shown a protective effect on immune-mediated, concanavalin A (Con A) induced hepatitis in mice. It could down-regulate the production of tumor necrosis factor (TNF-α) by T lymphocytes and macrophages, thereby reducing hepatic inflammation. Migration of CD4+ T lymphocytes from blood vessels and penetration of the subendothelial extracellular matrix was also inhibited. Allicin also inhibited TNF-α mediated T cells adhesion to the extracellular matrix and endothelial cells and attenuate the intercellular adhesion molecule-1 (ICAM-1) and vascular cell adhesion molecule-1 (VCAM-1) expression in endothelial cells. Allicin is reported to exert an immune modulatory effect on intestinal epithelial cells. It could suppress both the spontaneous and TNF- α -stimulated secretion of the chemokines IL-8, MIG and IP-10, as well as the secretion of IL-1b from intestinal epithelial cells. This hints at the further need of exploring immunomodulatory potential of allicin in various intestinal inflammatory diseases. Allicin was found partially effective in protecting the host against *Plasmodium yoelii*17XL through enhancement of innate and adaptive immune responses in rodent malaria model. The effect was due to the ability of allicin to enhance the pro-inflammatory immune response exhibited by the expansion of the populations of CD4+T cells, DCs and macrophages, as well as stimulation of DC maturation [61 - 63]. Many clinical trials have been conducted on allicin and allicin containing compounds for evaluating its therapeutic efficacy as confirmed from various pre-clinical studies. Instability of the compound allicin is one of the factors that have limited the progress of clinical studies and their respective applications. More research needs to be focused on developing techniques which can effectively deliver allicin to attain maximum therapeutic benefit [64].

Terminalia chebula Retz.

Terminalia chebula (Myrobalan) is a medicinal tree used in the traditional medicinal system, with well-documented history of safe and effective usage in the treatment of different diseases. Fruit rind is the most medicinally used part of this tree, as it contains the maximum therapeutically active constituents. Phytocompounds like gallic acid (GA) and chebulagic acid (CA) isolated from fruits of *T. chebula* were reported long back to possess immunomodulatory action as they inhibited the cytotoxic T cell mediated cytotoxicity in *in vitro* models [65]. Chebulagic acid could significantly suppress the onset and progression of collagen induced arthritis (CIA-experimental model of inflammatory joint disease that resembles the human disease rheumatoid arthritis) in mice. CD4+, CD25+ T cells which can control the disease progression in arthritis by inhibiting the functions of other pathogenic activated T cells, granulocytes, and macrophages. CA could exert immunosuppressive activity by induction of TNF- β, CD4+, CD25+ T cells in the knee joints of mice with CIA and thereby arrest the disease progression [66]. CA could exhibit potent anti-inflammatory effects due to its ability to inhibit LPS induced gene expression (TNF-a, IL-6, iNOS, 5-LOX and COX-2) in RAW 264.7 macrophages. Suppression of NF-κB activation and phosphorylation of mitogen activated protein kinases by CA facilitated this effect [67]. Phenolic compounds like Chebulinic acid and ellagic acid isolated from *T. chebula* extract showed considerable growth inhibition when tested on human sarcoma cell line through ATP assay [68].

GA has shown immunomodulatory effect against cyclophosphamide and cisplatin-induced myelosuppression in Swiss albino mice. Pre-treatment with gallic acid could reduce the immune suppression induced by the two cytotoxic drugs in mice. GA also facilitated the development of humoral immune response by improving the antibody titer. GA could significantly increase the weight of thymus a primary lymphoid organ responsible for initiating adaptive immune responses [69]. GA and ellagic acid (EA) have been reported to exhibit antileishmanial activity *in vitro* due to their high immunomodulatory potential. High immunomodulatory activity of both the compounds was evidenced by the increase in phagocytic capability, lysosomal volume, nitrite release, and intracellular calcium in murine macrophages [70]. A number of gallic acid derivatives have already been synthesized and are found to act as antimalarial and anti-cancerous compounds. Quantitative structure–activity relationship (QSAR), molecular docking studies could predict the immunomodulatory potential of these derivatives in terms of its high binding affinities with INFα-2, IL-4, and IL-6 [71].

Triphala is an important compound drug used in Indian traditional medicine, prepared by mixing dried fruit powder of *Terminalia chebula, Terminalia bellerica* and *Phyllanthus emblica* in the ratio of 1:1:1. Immunomodulatory activities are reported on *Triphala* and also its individual constituents (Chebulagic acid (CA), Chebulinic acid (CI) and Gallic acid (GA)), isolated from its fruit powder. CA, CI and GA inhibited the TNFα mediated angiogenesis and inflammation in the RF/6A cells, a microvascular endothelial cell line established from the choroid-retinal plexus of rhesus monkey foetus. The pro-angiogenic and pro-inflammatory activities in retinal capillary endothelial cells were exhibited by inhibition p38, ERK and NFkB phosphorylation by these compounds [72].

Piper longum L.

Piper longum commonly known as long pepper, is an important medicinal plant used in various systems of medicine. Fruit is the main useful part, but its roots are also mentioned as useful in traditional systems like Ayurveda. The fruit contains large number of alkaloids, the most abundant of which is piperine. It is also present in fruits of other species of piper genus like *Piper nigrum* (black pepper). Piperine influenced both humoral and cell-mediated immune responses in Balb/c mice. Piperine exerted a stimulatory effect on the humoral arm of immune system by increasing the circulating antibody titer and antibody forming cells. It could also affect stem cell proliferation by increasing the bone marrow cellularity and α-esterase positive cells. In *in vitro* models, it showed significant anti tumor activity by inhibiting the growth of solid tumor induced by Dalton's lymphoma ascites cells and ascites tumor induced by Ehrlich ascites carcinoma cells. Piperine displayed considerable immune-protective activity against cadmium induced suppressed immune activity and apoptosis in mice. Cadmium being a potent immune-toxicant, affects both humoral and cell mediated immunity, marked thymic atrophy and splenomegaly in rodents. Piperine supplementation could restore the apoptotic and necrotic cells of lymphoid organs in animal models. Pentacyclic oxindole group present in piperine is considered as the active molecule responsible for its immunomodulation activity. Another study comparing herbal compounds piperine, curcumin and picroliv found that, these compounds exert immunomodulatory activity through their multi-faceted activities such as anti-oxidative, anti-apoptotic and restorative ability against cell proliferative mitogenic response, thymic and splenic cell population and cytokine release. Maximum ameliorative response was shown by piperine in comparison to others, suggesting it to be an ideal drug of choice in immuno-compromised conditions. Piperine also showed anti-oxidative, anti-apoptotic and chemo-protective ability in Deltamethrin (DLM) induced thymic apoptosis. In molecular docking study, piperine could regulate various cellular events, as it could bind to the same active site where DLM binds with CD4 and CD8 receptors. It could also regulate the DLM induced oxidant anti-oxidant imbalance in murine thymocytes which resulted in oxidative stress in both *in vitro* and *in vivo* models. Internal administration of piperine decreased the extent of lipid peroxidation and increased the activities of enzymatic antioxidants (superoxide dismutase, catalase and glutathione peroxidase and non-enzymatic antioxidants (reduced glutathione, vitamin E and vitamin C) levels in Swiss albino mice. Piperine also caused a significant reduction in the caspase 3 (key mediators of apoptosis in the immune system) activity, which was induced by DLM [73 - 78].

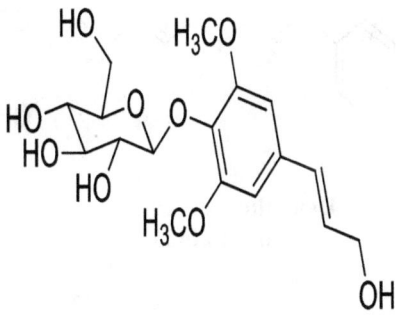

Syringin

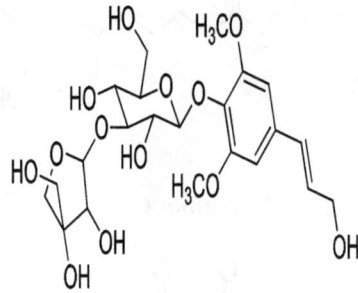

Cordifolioside A

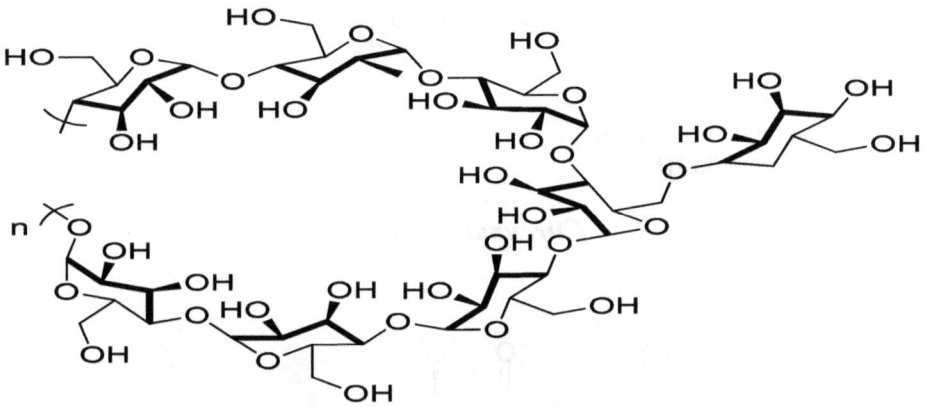

RR1

Tinospora cordifolia

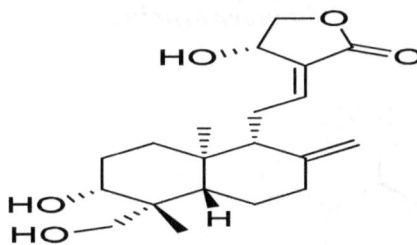

Andrographolide

(Fig. 2) contd.....

Andrographis paniculata

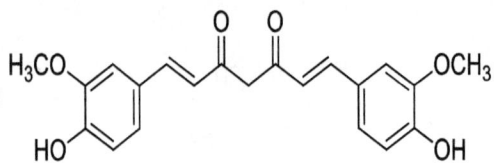 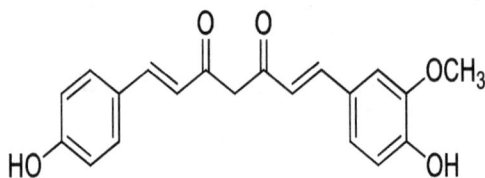

Curcumin I   **Demethoxycurcumin**
                                            Curcumin II

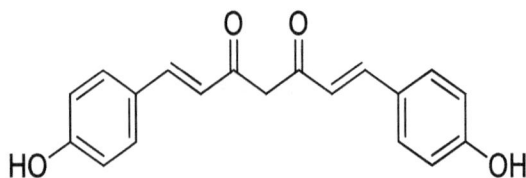 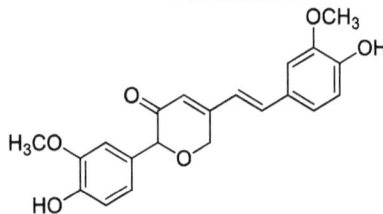

Bis-demethoxycurcumin   **Cyclocurcumin**
Curcumin III   **Curcumin IV**

Curcuma longa

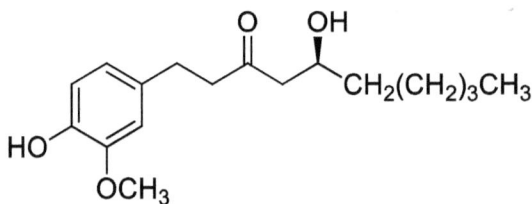

6-Gingerol

Zingiber officinale

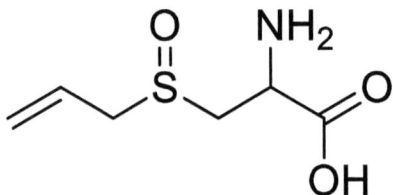 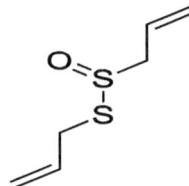

Alliin   **Allicin**

(Fig. 2) contd.....

Allium sativum

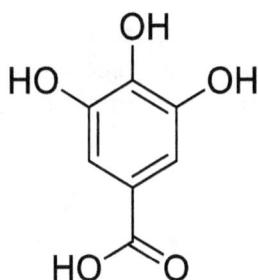

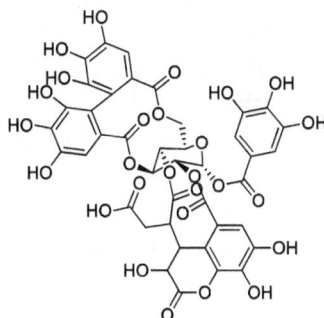

Gallic acid   Chebulagic acid

Terminalia chebula

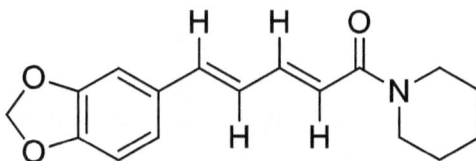

Piperine

Piper longum

Fig. (2). Immunomodulatory compounds of selected Ayurvedic Plants.

Piperine displayed protective activity against OVA induced allergic rhinitis in animal models by its potential to stabilize the mast cells and thereby inhibiting the release of mediators like histamine, IL-6, IL-1β, and IgE in serum [79]. Piperine at the dose of 15 μM could inhibit the B cells proliferation and thereby inhibit the secretion IgM antibody by murine B spleen cell *in vitro*. It could also decrease the cultured CD11c+ dendritic cells CD86, CD40 and MHC-II expression in a dose-dependent manner. But piperine was unable to modify *in vivo* thymus independent antigen induced antibody response [80]. Another piperine analogue butyl 4-(4-nitrobenzoate)-piperinoate (DE-07) displayed antitumor effect *via* oxidative and antiangiogenic actions. It also modulated the inflammatory response in the tumor microenvironment by inducing an increase on IL-1β and TNF-α levels, which might have regulated the generation of ROS and antiangiogenic effect. In animal models piperine also showed protective role against LPS induced mastitis by inhibiting the infiltration of neutrophils into mammary tissues and blocking inflammatory cytokine production. The activity was mediated through its potential of activating peroxisome proliferator activated receptor (PPARγ) and inhibiting the NF-KB signaling pathway [81]. Various clinical trials have been reported on piperine in digestive tract pathologies and skin diseases like vitiligo. Even though anti-tumour potential has been reported on piperine due to its apoptotic activity, no clinical study has been carried out on the same till date. Fixing safe therapeutic dose of pure piperine has been another hurdle, as in higher doses, it has been reported to have some negative effects on the liver and male fertility [82, 83, 84].

CONCLUDING REMARKS

Indian traditional medicine has a practice of using whole plant extract to stimulate immunomodulation, in which different contents of plant act synergistically to produce that therapeutic action. This might have been one of the factors which ensured safety of these drugs, as toxicity and therapeutic activity of individual constituents might have been balanced/modulated by others. But complexity of the chemical constituents in whole plant has made the full characterization and quality control of the crude extracts a difficult task. Hence identification, isolation, characterization and evaluation of therapeutic potentials of phytocompounds behind specific bioactivity became an important area of pharmaceutical research. This chapter highlights the immunomodulatory activities reported on Indian medicinal plant-based biomolecules of very varied chemistries for potential use in improving human health. Although significant immunomodulatory potential has been reported on phytocompounds isolated from these medicinal plants, many of them face constraints on clinical usage due to less bioavailability and non-fixation of safe therapeutic dosage to produce efficacy. Novel drug delivery systems, chemical modulation of the compounds, and techniques of mixing other compounds showing synergistic effect in fixed proportion may be developed for attaining desired therapeutic efficacy. Discovery of plant based immunomodulators devoid of toxic side effects and enhanced bioavailability can be a safer choice for long term administration.

CONSENT FOR PUBLICATION

Not applicable.

CONFLICT OF INTEREST

The authors declare no conflict of interest, financial or otherwise.

ACKNOWLEDGEMENTS

The authors are thankful to Dr. N. Srikanth, Director General, Central Council for Research in Ayurvedic Sciences, Ministry of AYUSH, Government of India, Dr. Deepak Bhatnagar, Professor and Head, School of Biochemistry, Devi Ahilya University, Indore, Dr. P.V.V. Prasad, Director, Central Ayurveda Research Institute, Kolkata and Dr. D. Sudhakar, Director, National Ayurveda Research Institute for Panchakarma, Kerala for their support, motivation and encouragement.

REFERENCES

[1]   MacGillivray DM, Kollmann TR. The role of environmental factors in modulating immune responses in early life. Front Immunol 2014; 5: 434.
[http://dx.doi.org/10.3389/fimmu.2014.00434] [PMID: 25309535]

[2]   Bascones-Martinez A, Mattila R, Gomez-Font R, Meurman JH. Immunomodulatory drugs: Oral and systemic adverse effects. Med Oral Patol Oral Cir Bucal 2014; 19(1): e24-31.
[http://dx.doi.org/10.4317/medoral.19087] [PMID: 23986016]

[3]   Lee SJ, Chinen J, Kavanaugh A, Diego S, Calif H. Immunomodulator therapy: Monoclonal antibodies, fusion proteins, cytokines, and immunoglobulins. J Allergy Clin Immunol 2010; 125(2) (Suppl. 2): S314-23.
[http://dx.doi.org/10.1016/j.jaci.2009.08.018] [PMID: 20036416]

[4]   Jantan I, Ahmad W, Bukhari SNA. Plant-derived immunomodulators: an insight on their preclinical evaluation and clinical trials. Front Plant Sci 2015; 6: 655.
[http://dx.doi.org/10.3389/fpls.2015.00655] [PMID: 26379683]

[5]   Behl T, Kumar K, Brisc C, *et al.* Exploring the multifocal role of phytochemicals as immunomodulators. Biomed Pharmacother 2021; 133: 110959.
[http://dx.doi.org/10.1016/j.biopha.2020.110959] [PMID: 33197758]

[6]   Nicholson LB. The immune system. Essays Biochem 2016; 60(3): 275-301.
[http://dx.doi.org/10.1042/EBC20160017] [PMID: 27784777]

[7]   Charles A, Janeway J, Travers P, Walport M, Shlomchik MJ. The components of the immune systemImmunobiology Immune System Health Diseases. 5th ed., New York: Garland Science 2001.https://www.ncbi.nlm.nih.gov/books/NBK27092/

[8]   Marshall JS, Warrington R, Watson W, Kim HL. An introduction to immunology and immunopathology. Allergy Asthma Clin Immunol 2018; 14(S2) (Suppl. 2): 49.
[http://dx.doi.org/10.1186/s13223-018-0278-1] [PMID: 30263032]

[9]   Medina KL. Overview of the immune system. Handb Clin Neurol 2016; 133: 61-76.
[http://dx.doi.org/10.1016/B978-0-444-63432-0.00004-9] [PMID: 27112671]

[10]   Nair A, Chattopadhyay D, Saha B. Plant-Derived Immunomodulators New Look to Phytomedicine: Advancements in Herbal Products as Novel Drug Leads. Elsevier Inc. 2018; pp. 435-99.
[http://dx.doi.org/10.1016/B978-0-12-814619-4.00018-5]

[11]   Grigore A. Plant Phenolic Compounds as Immunomodulatory Agents. Phenolic Compounds Biological Activity. InTech 2017.

[http://dx.doi.org/10.5772/66112]

[12]   Balasubramani SP, Venkatasubramanian P, Kukkupuni SK, Patwardhan B. Plant-based Rasayana drugs from Ayurveda. Chin J Integr Med 2011; 17(2): 88-94.
[http://dx.doi.org/10.1007/s11655-011-0659-5] [PMID: 21390573]

[13]   Dahanukar SA, Thatte UM, Rege NN. Immunostimulants in Ayurveda. Basel: Birkhäuser Basel 1999; pp. 289-323.
[http://dx.doi.org/10.1007/978-3-0348-8763-2_12]

[14]   Mahesh TS, Shreevidya M. A review on balya action mentioned in Ayurveda. J Ayurveda Integr Med 2014; 5(2): 80-4.
[http://dx.doi.org/10.4103/0975-9476.133796] [PMID: 24948857]

[15]   Doshi G, Une H, Shanbhag P. Rasayans and non-rasayans herbs: Future immunodrug - Targets. Pharmacogn Rev 2013; 7(14): 92-6.
[http://dx.doi.org/10.4103/0973-7847.120506] [PMID: 24347916]

[16]   Nishteswar K. Pharmacological expression of *Rasayanakarma*. Ayu 2013; 34(4): 337-8.
[http://dx.doi.org/10.4103/0974-8520.127672] [PMID: 24696568]

[17]   Agnivesha. Charaka samhita with Ayurveda deepika commentry. In: Trikamji Yadavji, editor. Reprint ed, Varanasi: Choukambha prakashan; 2013.

[18]   Wagner H. Leading structures of plant origin for drug development. J Ethnopharmacol 1993; 38(2-3): 93-104.
[http://dx.doi.org/10.1016/0378-8741(93)90004-O] [PMID: 8510457]

[19]   Kayser O, Masihi KN, Kiderlen AF. Natural products and synthetic compounds as immunomodulators. Expert Rev Anti Infect Ther 2003; 1(2): 319-35.
[http://dx.doi.org/10.1586/14787210.1.2.319] [PMID: 15482127]

[20]   Raveendran Nair PK, Rodriguez S, Ramachandran R, *et al.* Immune stimulating properties of a novel polysaccharide from the medicinal plant *Tinospora cordifolia*. Int Immunopharmacol 2004; 4(13): 1645-59.
[http://dx.doi.org/10.1016/j.intimp.2004.07.024] [PMID: 15454117]

[21]   Sharma U, Bala M, Kumar N, Singh B, Munshi RK, Bhalerao S. Immunomodulatory active compounds from *Tinospora cordifolia*. J Ethnopharmacol 2012; 141(3): 918-26.
[http://dx.doi.org/10.1016/j.jep.2012.03.027] [PMID: 22472109]

[22]   Singh D, Chaudhuri PK. Chemistry and Pharmacology of *Tinospora cordifolia*. Nat Prod Commun 2017;12:1934578X1701200.
[http://dx.doi.org/10.1177/1934578X1701200240]

[23]   Aranha I, Clement F, Venkatesh YP. Immunostimulatory properties of the major protein from the stem of the Ayurvedic medicinal herb, guduchi (*Tinospora cordifolia*). J Ethnopharmacol 2012; 139(2): 366-72.
[http://dx.doi.org/10.1016/j.jep.2011.11.013] [PMID: 22119223]

[24]   Bala M, Pratap K, Verma PK, Singh B, Padwad Y. Validation of ethnomedicinal potential of *Tinospora cordifolia* for anticancer and immunomodulatory activities and quantification of bioactive molecules by HPTLC. J Ethnopharmacol 2015; 175: 131-7.
[http://dx.doi.org/10.1016/j.jep.2015.08.001] [PMID: 26253577]

[25]   Aranha I, Venkatesh YP. Humoral immune and adjuvant responses of mucosally-administered *Tinospora cordifolia* immunomodulatory protein in BALB/c mice. J Ayurveda Integr Med 2020; 11(2): 140-6.
[http://dx.doi.org/10.1016/j.jaim.2017.10.006] [PMID: 30455069]

[26]   Li H, Li XL, Zhang M, *et al.* Berberine ameliorates experimental autoimmune neuritis by suppressing both cellular and humoral immunity. Scand J Immunol 2014; 79(1): 12-9.
[http://dx.doi.org/10.1111/sji.12123] [PMID: 24354407]

[27]   Hu Z, Jiao Q, Ding J, *et al.* Berberine induces dendritic cell apoptosis and has therapeutic potential for rheumatoid arthritis. Arthritis Rheum 2011; 63(4): 949-59.
[http://dx.doi.org/10.1002/art.30202] [PMID: 21162100]

[28]   Manne M, Goudar G, Varikasuvu SR, Khetagoudar MC, Kanipakam H, Natarajan P, *et al.* Cordifolioside: potent inhibitor against Mpro of SARS-CoV-2 and immunomodulatory through human TGF-β and TNF-α. 3 Biotech 2021; 11: 136.
[http://dx.doi.org/10.1007/s13205-021-02685-z]

[29]   Ajaya Kumar R, Sridevi K, Vijaya Kumar N, Nanduri S, Rajagopal S. Anticancer and immunostimulatory compounds from *Andrographis paniculata*. J Ethnopharmacol 2004; 92(2-3): 291-5.
[http://dx.doi.org/10.1016/j.jep.2004.03.004] [PMID: 15138014]

[30]   Puri A, Saxena R, Saxena RP, Saxena KC, Srivastava V, Tandon JS. Immunostimulant agents from *Andrographis paniculata*. J Nat Prod 1993; 56(7): 995-9.
[http://dx.doi.org/10.1021/np50097a002] [PMID: 8377022]

[31]   Iruretagoyena MI, Tobar JA, González PA, *et al.* Andrographolide interferes with T cell activation and reduces experimental autoimmune encephalomyelitis in the mouse. J Pharmacol Exp Ther 2005; 312(1): 366-72.
[http://dx.doi.org/10.1124/jpet.104.072512] [PMID: 15331658]

[32]   Qin LH, Kong L, Shi GJ, Wang ZT, Ge BX. Andrographolide inhibits the production of TNF-alpha and interleukin-12 in lipopolysaccharide-stimulated macrophages: role of mitogen-activated protein kinases. Biol Pharm Bull 2006; 29(2): 220-4.
[http://dx.doi.org/10.1248/bpb.29.220] [PMID: 16462022]

[33]   Calabrese C, Berman SH, Babish JG, *et al.* A phase I trial of andrographolide in HIV positive patients and normal volunteers. Phytother Res 2000; 14(5): 333-8.
[http://dx.doi.org/10.1002/1099-1573(200008)14:5<333::AID-PTR584>3.0.CO;2-D]   [PMID: 10925397]

[34]   Zhao Y, Huang P, Chen Z. Zheng S wei, Yu J yang, Shi C. Clinical application analysis of andrographolide. Med Sci 2017; 37: 293-9.
[http://dx.doi.org/10.1007/s11596-017-1730-z] [PMID: 28397057]

[35]   Wen T, Xu W, Liang L, *et al.* Clinical Efficacy of Andrographolide Sulfonate in the Treatment of Severe Hand, Foot, and Mouth Disease (HFMD) is Dependent upon Inhibition of Neutrophil Activation. Phytother Res 2015; 29(8): 1161-7.
[http://dx.doi.org/10.1002/ptr.5361] [PMID: 25960284]

[36]   https://clinicaltrials.gov/ct2/show/NCT03132623

[37]   https://www.centerwatch.com/clinical-trials/listings/117468/acute-exacerbation-of-chronic-bronc-itis-study-andrographolide n.d.

[38]   Catanzaro M, Corsini E, Rosini M, Racchi M, Lanni C. Immunomodulators inspired by nature: A review on curcumin. Molecules 2018; 23(11): 2778.
[http://dx.doi.org/10.3390/molecules23112778] [PMID: 30373170]

[39]   Kunnumakkara AB, Bordoloi D, Padmavathi G, *et al.* Curcumin, the golden nutraceutical: multitargeting for multiple chronic diseases. Br J Pharmacol 2017; 174(11): 1325-48.
[http://dx.doi.org/10.1111/bph.13621] [PMID: 27638428]

[40]   Kim GY, Kim KH, Lee SH, *et al.* Curcumin inhibits immunostimulatory function of dendritic cells: MAPKs and translocation of NF-kappa B as potential targets. J Immunol 2005; 174(12): 8116-24.
[http://dx.doi.org/10.4049/jimmunol.174.12.8116] [PMID: 15944320]

[41]   Momtazi-Borojeni AA, Haftcheshmeh SM, Esmaeili SA, Johnston TP, Abdollahi E, Sahebkar A. Curcumin: A natural modulator of immune cells in systemic lupus erythematosus. Autoimmun Rev 2018; 17(2): 125-35.

[http://dx.doi.org/10.1016/j.autrev.2017.11.016] [PMID: 29180127]

[42]   Srivastava RM, Singh S, Dubey SK, Misra K, Khar A. Immunomodulatory and therapeutic activity of curcumin. Int Immunopharmacol 2011; 11(3): 331-41.
[http://dx.doi.org/10.1016/j.intimp.2010.08.014] [PMID: 20828642]

[43]   Hewlings S, Kalman D. Curcumin. Foods 2017; 6(10): 92.
[http://dx.doi.org/10.3390/foods6100092] [PMID: 29065496]

[44]   Afolayan FID, Erinwusi B, Oyeyemi OT. Immunomodulatory activity of curcumin-entrapped poly d,l -lactic- *co* -glycolic acid nanoparticles in mice. Integr Med Res 2018; 7(2): 168-75.
[http://dx.doi.org/10.1016/j.imr.2018.02.004] [PMID: 29989030]

[45]   Gupta SC, Patchva S, Aggarwal BB. Therapeutic roles of curcumin: lessons learned from clinical trials. AAPS J 2013; 15(1): 195-218.
[http://dx.doi.org/10.1208/s12248-012-9432-8] [PMID: 23143785]

[46]   Bode AM, Dong Z. The amazing and mighty ginger Herb Med Biomol Clin Asp. 2nd ed. CRC Press 2011; pp. 131-56.
[http://dx.doi.org/10.1201/b10787-8]

[47]   Bhaskar A, Kumari A, Singh M, *et al.* [6]-Gingerol exhibits potent anti-mycobacterial and immunomodulatory activity against tuberculosis. Int Immunopharmacol 2020; 87: 106809.
[http://dx.doi.org/10.1016/j.intimp.2020.106809] [PMID: 32693356]

[48]   Amri M, Touil-Boukoffa C. *In vitro* anti-hydatic and immunomodulatory effects of ginger and [6]-gingerol. Asian Pac J Trop Med 2016; 9(8): 749-56.
[http://dx.doi.org/10.1016/j.apjtm.2016.06.013] [PMID: 27569883]

[49]   Tripathi S, Maier KG, Bruch D, Kittur DS. Effect of 6-gingerol on pro-inflammatory cytokine production and costimulatory molecule expression in murine peritoneal macrophages. J Surg Res 2007; 138(2): 209-13.
[http://dx.doi.org/10.1016/j.jss.2006.07.051] [PMID: 17291534]

[50]   de Lima RMT, dos Reis AC, de Menezes AAPM, *et al.* Protective and therapeutic potential of ginger (*Zingiber officinale*) extract and [6]-gingerol in cancer: A comprehensive review. Phytother Res 2018; 32(10): 1885-907.
[http://dx.doi.org/10.1002/ptr.6134] [PMID: 30009484]

[51]   Rahmani AH, Shabrmi FM, Aly SM. Active ingredients of ginger as potential candidates in the prevention and treatment of diseases *via* modulation of biological activities. Int J Physiol Pathophysiol Pharmacol 2014; 6(2): 125-36.
[PMID: 25057339]

[52]   Moutia M, Habti N, Badou A. *In Vitro* and *In Vivo* Immunomodulator Activities of *Allium sativum* L. Evid Based Complement Alternat Med 2018; 2018: 1-10.
[http://dx.doi.org/10.1155/2018/4984659] [PMID: 30008785]

[53]   Mikaili P, Maadirad S, Moloudizargari M, Aghajanshakeri S, Sarahroodi S. Therapeutic uses and pharmacological properties of garlic, shallot, and their biologically active compounds. Iran J Basic Med Sci 2013; 16(10): 1031-48.
[http://dx.doi.org/10.22038/ijbms.2013.1865] [PMID: 24379960]

[54]   Chandrashekar PM, Venkatesh YP. Identification of the protein components displaying immunomodulatory activity in aged garlic extract. J Ethnopharmacol 2009; 124(3): 384-90.
[http://dx.doi.org/10.1016/j.jep.2009.05.030] [PMID: 19505565]

[55]   Chandrashekar PM, Prashanth KVH, Venkatesh YP. Isolation, structural elucidation and immunomodulatory activity of fructans from aged garlic extract. Phytochemistry 2011; 72(2-3): 255-64.
[http://dx.doi.org/10.1016/j.phytochem.2010.11.015] [PMID: 21168173]

[56]   Chandrashekar PM, Venkatesh YP. Fructans from aged garlic extract produce a delayed

immunoadjuvant response to ovalbumin antigen in BALB/c mice. Immunopharmacol Immunotoxicol 2012; 34(1): 174-80.
[http://dx.doi.org/10.3109/08923973.2011.584066] [PMID: 21631395]

[57]   Fu E, Tsai MC, Chin YT, *et al.* The effects of diallyl sulfide upon *Porphyromonas gingivalis* lipopolysaccharide stimulated proinflammatory cytokine expressions and nuclear factor-kappa B activation in human gingival fibroblasts. J Periodontal Res 2015; 50(3): 380-8.
[http://dx.doi.org/10.1111/jre.12217] [PMID: 25203776]

[58]   Ho CY, Weng CJ, Jhang JJ, Cheng YT, Huang SM, Yen GC. Diallyl sulfide as a potential dietary agent to reduce TNF-α- and histamine-induced proinflammatory responses in A7r5 cells. Mol Nutr Food Res 2014; 58(5): 1069-78.
[http://dx.doi.org/10.1002/mnfr.201300617] [PMID: 24415531]

[59]   Salman H, Bergman M, Bessler H, Punsky I, Djaldetti M. Effect of a garlic derivative (alliin) on peripheral blood cell immune responses. Int J Immunopharmacol 1999; 21(9): 589-97.
[http://dx.doi.org/10.1016/S0192-0561(99)00038-7] [PMID: 10501628]

[60]   Quintero-Fabián S, Ortuño-Sahagún D, Vázquez-Carrera M, López-Roa RI. Alliin, a garlic (*Allium sativum*) compound, prevents LPS-induced inflammation in 3T3-L1 adipocytes. Mediators Inflamm 2013; 2013(1): 1-11.
[http://dx.doi.org/10.1155/2013/381815] [PMID: 24453416]

[61]   Bruck R, Aeed H, Brazovsky E, Noor T, Hershkoviz R. Allicin, the active component of garlic, prevents immune-mediated, concanavalin A-induced hepatic injury in mice. Liver Int 2005; 25(3): 613-21.
[http://dx.doi.org/10.1111/j.1478-3231.2005.01050.x] [PMID: 15910499]

[62]   Lang A, Lahav M, Sakhnini E, *et al.* Allicin inhibits spontaneous and TNF-? induced secretion of proinflammatory cytokines and chemokines from intestinal epithelial cells. Clin Nutr 2004; 23(5): 1199-208.
[http://dx.doi.org/10.1016/j.clnu.2004.03.011] [PMID: 15380914]

[63]   Feng Y, Zhu X, Wang Q, *et al.* Allicin enhances host pro-inflammatory immune responses and protects against acute murine malaria infection. Malar J 2012; 11(1): 268.
[http://dx.doi.org/10.1186/1475-2875-11-268] [PMID: 22873687]

[64]   Sarnelli G, Annunziata G, Magno S, Oriolo C, Savastano S, Colao A. Taste and the Gastrointestinal tract: from physiology to potential therapeutic target for obesity. Int J Obes Suppl 2019; 9(1): 1-9.
[http://dx.doi.org/10.1038/s41367-019-0012-6] [PMID: 31391920]

[65]   Hamada S, Kataoka T, Woo JT, *et al.* Immunosuppressive effects of gallic acid and chebulagic acid on CTL-mediated cytotoxicity. Biol Pharm Bull 1997; 20(9): 1017-9.
[http://dx.doi.org/10.1248/bpb.20.1017] [PMID: 9331989]

[66]   Lee SI, Hyun PM, Kim SH, *et al.* Suppression of the onset and progression of collagen-induced arthritis by chebulagic acid screened from a natural product library. Arthritis Rheum 2005; 52(1): 345-53.
[http://dx.doi.org/10.1002/art.20715] [PMID: 15641090]

[67]   Reddy DB, Reddanna P. Chebulagic acid (CA) attenuates LPS-induced inflammation by suppressing NF-κB and MAPK activation in RAW 264.7 macrophages. Biochem Biophys Res Commun 2009; 381(1): 112-7.
[http://dx.doi.org/10.1016/j.bbrc.2009.02.022] [PMID: 19351605]

[68]   Saleem A, Husheem M, Härkönen P, Pihlaja K. Inhibition of cancer cell growth by crude extract and the phenolics of Terminalia chebula retz. fruit. J Ethnopharmacol 2002; 81(3): 327-36.
[http://dx.doi.org/10.1016/S0378-8741(02)00099-5] [PMID: 12127233]

[69]   Shruthi S, Vijayalaxmi KK, Shenoy KB. Immunomodulatory effects of gallic acid Indian J Pharm Sci 2018; 80: 150-60.
[http://dx.doi.org/10.4172/pharmaceutical]

[70] Alves MMM, Brito LM, Souza AC, *et al.* Gallic and ellagic acids: two natural immunomodulator compounds solve infection of macrophages by Leishmania major. Naunyn Schmiedebergs Arch Pharmacol 2017; 390(9): 893-903.
[http://dx.doi.org/10.1007/s00210-017-1387-y] [PMID: 28643086]

[71] Yadav DK, Khan F, Negi AS. Pharmacophore modeling, molecular docking, QSAR, and *in silico* ADMET studies of gallic acid derivatives for immunomodulatory activity. J Mol Model 2012; 18(6): 2513-25.
[http://dx.doi.org/10.1007/s00894-011-1265-3] [PMID: 22038459]

[72] Shanmuganathan S, Angayarkanni N. Chebulagic acid Chebulinic acid and Gallic acid, the active principles of Triphala, inhibit TNFα induced pro-angiogenic and pro-inflammatory activities in retinal capillary endothelial cells by inhibiting p38, ERK and NFkB phosphorylation. Vascul Pharmacol 2018; 108: 23-35.
[http://dx.doi.org/10.1016/j.vph.2018.04.005] [PMID: 29678603]

[73] Kumar S, Kamboj J, Suman , Sharma S. Overview for various aspects of the health benefits of Piper longum linn. fruit. J Acupunct Meridian Stud 2011; 4(2): 134-40.
[http://dx.doi.org/10.1016/S2005-2901(11)60020-4] [PMID: 21704957]

[74] Sunila ES, Kuttan G. Immunomodulatory and antitumor activity of Piper longum Linn. and piperine. J Ethnopharmacol 2004; 90(2-3): 339-46.
[http://dx.doi.org/10.1016/j.jep.2003.10.016] [PMID: 15013199]

[75] Pathak N, Khandelwal S. Immunomodulatory role of piperine in cadmium induced thymic atrophy and splenomegaly in mice. Environ Toxicol Pharmacol 2009; 28(1): 52-60.
[http://dx.doi.org/10.1016/j.etap.2009.02.003] [PMID: 21783982]

[76] Pathak N, Khandelwal S. Comparative efficacy of piperine, curcumin and picroliv against Cd immunotoxicity in mice. Biometals 2008; 21(6): 649-61.
[http://dx.doi.org/10.1007/s10534-008-9150-y] [PMID: 18566892]

[77] Kumar A, Sasmal D, Sharma N. Immunomodulatory role of piperine in deltamethrin induced thymic apoptosis and altered immune functions. Environ Toxicol Pharmacol 2015; 39(2): 504-14.
[http://dx.doi.org/10.1016/j.etap.2014.12.021] [PMID: 25682002]

[78] Kumar A, Sasmal D, Sharma N. Mechanism of deltamethrin induced thymic and splenic toxicity in mice and its protection by piperine and curcumin: *in vivo* study. Drug Chem Toxicol 2018; 41(1): 33-41.
[http://dx.doi.org/10.1080/01480545.2017.1286352] [PMID: 28633599]

[79] Aswar U, Shintre S, Chepurwar S, Aswar M. Antiallergic effect of piperine on ovalbumin-induced allergic rhinitis in mice. Pharm Biol 2015; 53(9): 1358-66.
[http://dx.doi.org/10.3109/13880209.2014.982299] [PMID: 25868617]

[80] Bernardo AR, Barbosa Da Rocha JD, Freire De Lima ME, Decote-Ricardo D, Pinto-Da-Silva LH, Torres Peçanha LM, *et al.* Modulating effect of the piperine, the main alkaloid from Piper nigrum Rev Bras Med Vet 2015; 37: 209-16.

[81] Yu S, Liu X, Yu D. E C, Yang J. Piperine. Int Immunopharmacol 2020; 87
[http://dx.doi.org/10.1016/j.intimp.2020.106804] [PMID: 32707496]

[82] Stojanović-Radić Z, Pejčić M, Dimitrijević M, Aleksić A, Anil Kumar NV, Salehi B, *et al.* Piperine. Appl Sci (Basel) 2019; 9: 1-29.
[http://dx.doi.org/10.3390/app9204270]

[83] Periyasamy L, Chinta G, Coumar MS. Reversible testicular toxicity of piperine on male albino rats. Pharmacogn Mag 2017; 13(51) (Suppl. 3): 525.
[http://dx.doi.org/10.4103/pm.pm_405_16] [PMID: 29142409]

[84] Chinta G, Janarthanan R, Jesthadi D, Shanmuganathan B, Periyasamy L. Effect of piperine on goat epididymal spermatozoa: an *in vitro* study. Asian J Pharm Clin Res 2014; 7: 57-61.

CHAPTER 13

Pharmacological Properties of Bacterial Bioactive Molecules

Pallavi Kaushik[1], Prachi Jain[1], Sneha Keelka[1] and Mukesh Kumar Sharma[2,*]

[1] *Department of Zoology, University of Rajasthan, Jaipur-302004; Rajasthan, India*

[2] *Department of Zoology, SPC Government College, Ajmer-305001; Rajasthan, India*

Abstract: The pure or standardized extracts obtained from microbes like bacteria, fungi, actinomycetes, *etc.* are considered important sources of bioactive compounds. Some of the microbes show inhibitory action against the growth of certain bacteria, fungi, yeast, insects, *etc.* This provides opportunities for the development of newer drugs and enzymes or beneficial compounds. Large number of bacteria are responsible for producing different bioactive compounds like antibiotics, enzymes, and other secondary metabolites. Some compounds like Gallic acid, Amicoumacin, Prodigiosin, Nystatin, Spinosad, Milbemycin, Lipstatin, Subtilin, Albaflavenone, and Mollemycin A have been studied for their affectivity against bacterial, fungal, insects, pests, *etc.* These compounds are gaining increasing interest because of their unique composition and the possibility of wide industrial applications.

Keywords: Microbes, Bioactive compounds, Bacteria, Pharmaceutical, Drugs, Gallic acid, Amicoumacin, Prodigiosin, Nystatin, Spinosad, Milbemycin, Lipstatin, Subtilin, Albaflavenone, Mollemycin A.

INTRODUCTION

Bacteria play significant role in the production of a variety of bioactive compounds like alkaloids, steroids, terpenoids, peptides, polyketones, flavonoids, quinols and phenols, and natural antibiotics [1]. These compounds enable the interaction of the parent microbe with other microbes and other non-microbial systems. In case of **microbes–microbes interaction,** these compounds are involved in activities like; antimicrobial antibiotics, microbial regulators, growth factors and signaling compounds. In **microbe-lower animals (Invertebrates) interaction** the role of these compounds are as; miticidal, insecticidal, antiparasitic, Anti-feedants (invertebrates), anti-worm *etc.* In the **microbe-higher plants interaction,** the compounds play key roles being plant growth regulators,

---

* **Corresponding author Mukesh Kumar Sharma:** Department of Zoology, SPC Government College, Ajmer-305001; Rajasthan, India; Tel: +91-98291 99444; E-mail: mkshrma@hotmail.com

chlorosis inducing factors, and phytoalexins. Lastly in case of **microbe-mammalians** (Humans) interactions, these compounds show activities such as; Antitumor, antibiotics, enzyme inhibition and other pharmacologic activities [2]. Because of their outstanding chemical features, these bioactive compounds have functioned as scaffolds for the development of new products with huge therapeutic and industrial potential. These compounds have greater efficiency and specificity with target sites because of its co-evolution with biological systems [3]. Considering the looming crisis of antibiotic resistance that spreads among plant and bacterial pathogens as well as the increasing incidence of cancer, the hunt for novel, more efficient and less toxic drugs remains a priority. Studies on biochemical properties of natural products derived from microorganisms have elevated incredibly in the last few years because of increasing demand for the compounds having potential pharmaceutical applications or affordable value as cosmetics, drugs, fine chemicals and various personal-care products, potent drugs, and utilitarian home care products [4, 5]. Several bacteria derived compounds can contribute to manage host physiological and pathological states. Metabolomic profiling of gut bacteria can allow to decipher several molecules (among which short chain fatty acids vitamins, and other aromatic compounds controlling cholesterol synthesis, obesity, cardiovascular diseases, metabolic syndrome, *etc*.

The insights acquired within the last twenty years about human microbiota, and its fundamental role in maintaining a healthy physiological status, have opened a new approach to understand the complex reciprocal benefits between bacteria and humans.

Important Bioactive Compounds produced by Bacteria and Cyanobacteria

Gallic Acid

Gallic acid (3, 4, 5-trihydroxybenzoic acid) is produced by *Klebsiella pneumoniae* and *Corynebacterium* sp [6]. Alternatively, gallic acid can be produced by the microbial activity (hydrolysis) of tannic acid by an inducible enzyme tannase (tannin-acyl-hydrolase EC 3.1.1.20 [7].

It acts as a precursor for the commercial production of drug trimethoprim which is an antimicrobial drug. Gallic acid also has extensive variety of biological activities, which includes antibacterial, antiviral, analgesic properties. Gallic acid also contains antioxidant properties which protects human cells against oxidative damage [8]. Beside this gallic acid also performs cytotoxic activity against cancer cells, without damaging normal cells. Due to its therapeutic properties and various commercial applications, it is a compound of notable interest to pharmaceutical industries.

Amicoumacin

Amicoumacin was first recognized in 1980s from marine Gram-positive bacteria *Bacillus pumilus*. Later it was identified in other species of the genus *Bacillus*. It was recently studied that Amicoumacin is responsible for activation of different genes involved in various metabolic pathways. Amicoumacin uses a slightly different way of interaction with mRNA and 16S rRNA molecules. It interacts with mRNA stabilization at the E site rather than displacing it and imply a distinctive way of translation inhibition [9]. Early research of Amicoumacin confirmed that the main mode of action is aimed towards translocation [10].

Prodigiosin

Prodigiosin is a natural pigment produced by marine bacterium *Vibrio ruber,* which has a broad antimicrobial spectrum and is also responsible for inducing autolytic activity in the target cells (i.e., *Bacillus subtilis*). Prodigiosin is a red colored bioactive secondary metabolite produced by both gram-positive as well as gram-negative bacteria. The compound is characterized by pyrrolyl pyrromethene skeleton. Prodigiosins, which are isolated from bacteria and their synthetic derivatives, are identified as effective anti-cancer agents against various cancer cell lines. Prodigiosin contains numerous physiological functions that are associated with antibacterial, antifungal, or antiprotozoal activity [11, 12]. Beneficial effects of various bioactive constituents derived from bacterial source are mentioned in Fig. (**1**).

Geosmin

Geosmin is a bacteria derived odoriferous bioactive compound which imparts the muddy odor with great economic value. This is mainly produced by cyanobacteria. Although, the gene encoding for geosmin is present in other bacteria also like Actinobacteria, Delta and Gamma proteobacteria. The evolutionary history of geosmin gene shows the high sequence similarity of the cyanobacteria geosmin gene with fresh water and soil strains and it is also connected to niche adaptation [13]. Geosmin is highly associated with terrestrial environments. The bacterial species that are responsible for the Geosmin production in soil are actinomycetes – *Nocardia cummidelens; N. fluminea; Streptomyces luridiscabiei; S. albidoflavus* [14]. Geosmin in water bodies affect the migration of anadromous fishes as its presence or concentration in water current guides the glass eels towards the freshwater [15]. Geosmin is responsible for various functions such as predator aversion and also encourages organisms that disperse spores. It also acts as repellant for fruit flies, so that they do not harm the substances on which Streptomyces is growing [16].

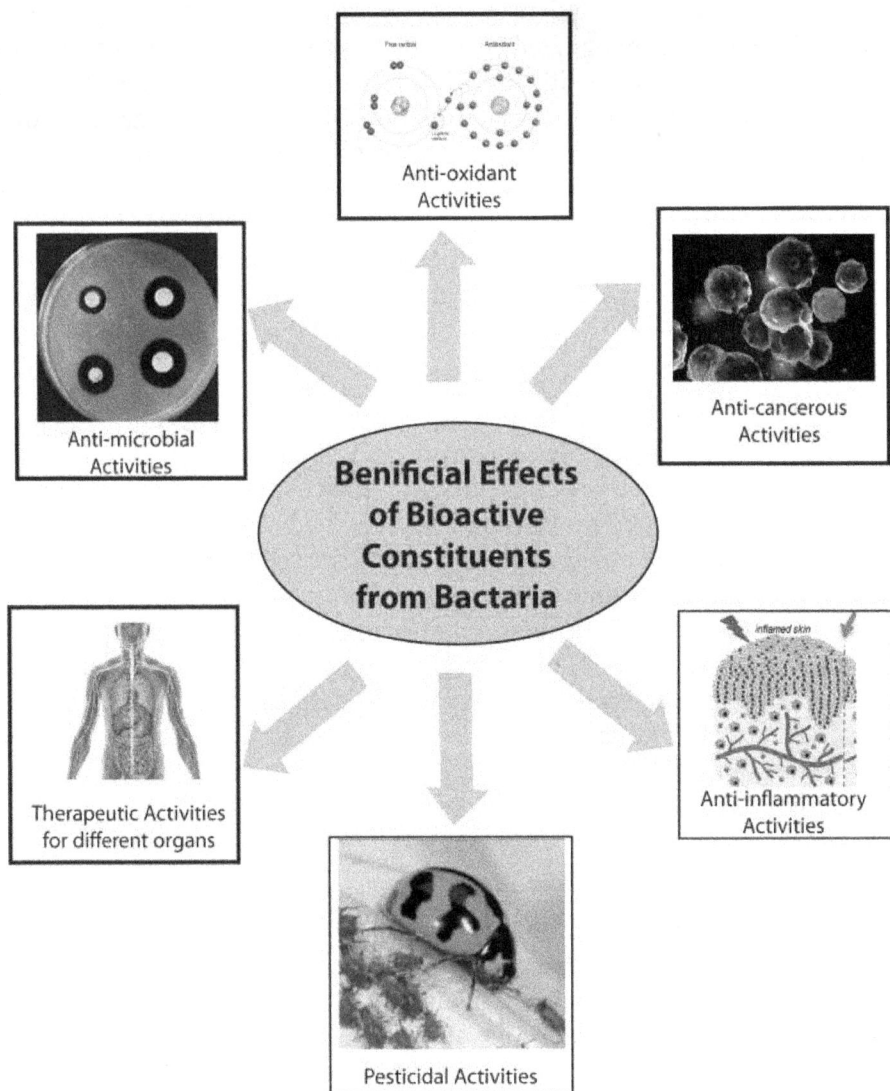

Fig. (1). Schematic diagram showing the beneficial effects of various bioactive constituents derived from bacterial source.

Nystatin

Nystatin, is the first isolated antifungal agent obtained from *Streptomyces noursei* in 1950 and is found to be effective against *Aspergillus* species [17]. Nystatin plays an important role as an antifungal agent in the treatment of oral, gastrointestinal, and genital candidiasis [18, 19]. The structure of this active compound is characterized as a polyene macrolide with a deoxysugar D-mycosamine, an aminoglycoside. The genomic sequence of nystatin reveals the presence of the polyketide loading module (nysA), six polyketide synthase modules (nysB, nysC, nysI, nysJ, and nysK) and two thioesterase modules (nysK and nysE). Oral nystatin is often used as a preventive treatment in people who are at risk for fungal infections, such as AIDS patients with a low CD4$^+$ count and people receiving chemotherapy. It has been investigated for use in patients after liver transplantation, but fluconazole was found to be much more effective for preventing colonization, invasive infection, and death. It is effective in treating oral candidiasis in elderly people who wear dentures [20].

Glycolipids:ieodoglucomide and ieodoglycolipid

Glycolipids ieodoglucomide C and ieodoglycolipid are obtained from marine bacterium *Bacillus licheniformis*. These compounds have been reported as antifungal agents against *Aspergillus niger*, *Rhizoctonia solani*, *Botrytis cinerea*, *Colletotrichum acutatum*, and *C. albicans* [21]. Ieodoglucomide C and ieodoglycolipid also perform antibiotic properties against various bacterial species such as *S. aureus*, *B. subtilis*, *B. cereus*, *S. typhi*, *E. coli* and *P. aeruginosa* and can also be established as a potential bioactive compound in production of new fungicides [22].

Erythromycin A

Erythromycin A is another important polyketide antibiotic with enormous medical applications that were first isolated from *S. erythraea* in 1952. Erythromycin A has antibiotic properties, so it is prescribed to deal with an extensive variety of bacterial infections [23]. Cytochrome P450 enzyme is used for the production of erythromycin [24]. It acts as a bacteriocin that inhibits the growth of bacteria at a higher concentration. This inhibition in bacterial growth is because of its binding to 50S subunit of ribosomal RNA, which is used for protein synthesis and is important for bacterial life and growth. Erythromycin also interferes in aminoacyl translocation and inhibits the transfer of tRNA from A site of rRNA to P site of rRNA [25]. Erythromycin is also used for the treatment of chlamydia infection, pelvic inflammatory disease and syphilis [26].

Spinosad

Spinosad is a commercial product derived from the mixing of naturally occurring spinosyns. The major component of spinosad is spinosyn A&D. Spinosyns are natural products that are isolated from *Saccharopolyspora spinosa* which are insecticidal in nature [27]. It controls various caterpillar pests that are harmful for agricultural production [28]. The insecticidal activity is suggested as a disruption of neural functions. The target site of action for spinosyn is suggested as $D\alpha6$ nicotinic receptor as per the knockdown studies on *Drosophila* [29]. This acts as a poison on insects by surface activity or in ingested form to control insect population [30]. Spinetorum is also a semisynthetic biological derivative of spinosyns. It was launched in 2007. It has productive results in terms of its insecticidal activity [31].

Milbemycin

Milbemycin is a natural product which is a fermentation product of actinomycetes in the genus *Streptomyces.* It is a 16-member macrocyclic lactone and was produced through fermentation by soil dwelling *Streptomyces hygroscopicus.* Milbemycin possesses a wide spectrum of insecticidal and parasiticidal properties [32, 33]. Milbemycins also undergo different molecular modifications with anti-helminthic activity [34]. Spinosad with milbemycin is used against roundworm and hookworm infection in dogs.

Lipstatin

Lipstatin is a natural compound produced by *Streptomyces toxytricini.* Its biosynthesis mechanism is still unknown, but it is explored that ACCase (acyl-coenzyme A carboxylase) helps in the biosynthesis of lipstatin. It is also studied that α-branched 3,5-dihydroxy fatty acid β-lactone component of lipstatin is derived from *S. toxytricini* by Claisen condensation between two fatty acid substrate by incomplete oxidative degradation of linoleic acid [35]. Lipstatin finds used as an anti-obesity medication purpose because it acts as an inhibitor of pancreatic lipase of humans. *The* β-lactone molecule of lipstatin helps in controlling the fat absorption in the small intestine and also manages the digestive activity of pancreatic lipases. Pancreatic lipase contains serine residue in its active site, so acylation of serine lipstatin inhibits its catalytic activity [36]. The IC_{50} of lipstatin for pancreatic lipase is 0.14 μM [37]. Lipstatin is of high cost due to its poor productivity, undetermined by the fact that it is a natural compound.

Subtilin

Subtilin is a compound produced by *Bacillus sps.* Different members of Bacillus have the ability to produce different bacteriocins and antimicrobial substances, including lipopeptides and peptides, which help them to kill other bacteria mostly gram-negative bacteria, as well as yeast and fungus. Thus it expresses a broad spectrum of inhibition. The bacteriocins of *Bacillus* are known as lantibiotics, these are considered as the most effective antibiotics according to genetic determinants, biosynthetic mechanism and peptide structure [38]. Lantibiotics contain thioether amino acids which add during post-translational modifications. Biosynthesis of subtilin is controlled by 2 component regulatory system SpaK/SpaR (histidine kinase and response regulator, respectively) and the alternative sigma factor H [39]. Subtilin has large industrial application in food preservation, health and medicine, acts as antibiotics, is also used as plant growth promoter and help as a bioprotectant in the decay of vegetables [40].

Albaflavenone

Albaflavenone is a secondary metabolite, also known as tricyclic sesquiterpene albaflavenone produced by *Streptomyces albidoflavus*. Its production was elucidated in *S. coelicolor*. The production of compound occurs by expression of genes known as sesquiterpene cyclase (SCO5222) and cytochrome P450 (CYP). These two genes are present in operon (SCO5223; CYP170A1). Biosynthesis of albaflavenone is by the allylic oxidation by CYP170A1 which converts *epi*-isozizaene to an epimeric mixture of albaflavenols and then converts to single ketone sesquiterpene albaflavenone [41]. This compound shows antibacterial effect on *Bacillus subtilis* and it is mostly produced during the germination period with a high antibacterial effect [42]. The synthesis of albaflavenone is completed in nine steps starting from 2-cyclopenten-1-one with high stereo control and it is not commercially available [43].

MollemycinA

Mollemycin A is a compound isolated from *Streptomyces sp.* also known as glyco-hexadepsipeptide-polyketide according to structure. This compound shows large inhibitory activity against different organisms like gram positive, gram negative bacteria and also against *Plasmodium falciparum* (parasite of malaria). The important promising feature is its effectivity at a very low dose (IC_{50}:10-50nM) and very low cytotoxicity [44].

Table 1. Different types of bioactive compounds derived from bacteria with their activities.

S.No.	Species Name	Bioactive Compounds	Activity	References
1	*Klebsiella pneumoniae* and *Corynebacterium* sp.	Gallic acid	Anti-microbial	[7]
2	*Bacillus pumilus*	Amicoumacin	Antibacterial	[9]
3	*Vibrio ruber*	*Prodigiosin*	Antibacterial, Antifungal, or Antiprotozoal	[11]
4	Cyanobacteria	Geosmin	Distract Predators Repel fruit flies	[14]

(Table 1) cont.....

5	*Streptomyces noursei*	Nystatin	Antifungal	[20]
6	*Bacillus licheniformis*	Ieodoglucomide C	Antifungal	[21]
7	*S. erythraea*	Erythromycin	Antibacterial	[23]
8	*Saccharopolyspora spinosa*	Spinosad	Insecticidal	[45]
9	*S. hygroscopicus*	Milbemycin	Insecticidal	[32]
10	*Streptomyces toxytricini*	Lipstatin	Antibacterial	[37]
11	*Bacillus subtilis*	Subtilin	Antibacterial	[46]
12	*Streptomyces albidoflavus*	Albaflavenone	Antimicrobial	[41]
13	*Streptomyces* sp	Mollemycin A	Antibacterial	[47]

Sequential methodology employed in screening and bulk production of bacteria derived bioactive compounds is mentioned in Fig. (**2**).

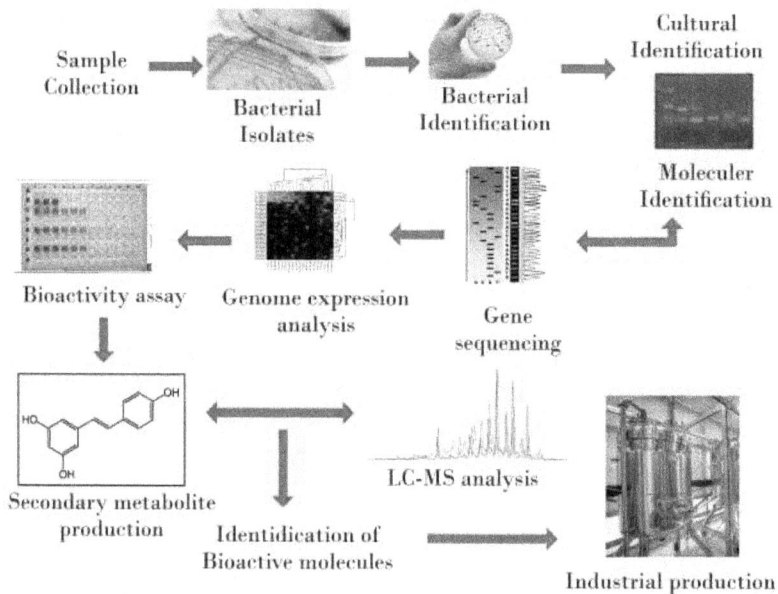

Fig. (2). The figure shows the sequential methodology employed in screening and bulk production of bacteria derived bioactive Bioactive compounds.

Thus, the study of bioactive compounds of bacterial origin with their therapeutic application seems important. Some important bioactive compounds produced by bacteria are described in this chapter (Fig. **3**).

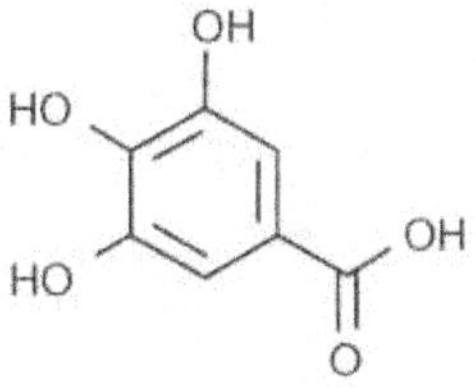

Gallic Acid

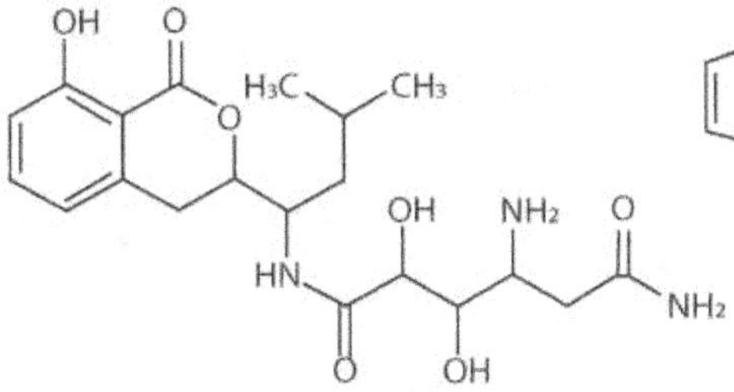

Amicoumacin

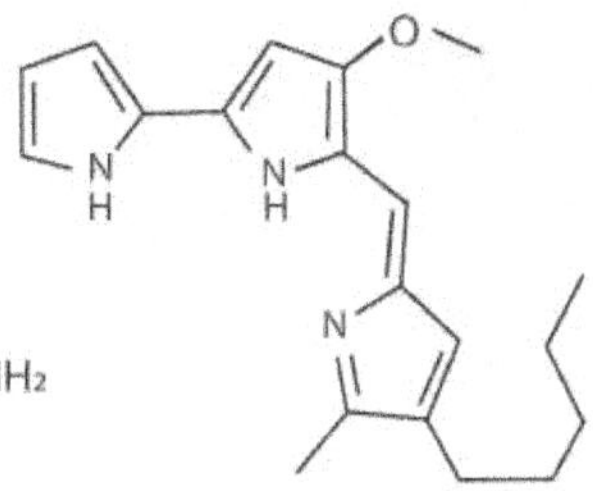

Prodiogiosin

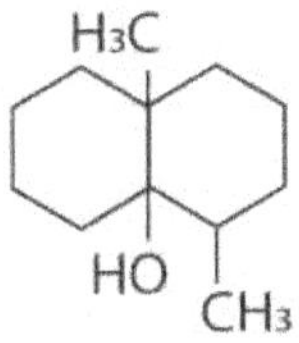

Geosmin

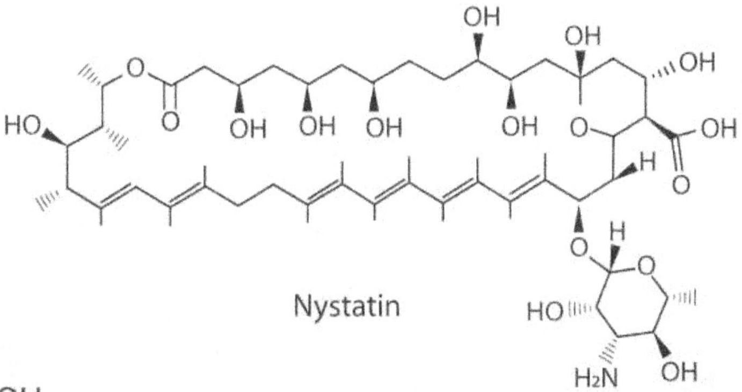

Nystatin

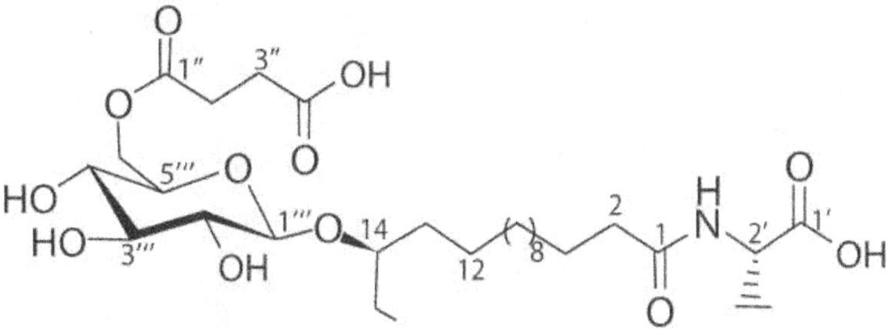

Ieodoglucomide C

(Fig. 3) contd.....

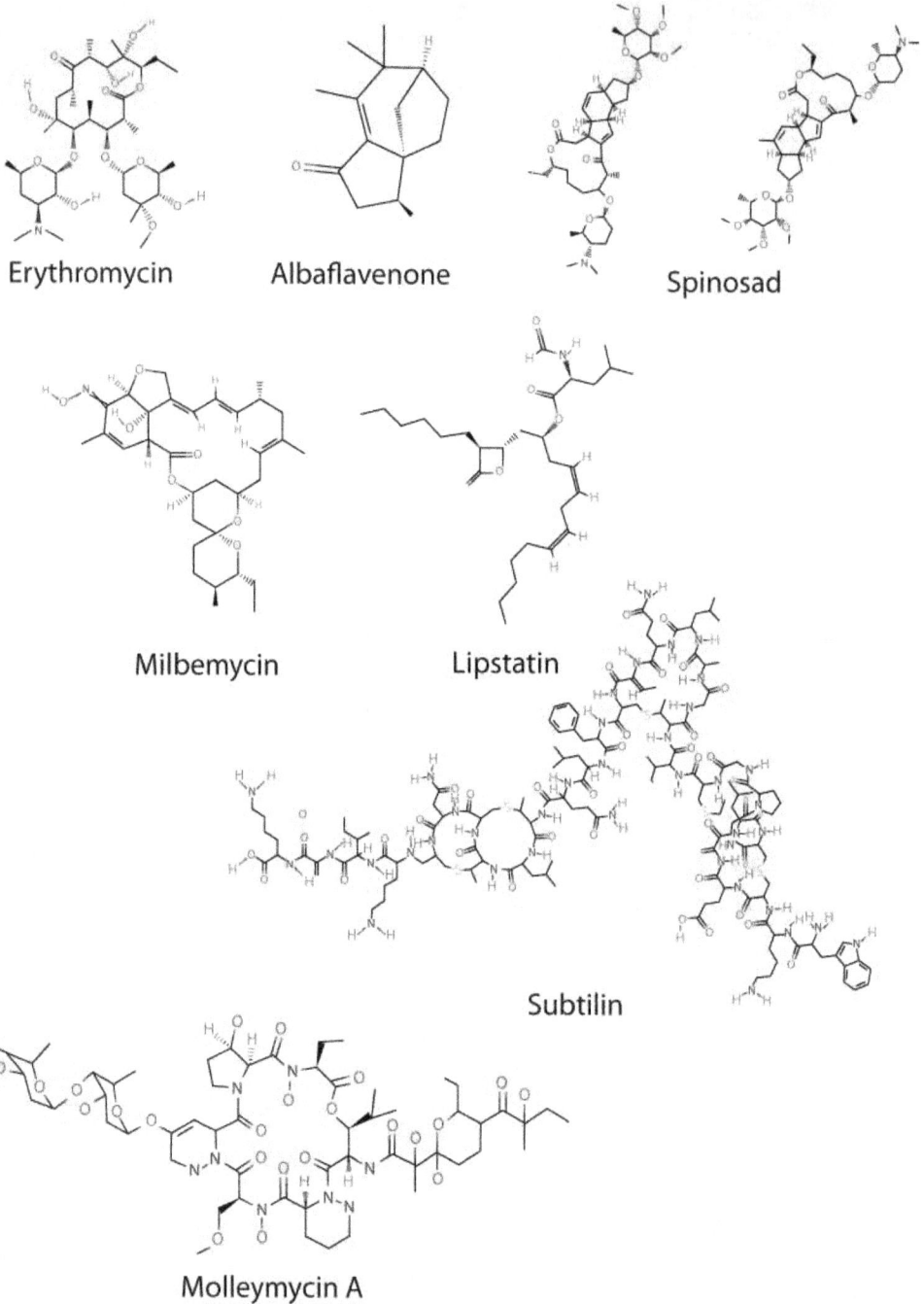

Erythromycin   Albaflavenone   Spinosad

Milbemycin   Lipstatin

Subtilin

Molleymycin A

Fig. (3). Structures of bioactive compounds derived from Bacteria.

CONCLUSION

Natural compounds are crucial and important resource of bioactives which can be harnessed for the benefit of mankind. Microbes which have evolved in diverse habitats express unique secondary metabolites which enable their survival in adverse conditions. The standardized or pure extracts from such microbes have been evaluated for their applicability in medicine and industry. Thus, the research and development in this field seem promising for the development of newer drugs and insecticides, pesticides, parasiticidal, repellents, *etc.* Overall, bacteria based natural products need to be further studied to expand the current knowledge as well as to encounter future requirements. But, the side effects, including toxicity to non-target cells or community shall be addressed with care. Moreover, the semi-synthetic derivatives of natural compounds are also produced with high affectivity and nominal toxicity, are also considered promising. Once the standardization of the compound is done, the increased production can be performed using recombinant DNA technologies and engineering strategies. Current advanced technologies like CRISPR/Cas (Clustered Regularly Interspaced Short Palindromic Repeats/CRISPR associated protein) can be used for further advancement in the field of microbial natural products, which remain a reliable source for novel compounds in drug discovery.

CONSENT FOR PUBLICATION

Not applicable.

CONFLICT OF INTEREST

The authors declare no conflict of interest, financial or otherwise.

ACKNOWLEDGEMENTS

The authors extend their gratitude to the UGC, for providing financial assistance in the form of UGC-JRF to Sneha Keelka (UGC Ref. No.:776/CSIR-UGC NET DEC. 2018).

REFERENCES

[1]   Singh M, Kumar A, Singh R, Pandey KD. Endophytic bacteria: a new source of bioactive compounds. 3 Biotech. 2017 Oct;7(5):315.

[2]   Shukla R. Studies on bioactive compounds from different microorganisms. Int J Sci Eng 2015; 6(6): 9.

[3]   Simmons TL, Andrianasolo E, McPhail K, Flatt P, Gerwick WH. Marine natural products as anticancer drugs. Mol Cancer Ther 2005; 4(2): 333-42.
[http://dx.doi.org/10.1158/1535-7163.333.4.2] [PMID: 15713904]

[4]   Andersen RJ, Williams DE. Chemistry in the marine environment. Cambridge, UK: Pharmaceuticals from the Sea The Royal Society of Chemistry 2000; pp. 55-79.

[5] Mazzoli R, Bosco F, Mizrahi I, Bayer EA, Pessione E. Towards lactic acid bacteria-based biorefineries. Biotechnol Adv 2014; 32(7): 1216-36.
[http://dx.doi.org/10.1016/j.biotechadv.2014.07.005] [PMID: 25087936]

[6] Bajpai B, Patil S. A new approach to microbial production of gallic acid. Braz J Microbiol 2008; 39(4): 708-11.
[http://dx.doi.org/10.1590/S1517-83822008000400021] [PMID: 24031294]

[7] Aissam H, Errachidi F, Penninckx MJ, Merzouki M, Benlemlih M. Production of tannase by Aspergillus niger HA37 growing on tannic acid and Olive Mill Waste Waters. World J Microbiol Biotechnol 2005; 21(4): 609-14.
[http://dx.doi.org/10.1007/s11274-004-3554-9]

[8] Treviño-Cueto B, Luis M, Contreras-Esquivel JC, Rodríguez R, Aguilera A, Aguilar CN. Gallic acid and tannase accumulation during fungal solid state culture of a tannin-rich desert plant (Larrea tridentata Cov.). Bioresour Technol 2007; 98(3): 721-4.
[http://dx.doi.org/10.1016/j.biortech.2006.02.015] [PMID: 16574410]

[9] Polikanov YS, Osterman IA, Szal T, *et al.* Amicoumacin a inhibits translation by stabilizing mRNA interaction with the ribosome. Mol Cell 2014; 56(4): 531-40.
[http://dx.doi.org/10.1016/j.molcel.2014.09.020] [PMID: 25306919]

[10] Maksimova EM, Vinogradova DS, Osterman IA, *et al.* Multifaceted Mechanism of Amicoumacin A Inhibition of Bacterial Translation. Front Microbiol 2021; 12: 618857.https://www.frontiersin.org/articles/10.3389/fmicb.2021.618857/full
[http://dx.doi.org/10.3389/fmicb.2021.618857] [PMID: 33643246]

[11] Anita K. MazaheriAssadi M, Fakhr F. Review of Prodigiosin Online J Biol Sci 2006; 6.

[12] Darshan N, Manonmani HK. Prodigiosin and its potential applications. J Food Sci Technol 2015; 52(9): 5393-407.
[http://dx.doi.org/10.1007/s13197-015-1740-4] [PMID: 26344956]

[13] Churro C, Semedo-Aguiar AP, Silva AD, Pereira-Leal JB, Leite RB. A novel cyanobacterial geosmin producer, revising GeoA distribution and dispersion patterns in Bacteria. Sci Rep 2020; 10(1): 8679.
[http://dx.doi.org/10.1038/s41598-020-64774-y] [PMID: 32457360]

[14] Schrader KK, Davidson JW, Rimando AM, Summerfelt ST. Evaluation of ozonation on levels of the off-flavor compounds geosmin and 2-methylisoborneol in water and rainbow trout Oncorhynchus mykiss from recirculating aquaculture systems. Aquacult Eng 2010; 43(2): 46-50.
[http://dx.doi.org/10.1016/j.aquaeng.2010.05.003]

[15] Tosi L, Sola C. Role of Geosmin, a Typical Inland Water Odour, in Guiding Glass Eel Anguilla anguilla (L.) Migration. Ethology 1993; 95(3): 177-85.
[http://dx.doi.org/10.1111/j.1439-0310.1993.tb00468.x]

[16] Stensmyr MC, Dweck HKM, Farhan A, *et al.* A conserved dedicated olfactory circuit for detecting harmful microbes in Drosophila. Cell 2012; 151(6): 1345-57.
[http://dx.doi.org/10.1016/j.cell.2012.09.046] [PMID: 23217715]

[17] Stanley VC, English MP. Some effects of nystatin on the growth of four Aspergillus species. J Gen Microbiol 1965; 40(1): 107-18.
[http://dx.doi.org/10.1099/00221287-40-1-107] [PMID: 5323080]

[18] Santelmann H, Laerum E, Roennevig J, Fagertun HE. Effectiveness of nystatin in polysymptomatic patients. A randomized, double-blind trial with nystatin versus placebo in general practice. Fam Pract 2001; 18(3): 258-65.
[http://dx.doi.org/10.1093/fampra/18.3.258] [PMID: 11356731]

[19] Zhang X, Li T, Chen X, Wang S, Liu Z. Nystatin enhances the immune response against *Candida albicans* and protects the ultrastructure of the vaginal epithelium in a rat model of vulvovaginal candidiasis. BMC Microbiol 2018; 18(1): 166.

[http://dx.doi.org/10.1186/s12866-018-1316-3] [PMID: 30359236]

[20]   Lyu X, Zhao C, Hua H, Yan Z. Efficacy of nystatin for the treatment of oral candidiasis: a systematic review and meta-analysis. Drug Des Devel Ther 2016; 10: 1161-71.
[http://dx.doi.org/10.2147/DDDT.S100795] [PMID: 27042008]

[21]   Tareq FS, Lee HS, Lee YJ, Lee JS, Shin HJ. Ieodoglucomide C and Ieodoglycolipid, New Glycolipids from a Marine-Derived Bacterium *Bacillus licheniformis* 09IDYM23. Lipids 2015; 50(5): 513-9.
[http://dx.doi.org/10.1007/s11745-015-4014-z] [PMID: 25893812]

[22]   Pham JV, Yilma MA, Feliz A, *et al.* A Review of the Microbial Production of Bioactive Natural Products and Biologics. Front Microbiol 2019; 10: 1404.https://www.frontiersin.org/articles/10.3389/fmicb.2019.01404/full
[http://dx.doi.org/10.3389/fmicb.2019.01404] [PMID: 31281299]

[23]   Cobb RE, Luo Y, Freestone T, Zhao H. Drug Discovery and Development via Synthetic Biology.Synthetic Biology. Boston: Academic Press 2013; pp. 183-206.https://www.sciencedirect.com/science/article/pii/B9780123944306000108 [Internet]
[http://dx.doi.org/10.1016/B978-0-12-394430-6.00010-8]

[24]   Hunt CM, Watkins PB, Saenger P, *et al.* Heterogeneity of CYP3A isoforms metabolizing erythromycin and cortisol. Clin Pharmacol Ther 1992; 51(1): 18-23.
[http://dx.doi.org/10.1038/clpt.1992.3] [PMID: 1732074]

[25]   Siibak T, Peil L, Xiong L, Mankin A, Remme J, Tenson T. Erythromycin- and chloramphenicol-induced ribosomal assembly defects are secondary effects of protein synthesis inhibition. Antimicrob Agents Chemother 2009; 53(2): 563-71.
[http://dx.doi.org/10.1128/AAC.00870-08] [PMID: 19029332]

[26]   Farzam K, Nessel TA, Quick J. Erythromycin.StatPearls. Treasure Island, FL: StatPearls Publishing 2021.http://www.ncbi.nlm.nih.gov/books/NBK532249/ Internet

[27]   Geng C, Watson GB, Sparks TC. Nicotinic acetylcholine receptors as spinosyn targets for insect pest management. Cohen E. Advances in Insect Physiology 2013; 101-210. https://www.sciencedirect.com/science/article/pii/B978012394389700003X

[28]   Miles M, Mayes M, Dutton R. The effects of spinosad, a naturally derived insect control agent, to the honeybee (Apis melifera). Meded Fac Landbouwkd Toegep Biol Wet 2002; 67(3): 611-6.
[PMID: 12696428]

[29]   Perry T, McKenzie JA, Batterham P. A Dα6Dα6 knockout strain of Drosophila melanogaster confers a high level of resistance to spinosad. Insect Biochem Mol Biol 2007; 37(2): 184-8.
[http://dx.doi.org/10.1016/j.ibmb.2006.11.009] [PMID: 17244547]

[30]   Salgado VL. Studies on the Mode of Action of Spinosad: Insect Symptoms and Physiological Correlates. Pestic Biochem Physiol 1998; 60(2): 91-102.
[http://dx.doi.org/10.1006/pest.1998.2332]

[31]   Sparks TC, Crouse GD, Dripps JE, *et al.* Neural network-based QSAR and insecticide discovery: spinetoram. J Comput Aided Mol Des 2008; 22(6-7): 393-401.
[http://dx.doi.org/10.1007/s10822-008-9205-8] [PMID: 18344004]

[32]   Copping LG, Duke SO. Natural products that have been used commercially as crop protection agents. Pest Manag Sci 2007; 63(6): 524-54.
[http://dx.doi.org/10.1002/ps.1378] [PMID: 17487882]

[33]   Poppenga RH, Oehme FW. Pesticide Use and Associated Morbidity and Mortality in Veterinary Medicine.Hayes' Handbook of Pesticide Toxicology. 3rd ed. New York: Academic Press 2010; pp. 285-301.https://www.sciencedirect.com/science/article/pii/B9780123743671000070 [Internet]
[http://dx.doi.org/10.1016/B978-0-12-374367-1.00007-0]

[34]   Sharma S, Anand N. Natural Products.Pharmacochemistry Library. Elsevier 1997; pp. 71-123.https://www.sciencedirect.com/science/article/pii/S0165720897800256 [Internet]

[35]   Bai T, Zhang D, Lin S, *et al.* Operon for biosynthesis of lipstatin, the Beta-lactone inhibitor of human
        pancreatic lipase. Appl Environ Microbiol 2014; 80(24): 7473-83.
        [http://dx.doi.org/10.1128/AEM.01765-14] [PMID: 25239907]

[36]   Kumar P, Dubey KK. Current trends and future prospects of lipstatin: a lipase inhibitor and pro-drug
        for obesity. RSC Advances 2015; 5(106): 86954-66.
        [http://dx.doi.org/10.1039/C5RA14892H]

[37]   Weibel EK, Hadvary P, Hochuli E, Kupfer E, Lengsfeld H. Lipstatin, an inhibitor of pancreatic lipase,
        produced by Streptomyces toxytricini. I. Producing organism, fermentation, isolation and biological
        activity. J Antibiot (Tokyo) 1987; 40(8): 1081-5.
        [http://dx.doi.org/10.7164/antibiotics.40.1081] [PMID: 3680018]

[38]   Abriouel H, Franz CMAP, Omar NB, Gálvez A. Diversity and applications of *Bacillus* bacteriocins.
        FEMS Microbiol Rev 2011; 35(1): 201-32.
        [http://dx.doi.org/10.1111/j.1574-6976.2010.00244.x] [PMID: 20695901]

[39]   Stein T, Heinzmann S, Düsterhus S, Borchert S, Entian KD. Expression and functional analysis of the
        subtilin immunity genes spaIFEG in the subtilin-sensitive host Bacillus subtilis MO1099. J Bacteriol
        2005; 187(3): 822-8.
        [http://dx.doi.org/10.1128/JB.187.3.822-828.2005] [PMID: 15659659]

[40]   Caulier S, Nannan C, Gillis A, Licciardi F, Bragard C, Mahillon J. Overview of the Antimicrobial
        Compounds Produced by Members of the *Bacillus subtilis* Group. Front Microbiol 2019; 10: 302.
        [http://dx.doi.org/10.3389/fmicb.2019.00302] [PMID: 30873135]

[41]   Moody SC, Zhao B, Lei L, *et al.* Investigating conservation of the albaflavenone biosynthetic pathway
        and CYP170 bifunctionality in streptomycetes. FEBS J 2012; 279(9): 1640-9.
        [http://dx.doi.org/10.1111/j.1742-4658.2011.08447.x] [PMID: 22151149]

[42]   Čihák M, Kameník Z, Šmídová K, *et al.* Secondary Metabolites Produced during the Germination of
        Streptomyces coelicolor. Front Microbiol 2017; 8: 2495.
        [http://dx.doi.org/10.3389/fmicb.2017.02495] [PMID: 29326665]

[43]   Kobayashi T, Kon Y, Abe H, Ito H. Concise total synthesis of albaflavenone utilizing sequential
        intramolecular aldol condensation: determination of absolute configuration. Org Lett 2014; 16(24):
        6397-9.
        [http://dx.doi.org/10.1021/ol503202d] [PMID: 25469861]

[44]   Raju R, Khalil ZG, Piggott AM, *et al.* Mollemycin A: an antimalarial and antibacterial glyco-
        hexadepsipeptide-polyketide from an Australian marine-derived Streptomyces sp. (CMB-M0244). Org
        Lett 2014; 16(6): 1716-9.
        [http://dx.doi.org/10.1021/ol5003913] [PMID: 24611932]

[45]   Sanchez S, Guzman-Trampe S, Ávalos M, Ruiz B, Rodríguez-Sanoja R, Jimenez-Estrada M.
        Microbial natural products. Hoboken, NJ: John Wiley & Sons, Inc. 2012.
        [http://dx.doi.org/10.1002/9781118391815.ch3]

[46]   Qin Y, Wang Y, He Y, Zhang Y, She Q, Chai Y, *et al.* Characterization of Subtilin L-Q11, a Novel
        Class I Bacteriocin Synthesized by Bacillus subtilis L-Q11 Isolated From Orchard Soil. Front
        Microbiol 2019. Available from: https://www.frontiersin.org/articles/10.3389/fmicb.2019.00484/full

[47]   Blunt JW, Copp BR, Keyzers RA, Munro MHG, Prinsep MR. Marine natural products. Nat Prod Rep
        2016; 33(3): 382-431.
        [http://dx.doi.org/10.1039/C5NP00156K] [PMID: 26837534]

SUBJECT INDEX

A

Absorption 1, 39, 75, 97, 103, 122, 169, 212
  fat 267
  intestinal 1
  process 97
Acanthophora spicifera 37
Acaricidal activity 141, 143, 160
Accumulation 9, 12, 16, 142, 182
  elicitor-stimulated 182
Acentric chromosome fragments 208
Acetylcholinesterase 8
Acetylglucosamine 47, 50
Acid(s) 9, 32, 52, 47, 48, 52, 54, 55, 67, 71, 78, 80, 82, 96, 100, 101, 103, 106, 111, 120, 121, 124, 137, 138, 139, 140, 144, 146, 147, 158, 159, 160, 161, 181, 182, 183, 191, 192, 229, 249, 250, 254, 262, 263, 267, 268
  arachidonic 144, 146
  ascorbic 71, 96, 106
  asiatic 47
  bile 147
  caffeic 48, 55, 78, 82, 101, 158, 183
  chebulagic 249, 250, 254
  chebulinic 250
  chlorogenic 96
  cinnamic 182
  corosolic 47, 52
  coumaric 158
  decanoic 181, 182
  dodecanoic 181, 182
  ellagic 48, 55, 80, 100, 250
  ferulic (FA) 54, 101, 103, 111, 158, 182, 183
  gallic (GA) 48, 55, 158, 160, 182, 183, 249, 250, 254, 262, 263, 268
  gastric 147
  gentisic 183
  glucuronic 54
  glycyrrhizic 74
  hemidesmusoic 185, 189, 192
  heptacosanoic 47, 52
  hexadecanoic 181, 182, 192

  hydroxybenzoic 121
  linoleic 267
  maslinic 160
  nicotinic 137, 139
  octacosanoic 191
  octadecanoic 181
  octadecenoic 138
  octanoic 181
  organic 158
  palmitic 181, 182
  perchloric 183
  peroxyacetic 67
  phenolic 158
  protocatechuic 182, 183
  tannic 9, 161, 263
  ursolic 32, 52, 159
  vanillic 182, 183
  xanalteric 229
Acinetobacter baumannii 43, 45, 46, 50
Acorus calamus 26
Actinidia deliciosa 46, 48
Actinomycetes 262, 264, 267
Activation 9, 14, 35, 43, 76, 98, 103, 121, 239, 242, 246, 248, 264
  cytokine release 35
  enzyme 43
  macrophage 242
  microglia 9
Active Anti-diabetic Compounds 196
Activities 141, 142, 144, 147, 250, 227, 239, 263, 264, 267
  anticancer 247
  antifungal 141, 144
  anti-helminthic 267
  antileishmanial 250
  anti-malignant 227
  antiprotozoal 264
  catalytic 267
  cytotoxic 263
  digestive 267
  immunosuppressive 250
  nematicidal 142, 147

phagocytic 239
Acute respiratory distress syndrome 71
Adaptive defence mechanisms 237
Adenocarcinoma 33
Adipocytes 248, 249
Aerobic respiration 8
Agents 9, 28, 29, 36, 57, 80, 95, 118, 119, 123, 141, 148, 158, 208, 227, 236, 237, 264
  anti-bacterial 118
  anticoccidial 158
  anti-coronavirus 80
  antioxidative 9
  anti-tumour 227
  antiviral 123
  effective anti-cancer 264
  flavoring 141, 148
  genotoxic 208
  hygroscopic 119
  hypomethylating 28
  oxidizing 95
Ajwain ayurvedic formulations 137
Alanine amino transferase 143
Albaflavenone 262, 268
  single ketone sesquiterpene 268
Aldose reductase inhibitors 197
Alkaline Phosphatase (ALP) 143, 197
Allium sativum 107, 110, 210, 236, 242, 247, 254
Aloe barbadensis 111
Alternaria brassicicola 226
Alzheimer's 2, 5, 11
  brain 11
  disease 2, 5
Amaranthus gangeticus 55
Ameliorate insulin resistance 98
Aminoglycoside 266
Amino transferase (ALT) 143
Anaphylactic reaction 244
Andrographolide sulfonate 244
Angiogenesis 25, 32, 132
  activity 32
  impairing 123
Animal 155
  waste 155
  welfare 155

Anthelmintic activity 142, 148
Antherogenecity 120
Anthocyanidins 6, 8
Anthocyanins 4, 13, 31, 107, 110, 158
  vasicinol Mangiferin 110
Anthraquinone glycoside 98
Anti-amyloidogenic effect of flavonoids 9
Anti-amyloid study Secretases inhibition 3
Antiangiogenic actions 254
Antiangiogenic effect 255
Antibacterial 52, 53, 141, 143, 160, 165, 268
  activity 52, 141, 143
  effect 160, 268
  properties 165
  resistance 53
Anti-biofilm activity 43, 45, 46, 48, 49, 51, 53, 54, 55, 56
  activity of cinnamaldehyde 49
  assay 49
  bioactives 45, 49, 58
  efficacy 54, 56
Antibiotic(s) 44, 45, 50, 51, 52, 54, 55, 58, 156, 162, 163, 164, 262, 263, 268
  conventional 54, 55, 58
  natural 262
  sensitivity 52
  microbes 164
Antibodies 67, 71, 81, 238, 242, 243, 251
  natural 242
Antibody secreting 238, 239
  cells 238
  plasma cells 239
Anticancer 24, 25, 29, 33, 148
  effects 33, 148
  properties 25, 29
  therapeutics 24
Anti-cholinesterase 8
  activity 8
  effects 8
Anticoccidial activity 160
Antidiabetic 56, 96, 103, 105, 106, 107, 112, 135, 141, 144, 145, 179, 195, 196, 197
  activity 103, 107, 141, 144, 196, 197
  agent 145
  effects 106, 107, 112, 196

www.ingramcontent.com/pod-product-compliance
Lightning Source LLC
Chambersburg PA
CBHW061340210326
41598CB00035B/5833